THE WEARINESS OF THE SELF

The Weariness of the Self

Diagnosing the History of Depression
in the Contemporary Age

ALAIN EHRENBERG

McGill-Queen's University Press
Montreal & Kingston · London · Ithaca

9/15/10
Lan
 # 29.95

ISBN 978-0-7735-3625-8

Legal deposit first quarter 2010
Bibliothèque nationale du Québec

Printed in Canada on acid-free paper that is 100% ancient forest free
(100% post-consumer recycled), processed chlorine free.

McGill-Queen's University Press acknowledges the support of the Canada
Council for the Arts for our publishing program. We also acknowledge
the financial support of the Government of Canada through the Book
Publishing Industry Development Program (BPIDP) for our publishing
activities.

Originally published as *La fatigue d'être soi: Dépression et société*,
© Éditions Odile Jacob, 1998. Translation of this book has been made
possible by a grant from DREES-MIRE

Translated by Enrico Caouette, Jacob Homel, David Homel,
and Don Winkler, under the direction of David Homel

Library and Archives Canada Cataloguing in Publication

Ehrenberg, Alain
   The weariness of the self: diagnosing the history of depression
in the contemporary age/Alain Ehrenberg.

   Translation of: La fatigue d'être soi.
   Includes bibliographical references and index.
   ISBN 978-0-7735-3625-8

   1. Depression, Mental – Social aspects. 2. Depression, Mental – History.
3. Social psychology. I. Title.

RC537.E3713 2010   616.85'27   C2009-906796-X

Typeset in New Baskerville 10.5/13
by Infoscan Collette, Quebec City

For Pierre Chambat.
For Antonin, Jonathan, and Judith.
For Corinne.

Contents

Acknowledgments

Claude Barazer, Pierre Chambat, Jacques Cloarec, Jacques Donzelot, Corinne Ehrenberg, Olivier Mongin, Édouard Zarifian, and Patrick Zylberman all gave of their time to comment on different versions of this book. Anne Lovell also contributed a number of helpful suggestions.

Nicole Phelouzat gave me remarkable research support and helped me improve this work. I would also like to thank Christophe Guias for his editorial contributions.

Foreword

The publication of *La fatigue d'être soi: Dépression et société* in an English translation will be welcomed by scholars and clinicians familiar with the French edition and eager to have Alain Ehrenberg's vision of the history and sociology of depression made available to anglophone audiences. Ehrenberg's book is already familiar to European readers through German, Italian, and Spanish editions. The book will be "unfamiliar" to most anglophone readers not only because it is newly translated but also because it is at odds with the conventional understanding of depression and sociology in North America. In his illuminating introduction, written for this edition, Ehrenberg distances himself from the epistemologies and intellectual traditions underpinning the recent claims of American social scientists regarding depression and bipolar depressive disorder: (1) the claim that depression, as distinct from normal sadness, is objectively given, and (2) that depression, as distinct from its psychiatric formulation, is essentially subjective (in the sense of being self-centred). The differences are partly intellectual: Ehrenberg's debt to Durkheim and Wittgenstein sets him apart from the American authors and the objective-versus-subjective contretemps. But there are also important cultural differences: Ehrenberg's understanding of society, the self, the meaning of depression, and the human condition are profoundly *foreign* with respect to epistemology.

It would be a mistake to think of these differences as being "merely" cultural: that is, something optional, on the surface, enactive, equivalent to a "lifestyle." Ehrenberg argues that modern psychiatry possesses an *intrinsic* culture and is otherwise inconceivable. Indeed, global psychiatry has multiple cultures, differentiated by their practices and institutions and, likewise, by their imaginaries. *The Weariness of the Self* embeds French psychiatry and, more specifically, depression in the continuously evolving society, culture, and history of France. And, in this way, the book permits a comparison of two psychiatric cultures and their epistemologies (overlapping and equally scientific but different) through which attentive anglophone readers will be able to recognize and consider what might otherwise be invisible and inaccessible – their taken-for-granted beliefs about the normal and the pathological.

Ehrenberg's book is distinctive in one more way. Its author advocates nothing other than a satisfying ethnographic account of his subject. Each of the books mentioned in the introduction has a mission: on the one hand, to help "victims" understand and acknowledge their distinctiveness and efficaciously pursue the potential fullness of their lives; on the other hand, to help psychiatric science penetrate the haze of culture, contingency, and conventional wisdom. In both cases, the writer's goal is the recovery of a kind of authenticity that now lies buried beneath history and culture and social institutions. These are popular themes in North American culture, and books that replicate these themes are likewise popular. Many readers are pleased to discover in learned works what they already believe. *The Weariness of the Self: Diagnosing the History of Depression in the Contemporary Age* delivers a different kind of pleasure.

Allan Young
McGill University

Listening to the Spirit of Depression:
A Tale of Two Continents

Even a complaint, making a complaint, can give life some spice and make it endurable: there is a small dose of revenge in every complaint.[1]

Nietzsche, *Twilight of the Idols,* 1889

When we speak of depression and, in a more general way, mental health, we are immediately cast into a world of controversy. The reasons for this are many, but one of them is stronger than the others: we are approaching the delicate border between mind and body. This old question is no longer the domain of philosophers, neurobiologists, and psychoanalysts. It concerns all of us because, at least in the West, mental health issues have had a central role in our societies since the 1970s. Mental health concerns not only health but also the socialization of the modern individual. It challenges the essential elements of individualist societies, like self-value, the opposition between responsibility and illness, the ability to succeed in life, the ability to educate one's children, and so on. The Surgeon General's report on mental health published in 1999 sets down this fact with the greatest clarity: "From early childhood until death, mental health is the springboard of thinking and communication skills, learning, emotional growth, resilience, and self-esteem. These are the ingredients of each individual's successful contribution to community or society. Americans are inundated with messages about success ... without appreciating that successful performance rests on a foundation of mental health."[2] What else are we speaking of in this relationship, as in so many others, if not our social ideals?

Depression plays a major roll in these ideals as it brings together in one pathological entity all the obstacles that prevent us from realizing them. No other mental pathology occupies such a position both in medicine and in society. From the beginning of the 1970s, it designates a spectrum of problems, ranging from the slowed individual whom we have to pump up like a tire so he or she can live a normal social life to the psychosis of melancholia marked by guilt delirium so severe that the person who suffers from it is filled with a desire for death – a desire that he or she often fulfills. Depression's medical and social situation has led me to study it as an attitude, as a state of mind inherent to contemporary individualism.

When I began working on this book in 1995, I was astonished by the absence of the social history and historical sociology of depression in Great Britain and the United States.[3] In the hope of giving the reader a glimpse of the different paths open to sociology and anthropology in examining the relations between mental pathology and social life, I first look at the questions raised by antidepressants. I then situate my own work regarding the North American discussions by focusing on three books on depression and bipolar disorders, all of which have been published over the last twelve years: David A. Karp, *Speaking of Sadness: Depression, Disconnection, and the Meanings of Illness* (1996); Emily Martin, *Bipolar Expeditions: Mania and Depression in American Culture* (2007); and Alan V. Horwitz and Jerome Wakefield, *The Loss of Sadness: How Psychiatry Transformed Normal Sorrow into Depressive Disorder* (2007). These works enable me to speak of the social content of depression.

THE SOUL OF THE ANTIDEPRESSANT

Since the launch of Prozac at the end of the 1980s, public opinion on antidepressants has been polarized. We saw abundant works on the medicalization of mental anguish and emotional states as well as on the moral, political, and social issues raised by the massive prescribing of medications for maladies whose status as illnesses is unclear. Are these prescribed drugs not close to the illicit drugs that modify not only a troubled mood but also the patient's very personality? How can we distinguish between the troubled mood we *have* and the troubled personality we *are*? Should antidepressants be limited to certain types of depressions or be prescribed as soon as a depressive symptomology is diagnosed? The debate begins with the discovery of antidepressants in 1957, and it features the two opposing views of their discoverers: the Swiss Roland Kuhn, for whom they were correctors of troubled moods, and the American

Nathan Kline, for whom they were "psychic energizers." In the same way, we can see, from that time onward, how psychiatrists questioned the effectiveness of antidepressants on various types of depressions and even on depression in general. Diagnostic chaos reigned, and the reason for this had to do with the very nature of the depressive phenomenon: that is, its incredible heterogeneity. The concept of "masked depression" was invented to help general practitioners recognize and diagnose depression. Is the fact that antidepressants were once prescribed for ill people but are now given to well people not worrisome? From 1958 on, psychiatrists were optimistic that psychotropic drugs would restore the joy of life to those whom "modern life" had infected. "Do we not see patients every day who, with or without an organic syndrome, see their lives dominated by their psychic condition?" asked certain Dr Coirault at a 1962 symposium. "Depression seems to run modern man's entire life. The fact is cause for concern." (For these points, see Chapter 3.)

For a long time, today's many controversies were just technical, practical, and conceptual discussions in psychiatry. The sociologist who dives into the psychiatric literature can only admire the wealth and quality of these discussions, which began anew when selective serotonin reuptake inhibitors (SSRIS) came on the scene. Then, controversies over antidepressants became a public issue that resulted in constant polemics not only over the morality of prescribing antidepressants but also over the medication's ability to relieve depression.[4] Peter Kramer pointed out the ambivalence of his patients:[5] some thought they had finally become themselves thanks to the medication, while others believed they had become someone else.[6] He pointed to the dilemma of the modern individual, for whom a particular molecule can facilitate the ideals of autonomy, self-realization, and the ability to act by oneself. And therein lies a decisive point: antidepressants, both new and old, certainly act on sadness, but they also act on mental anguish, that dejection of the self that slows the depressed person to the point of immobility. They remove inhibition, which is a major obstacle for modern individuals, something that makes it difficult for them to act and thus prevents them from making something of themselves. Inhibition has taken on a major role in our society, which emphasizes individual flexibility and the value of competition. In psychiatry, the concern over inhibition characterizes what I call the second age of depression. In the first age of depression, between the discovery of sismotherapy at the end of the 1930s and the nosographical revolution of the third *Diagnostic and Statistical Manual of Mental Disorders* (DSM-III) initiated in 1980, depression was a subfield of Freudian neurosis. The second age of depression witnessed both the freeing of depression from neurosis and a major displacement of the concept of depression. Depression came to be seen as a slowing of action, and antidepressants were seen as addressing this problem. To echo the 1980 statement of Daniel Widlöcher, one of the leaders of French psychiatry, depression is a style of action rather than a subjective state. The depressed person is in a state of breakdown. He or she personifies the inadequate individual with regard to the norms of action. Today, depression concerns the spirit in which we act. Two key words are attached to antidepressants: "enhancement" and "empowerment." They are also two key words in American society.

Action undertaken by oneself is at the very heart of the idea of democracy because democracy is the social form that gives any given individual a chance to progress and to make something of herself thanks to her own initiative.[7] The individual who makes her way by herself is plagued by the worry that is concomitant with that kind of life. She is like the Puritan who is continually harassed by the question: Am I chosen or am I damned? Faced with action, the modern individual is harassed by the questions: Why me? Why not me? Am I up to the demands? Her inadequacy makes her feel guilty, and she begins to doubt her capacities. Illness can follow.

This creator of action, the modern individual, is "the frail athlete of life" of whom Charles Baudelaire speaks in "The Spirit of Wine." To make something of himself, the individual must have, in his everyday life, the right stuff. Ordinary heroism, democratic heroism, is essential as much for Baudelaire[8] as for Emerson.[9] In 1860, Baudelaire gave his celebrated essay "Artificial Paradise" the subtitle "On Hashish and Wine as Means of Expanding Individuality." He describes how "hashish causes an intensification of one's individuality,"[10] something ordinary man does in order to reach divinity, whereas the poet reaches it through poetry. According to Baudelaire, "Hashish reveals to the individual no more than the individual himself."[11] *Listening to Prozac* is the distant heir of Baudelaire's theme of intensifying the self, of enhancing and empowering the creator of action.

On 26 March 1990, *Newsweek* put Prozac on its cover and revealed to the general public that people, claiming to be depressed, were flocking to their doctors to get this action pill. Twenty years later, has the United States burned the idol it once worshipped? Instead, I think the country has opted for a collective representation of its moral dilemmas, becoming a pill-taking society, and everyone knows it will not retreat from that path. Antidepressants have reinforced postmodern irony, which is sometimes elegant, but generally without practical consequences.

Antidepressants have resulted in moral, political, and social debates over depression. Yet depression goes far beyond medication. Considered by psychiatric epidemiology as the most common mental disorder since 1970, it has a vaster and more complex history than simply as an emblem of psychopharmacology. And it is at the heart of the tensions of modern individualism. This is why we need to listen less to the antidepressant and more to the spirit of depression.

AMERICAN DEPRESSIONS

The works of Karp and Martin arise from a particular tradition of American social inquiry. On the one hand, they describe a sociological problem; on the other, they fight the stigma associated with mental illness. Sociological and moral inquiries are linked in that they both describe how patients are victims not only of the illness that affects them but also of society's intolerance. These works are informed by a self-help dimension, an attempt to empower individuals.[12] Horwitz and Wakefield's The Loss of Sadness embodies an analytical spirit that brings together facts and organizes arguments and counter-arguments to form a dossier. Karp and Martin find their criteria for truth in culture, while Horwitz and Wakefield find theirs in nature.

The Attachment to Experience

American sociological and anthropological work is often accompanied by a desire to reduce the shame and guilt of people affected by a certain problem. Mental disorder is certainly regularly identified with a weakness of character, but there is nothing specifically American about that. On the other hand, what sets the United States apart, and constitutes a practical supplementary motivation for worrying about stigmatization, is the absence of universal health insurance. This institutional situation has practical consequences that stigmatize the psychiatric patient in a very concrete way: there is no parity between the reimbursement of costs pertaining to mental illness and those pertaining to somatic illness.[13] Certainly, as Horwitz and Wakefield point out, "the reality is that clinicians always have found and always will find ways of responding to their patients' needs consistent with diagnostic definitions so that they receive reimbursement for treatment."[14] But a situation that is dependent upon doctors is not a situation that is institutionally applicable to all. Americans have more *social* reasons to be "brain-centred" than do the French, who, once they have been diagnosed by a physician, have health insurance for all types of pathologies.

The neurosciences and the cognitive sciences are equally in fashion in France, but they are the subjects of violent controversies that we do not see elsewhere: there is talk of "the death of the self," and "cognitive drill," and "Anglo-Saxon imperialism." If our system of social protection does not move us to adopt neuroscientific perspectives, we should not forget that France is, without a doubt, the last bastion of psychoanalysis in Europe. Since the beginning of the twenty-first century, we've seen a war over the self – a battle between the supporters of the "talking self" (who believe that neurosciences are a danger for humankind's humanity) and the supporters of the "cerebral self" (who believe that neurosciences can result in no longer loading guilt onto patients and their parents).[15] In the United States, only the "cerebral self" counts since the "talking self" has more or less disappeared. Besides, in the United States, psychoanalysis never had the intellectual and political pretensions that it did in France. All it wants to do is keep a place for analytic or analysis-inspired psychotherapies within general support mechanisms; it does not want to reform the entire society.

Emily Martin's valuable empirical work, a mixture of interviews and participant observations of contrasting terrains, helps us to understand the different experiences of people affected by bipolar disorders. The quality of the descriptions, whether they deal with receiving a diagnosis or with the ambivalent relations between people and medication, is impressive. And therein lies the strength of Martin's book.[16] She justifies using the classical term "manic-depression," rather than "bipolar," "because it leaves open the question whether the condition is to be understood only as an illness or also as a psychological style."[17] Notice that she does not discuss a fundamental point, which is that psychiatrists once spoke of a manic-depressive *psychosis,* emphasizing the delirium aspect of the problem. Of course, today the term is "bipolar disorder," which, rightly or wrongly (and here is not the forum for such a discussion), extends the category beyond "madness." The historical elements she provides do not allow us to understand how manic-depressive psychosis was transformed into bipolar disorder. Martin points out that she deliberately uses "the phrase 'living under the description of manic-depression (or bipolar disorder)' to refer to people who have received the medical diagnosis. The phrase is meant to reflect that they have been given a diagnosis. At the same time, it calls attention to another social fact: the diagnosis is only one description of a person among many."[18]

The problem is that it is not only one description among others: to see the issue that way is to set aside the fact that people are *really* suffering from this disorder, however it is described. The distinction between normal and pathological is not only an issue of varying social and cultural norms; it is also a practical issue of psychopathology, which involves psychic norms. Certainly, hypomania fits with American norms of success, self-realization, and so on. But hypomania can be transformed into mania, moving all the way to delirium, before retreating into a depression that is often deep. There is a real solidarity between mania and depression in the *reality* of the pathology. Martin does not deny the reality of the suffering; she tends to think that its form of expression is a cultural fact: "The 'reality' of manic-depression lies in the cultural contexts that give particular meanings to its oscillations and multiplicities."[19] But this oscillation *is* the illness, and it is independent of the cultural context. The risk is making the psychopathology disappear. The psychopathological reality – without quotation marks – must in itself be part of the sociological account. People do not only live "under a description," except perhaps in self-help groups whose purpose is to bind them together and to help them live better.[20] Defining the entity that has affected the person as a lifestyle rather than as simply an illness is a central contribution of these groups. More important, they also contribute to a better acceptance of mental pathology. But is the anthropologist obliged to propagate the values of self-help groups?[21] Shouldn't he or she situate them and extrude their social significance within the American context? Choosing the first alternative has the epistemological consequence of reducing a psychopathological fact to a case of suffering whose elements are social (even though Martin does point to their biological origins). But is there nothing in between biology and culture? This reduction appears at its most obvious when Martin mentions psychotropic medication (i.e., mood regulators and antidepressants): "These agents ease suffering. A cure, however, is another matter. A cure implies healing, and healing would have to address not just people's experience, crucial as that is. Healing would have to address the strong but not invincible barriers to our ability to flourish, as individuals and as part of collectivities."[22] These barriers – race, gender, class – are what would have to be lifted in order to cure manic-depressive disorder. Whatever its etiology, its solution is social: it depends on the manic-depressive self being reunited with the community.

Speaking of Sadness is built as an inquiry based on in-depth interviews with some fifty people. The theme that emerges from the interviews is this: depression is "a disease of disconnection."[23] Sociology's overall goal, like Martin's, is "to provide a forum for those whose voices are either stilled or not well understood."[24] Karp also attempts to sum up the impressive argumentation surrounding depression in the United States. He believes that it stems from a cultural context that results in "our collective vulnerability to emotional distress."[25] His thesis? There has been a personal dislocation due to the triple movement of medicalization, disconnection, and postmodernization. These "increasingly loose human connections" contribute to an increase in depression. The loss of the social bond, of community, gives depression its deep – that is, sociopolitical – meaning. "Most people suffering from depression, like street pedestrians, are only dimly aware of how culture might be contributing to their depressed conditions."[26] Karp joins the line begun by Phillip Rieff in *The Triumph of the Therapeutic* (1966), then continued by Richard Sennett in *The Fall of Public Man* (1979), Christopher Lasch in *The Culture of Narcissism* (1979), and Robert Bellah et al. in *The Habits of Heart* (1985). Karp, like these authors,[27] and like Martin, ends his book by declaring his "faith that we will be smart enough to redefine ourselves in *relational* rather than individualistic terms."[28]

From the very first pages of their respective books, Karp and Martin admit to their own chronic depression and bipolarity.[29] It would not occur to a French sociologist to lay claim to such a private state in a public forum. (It's quite different for writers in France who, in the auto-fiction fashion, tend to turn themselves into a literary genre and wipe away the distinction between autobiography and fiction.) This is not an issue of personal psychology but, rather, of seeing things within a social perspective. Allowing the individual voice to express itself and to join the collective voice, allying the personal or private self with the shared self: these are self-central themes in American culture. Martin and Karp follow Emerson's model, which fuses the personal and the historic, the pursuit of private happiness and public happiness: they proclaim their faith in a rebirth of America, which is always a rebirth of the community. This accounts for why, in the United States, we often see the proximity of sociology/anthropology and the literature of resilience. The latter is characterized by turning the negative value of the stigma into a positive lifestyle value, giving dignity not only to a depressive and bipolar life but also to autism, hyperactivity, phobia,[30] and so on.

But one tricky issue remains, and I am leaving it open. If it is true that a mental pathology is mental because it disturbs our emotions and our relational life, does not the struggle against stigmatization soon reach its limits? Is it fair, on the descriptive level as well as on the moral level, to consider that being affected by a serious psychiatric disorder is the same as being affected by diabetes?[31] Should diabetes be considered a lifestyle? And, if it should, is it a lifestyle in the same way that bipolar disorder is a lifestyle? How many psychiatric patients wish to see themselves as having a sort of mental diabetes? And if this does come to pass, will it improve their relationships? Or is this just one more description with no practical consequences?

All these stories give an account of what these lives are like, and, at the same time, they defend a pluralist view of social normality, reminding the United States of its ideals of freedom and pluralism. Like Tracy Thompson says in her autobiography of depression *The Beast: A Journey through Depression,* the task of the sociologist "is not blaming the victim: it is – to use a trendy phrase – empowering the victim."[32] This literature is what has been handed down by the Puritan tradition of the exemplary biography and the examination of the self, taken up again by American romanticism.[33] Stories of illness (and, to a lesser extent, sociology) have contributed to a major change in the social status of mental pathologies: they are now both illness and lifestyle. In order for the winds of freedom to blow, the American Founding Fathers thought that a multiplicity of beliefs was best. In today's world, lifestyles are flowering so that each individual may reach that level of self-reliance without which the United States would lose the energy that other countries so admire.

As for the French sociologist, his tendency would be to fold the private realm into the public realm, from his point of view the only one with any value. Yet there is a French equivalent to this American emphasis on the self. It does not focus on syndromes such as depression, bipolar disorders, attention deficit hyperactivity disorder, or Asperger's syndrome but, rather, on "social suffering," those social problems that do not necessarily express themselves through pathologies. In the United States, the tendency is towards a multiplicity of syndromes; in France, the tendency is towards bringing everything together under the same category. From the beginning of the 1990s, a growing number of sociologists and anthropologists have been trying to create "a clinic for broken social bonds" – social bonds damaged by mass unemployment, an insecure workforce, urban ghettos, and global capitalism's new forms of exploiting subjectivity. These anthropologists/sociologists unite research and political action. Their ancestors are Pierre Bourdieu and Axel Honneth, who saw recognition as the solution to suffering. Unlike the Americans, they do not try to unite the personal and the collective, they do not believe in allying the pursuit of personal happiness and the pursuit of public happiness; rather, they believe in the tradition of the Social Question (defined as the poverty of the masses) that flows from the French Revolution. What French sociologists and anthropologists want is less emphasis on human rights and more emphasis on the rights of the poor; less emphasis on people brought together to discuss the different concerns of various interest groups and more emphasis on people united in their suffering.[34] These anthropologists/sociologists are concerned with the people whom the state has abandoned to market forces. Both French and American social sciences sometimes tend to succumb to what French Indianist Francis Zimmerman has called "the mourning paradigm."[35] But they both do it according to their respective national styles.

The Expansion of the Diagnosis: Subjectivity versus Objectivity

Horwitz and Wakefield's *Loss of Sadness* is situated squarely in the eye of the storm, which consists of the polemics and controversies surrounding the DSM-III since it was published in 1980. They try to solve the thorny problem of mental health. How can we distinguish between normal suffering, even when it is intense, and a disorder, an authentic pathological condition?

Their book is to be recommended. Without sentimentality, it takes us firmly into the main issues and debates regarding the medicalization of depression and the blurring of the borders between what is normal and what is pathological.[36] They take on these tricky problems, providing solid arguments and displaying their cultural sophistication. One of the virtues of *Loss of Sadness* is that it responds to potential counter-arguments. Showing a true spirit of synthesis, it reviews the many factors that have led to the expansion of the diagnosis of depression.

According to Horwitz and Wakefield, the expansion of the diagnosis of depression arises from various socio-cultural changes; however, it arises especially from the DSM-III itself (and then the DSM-IV), whose criteria do not tie a pathological condition to solid factors: "The 'Age of Depression' results from a faulty definition of depressive disorder" (6). Symptom-based diagnoses indicate a kind of progress, but one of their effects is that the ordinary problems of life become classified as mental disorders. Though one of Horwitz and Wakefield's chapters is concerned with the concept of depression found in the DSM, I focus my comments on their critique of the social sciences. The heart of their argument involves the role of context: if depression results from a context (e.g., loss of a job, difficult living conditions, etc.), we have normal suffering; if that suffering lasts longer than the context within which it occurred, we have a disorder.

Horwitz and Wakefield's first attack is on culturalist approaches to depression, which make any serious critique of the DSM impossible. They review two anthropological schools: (1) the culture and personality anthropology of Ruth Benedict and (2) the more recent cross-cultural psychiatric anthropology of Arthur Kleinman. They criticize the relativism of both schools, according to which what is true here may be false elsewhere. For Horwitz and Wakefield, the biological body is universal; cultural content and the forms of emotional expression are variable. As a consequence, diseases are the same everywhere; only illnesses are different. The mistake of relativism is that, unlike the DSM, it offers only soft criteria and, as a result, is not able to limit the expansion of the diagnosis. In the end, culturalism has nothing to say about what objectively distinguishes (at least, independently of the collective preferences of any given society) normal intense sadness from authentic depression.

As for the methods used by sociologists – and epidemiologists – to measure depression in the general population, these, according to Horwitz and Wakefield, have worsened the mistakes of the DSM. Sociologists are interested in social stress factors in the community, whereas the DSM is interested in clinical populations. Horwitz and Wakefield show that three processes drive individuals into distress: (1) low social status, (2) the loss of valued attachments, and (3) the inability to reach important goals. These are normal causes for distress, not pathological conditions. The instrument of inquiry favoured by sociologists – the Center for Epidemiological Studies Measure of Depression (CES-D) – promotes the confusion between normal distress and depression because its criteria are less constraining than are those of the DSM (e.g., in the former, the symptoms need only last a day, while in the latter they must last two weeks). Sociologists "fail to distinguish whether high scores on symptom scales stem from persons with chronic and recurrent conditions that fluctuate independently of social conditions or from those with transitory and situationally induced stress."[37] They tend to study normal responses to stress factors and not the "internal psychological dysfunctions" that last beyond the traumatic event.[38] Their position is that a disease can be caused by social factors but be characterized by long-term psychological dysfunction. The criterion regarding the duration of the pathological character is this: in an improved environment, the problem persists. If it does not, then we are dealing with a form of distress that is not pathological. This position is in line with common sense since it does not reject supporting this distress through medical care.

How do Horwitze and Wakefield resolve the problem?

They contend that, to go beyond cultural relativism, we need to address the "universals of human nature [that are] due to our common evolutionary heritage and the role these universals play in identifying normal and disordered conditions."[39] Cultural variation rests on a universal material foundation, which is biological. Biology is the hard fact upon which lies the soft fact of culture. This hard fact is universal and allows us to distinguish between normality and abnormality and, thereby, to avoid the errors and limitations of cultural relativism. First comes the biological basis, then comes cultural variation. If anthropologists do not recognize this point, "they will not be able to develop strong concepts of either normality or disorder or strong theories for the factors that determine cultural expressions of depressive conditions."[40]

To those who state that mental pathology is value-laden, which Horwitz and Wakefield do not deny (and this is one of their strengths), these authors reply that cultural responses to loss are a matter of evolutionary selection and that "the *categories* that trigger sadness responses – losses of intimate attachments, low or declining social status, or the failure to achieve desired goals – are universals."[41] Universalism is thus bound to evolutionary selection. For Horwitz and Wakefield, the choice is clear: it is either evolution or it is value judgments. And their solution is elegant: we need to base our criteria more objectively on biology, whose central concept is function, which, in turn, can be supported by evolution.

We owe this solution to Wakefield, who holds that mental disorders stand at the border between value judgments (which are cultural) and science (which is value-free). In an article that philosophers know well, he proposes "a hybrid account of disorder as harmful dysfunction, wherein *dysfunction* is a scientific and factual term based in evolutionary biology that refers to a failure of an internal mechanism to perform a natural function for which it was designed and *harmful* is a value term referring to the consequences that occur to the person because of the dysfunction and are deemed negative by sociocultural standards."[42] It would then be possible to take account of values while remaining value-free: "Only dysfunctions that are socially disvalued are disorders."[43] The argument's simplicity accounts for its elegance.

THE CLAIM OF HUMAN NATURE

The point at which I open a discussion with the work of Horwitz and Wakefield, which is remarkable in its rigour and its refusal to bury any problems, can be formulated as follows. The limit of their response to the harness of cultural relativism and of the sociology of stress factors arises, in my opinion, from the fact that, to the subjectivity of cultural variation, they oppose the objectivity of the biological species, supported by the argument of function as selected by evolution. Objectivity is the mirror of subjectivity. The consequence: it reproduces the problem instead of solving it. Why?

The problem raised by this alternative arises from the erroneous idea – albeit very common in anthropology – of value (or value judgment) and human nature. We need to isolate this point since it leads us into the natural criterion for the distinction between normal sadness (even if intense) and pathology. The evolutionary concept of "harmful dysfunction" responds to the concept of judgment as personal preference (people find it undesirable to have "negative emotions") or as collective preference – that is, as social construct. The concept of value is intertwined with the concept of nature, as long as we had the adjective "human."

The pragmatist philosopher Stanley Cavell sheds much light on this point. The opposition between the conventional and the natural is generally stated as an opposition between an arrangement created by society – between, on the one hand, what *we* (or some founders) have accepted and that has no necessity outside of what we have signed into being (i.e., a social contract) and, on the other, that which does not move (i.e., nature in the ecological sense and the body in the biological sense). Cavell comes up with an example that clearly indicates the limits of this dualism: "Someone *may* [emphasis Cavell's] be bored by an earthquake or by the death of his child or the declaration of martial law, or may be angry at a pin or a cloud or a fish, just as someone may quietly (but comfortably?) sit on a chair of nails. That human beings *on the whole* [emphasis mine] do not respond in these ways is, therefore, seriously referred to as conventional; but now we are thinking of convention not as the arrangements a particular culture has found convenient, in terms of its history and geography, for effecting the necessities of human existence, but as those forms of life which are normal to any group of creatures we call human."[44] Convention is not a social construct but, rather, a feature inherent to human nature itself. The concept of nature used by Horwitz and Wakefield, and also by the followers of the philosophy of naturalism, is not that of *human* nature. Human nature is conventional, says Cavell. What does that mean? Not "what is true here is false elsewhere," a proposition that falls before Horwitz and Wakefield's critique. But more like what follows.

The conventionality of human nature can be clearly understood thanks to a distinction Wittgenstein makes between two forms of the forbidden: "You must not put your hand on the element or you'll get burned" is not equivalent to "You must not sleep with your sister." In the first case, what is designated is a causal relation – a fact born of experience – and, in the second, what is designated is an authoritative argument that precedes and precludes all explanation and personal experience. With regard to the first case, Wittgenstein speaks of causal conditioning; with regard to the second, he speaks of logical conditioning, which means that the proposition relies on language. We don't need to define what getting burned means (we can show it, or imitate an expression of pain, etc.); however, in order to permit or forbid sleeping with one's sister, we must first define "sister." And "sister" can be defined only through a system of rules and relations that is meaningful for everyone involved. To define is to give meaning. Individuals living according to particular customs or rules inevitably know their meanings.[45] Biological fact involves functions; social fact involves meanings. And function is subordinate to meaning. That is why adopting a convention is a natural and practical necessity. Social life presupposes values: it is normative from one end to the other. Social fact is, then, a fact of value. It is as hard as a biological fact but is in another category of hardness. Must we accept a single concept of value and a single concept of fact? I see no serious argument for doing so.

Horwitz and Wakefield are correct in urging sociology and anthropology to stop reasoning in terms of "culture and depression" because these terms are relativist and, therefore, without consequence. Using them is like talking in order to say nothing. Besides, criticizing the DSM, like criticizing Big Pharma, has become an inexhaustible literary genre both in France and in the United States. Anthropologists and sociologists confuse biological nature and human nature, thus essentializing the opposition between nature and culture, between facts and values. They fall into this trap (which is rooted in the philosophy of mind) because their basic hypothesis separates facts (which arise from science) and values (which arise from opinion).

The nature of the social fact is that opinion and representation are not outside the object but, rather, are a property of it. For example, when we speak of absence of guilt in conduct disorders or, in the other direction, excessive guilt in melancholia are we not making an evaluation? Are we not judging? Are we not granting a value to a fact without which there would be no fact? If we did not speak of excess guilt in melancholia or the absence of guilt in conduct disorders, neither the fact of melancholia nor the fact of conduct disorder would exist. This intertwining of fact and value cannot be integrated within Horwitz and Wakefield's concept of nature. The fact/value dualism is pure metaphysics.[46] In the footsteps of Hilary Putnam, another great American pragmatist philosopher, I would say that "the picture of our language in which nothing can be *both* a fact *and* value-laden is wholly inadequate and that an enormous amount of our descriptive vocabulary is and has to be 'entangled.'"[47]

Horwitz and Wakefield inhabit a public health perspective: they want to rationalize a chaotic and costly situation. But the consequence of their naturalist approach to depression remains theoretical, and their attempt to find a criterion through which to rationalize the situation does not work. The reason is simple: it is not a methodological problem. The expansion of the diagnosis of depression arises less from the instruments for measuring suffering (and the absence of solid criteria to distinguish the normal from the pathological) and more from the complex recomposition of relations between illness, health, and life and their relation to individual autonomy.

The History of Depression and the History of the Individual

The work you are about to read positions itself between the culturalist and the naturalist temptations. As the Introduction indicates its hypotheses, objectives, and methods, there is no need to set them out here. Allow me simply to point out the spirit in which *The Weariness of the Self* was written.

At the risk of surprising the reader, I'll say it straight off: this book denounces nothing, does not seek to do good, does not think that depression is a problem of distinguishing the normal from the pathological, does not aim to provide constructive criticism. It attempts to *clarify* and to realistically *describe* the history of depression in the twentieth century. Sociology must account for the dilemmas of human life as social life – that is, it must be normative. It transforms experience into language and thus makes it accessible. This is what Martin does in her ethnographic observations, and this is why her book bears the seal of conviction.

I conceived of this book as a dossier. But my approach, unlike that of Horwitz and Wakefield, does not aim to determine a solid criterion that might allow me to reestablish a *medical* truth for pathology by stripping away its social reasons and removing the weight of its values. Instead, I try to account for the concept of depression *such as it exists today* in all its extensions and diversity. The very confusion into which these extensions lead us is part of the problem of depression as a social fact. In the history of depression in the twentieth century, change occurs at all levels: the status of depression, of antidepressants, of psychotherapies, and of medicine in general (which is no longer concerned just with illness but also with health, with enhancement and empowerment, and with social normativity itself).[48]

This is why my goal is to give readers an overall picture of depression in all its psychiatric and anthropological dimensions. I want to give an account of depression's medical and social success. This implies a historical perspective that will help the reader understand, for example, how depression, and not anxiety, ended up being the label that includes all of modern humanity's suffering. I show, in chapter 7, how anxiety was folded into depression during the 1980s. Depression speaks to us of illness, unhappiness, misfortune, and failure. I pay close attention to psychiatric reasoning and include psychoanalysis as well as biological psychiatry and psychopharmacology in my study. Psychiatry is far from being a nosographic practice that labels individuals with social constructs. As a profession, it has practical problems to work out. What is the matter with the patient? How can he or she be treated? What treatments flow from the diagnosis? Why does the treatment work or not work? Is suicide a risk? These are the issues that I address.

I worked on this book, keeping in mind one of Wittgenstein's propositions in his *Philosophical Investigations*: "A philosophical problem has the form: 'I don't know my way about.'"[49] With depression, we all have trouble seeing clearly and finding a way out of our confusion. That is the problem Horwitz and Wakefield had. But my path is quite different from theirs. First off, I was quite surprised by their preoccupation with sadness since depression goes far beyond that.[50] Mental pain, the self-disgust that inhibits action, is as central to depression as is sadness. We have trouble seeing clearly because depression, far from being a problem of distinguishing the normal from the pathological, brings together such a diversity of symptoms that the difficulty of defining and diagnosing it is a constant fact of psychiatry. Jacques Lacan believed that anxiety does not deceive. On the other hand, depression is the illness of deception (see chapter 3, section entitled "An Impossible Definition"). And this must be our point of departure. How do we give form to the magma of depression?

I assume that depression is of anthropological interest and that it can be explored through the provision of a historical perspective.

In saying that depression is of "anthropological interest," I mean that its medical and social success is linked to a major change in the idea that humanity has of itself. In their celebrated and magnificent work *Saturn and Melancholy*, Klibansky, Panofski, and Saxl wrote that melancholia is closely bound to the Western history of self-consciousness; it is its exacerbation. Indeed, according to Klibansky, "to give an overall perspective [on melancholia] ... would mean writing the history of contemporary man."[51] It is the exacerbation of self-consciousness in the form of the autonomous individual (insofar as we are social beings trained to conceive of ourselves and to act as the agents of our own destiny) trained according to the logical conditioning I mentioned earlier. In the sixteenth century, melancholia was the elective illness of the exceptional man, of he who had nothing above him. During the Romantic period, it stood at the crossroads of creative genius and madness. Today, it is the situation of every individual in Western society. I want to provide a glimpse of this history while showing that contemporary depression is the marriage between the traditional melancholia of the exceptional person and the modern egalitarian idea that anyone can be exceptional. Unlike Karp (and Sennett and Lasch when they speak of narcissistic pathologies), I do not approach depression as a weakening of social bonds but, rather, as an attitude, a mindset heavy with multiple social practices and representations of ourselves in a society in which values associated with autonomy (e.g., personal choice, self-ownership, individual initiative) have been generalized.[52] Depression, then, is a pathology of grandeur (for Freud, remember, melancholia was the delusion of inferiority). Thus, depression brings together all the tensions of the modern individual.

"Then we find, as the ripest fruit on that tree, the *sovereign individual,* something which resembles only itself."

Friederich Nietzsche, *Genealogy of Morals,* 1887

"It is easy, as we can see, for a barbarian to be healthy; for a civilized man the task is hard."

Sigmund Freud, *An Outline of Psychoanalysis,* 1938

"The image keeps returning of a man in movement, with no guide; his honour is to think and speak without yielding to nihilism."

Claude Lefort, *Écrire. À l'épreuve du politique,* 1992

The Sovereignty of the Self
or the Return of Nervousness

Today, depression represents the different facets of our unhappiness. During the 1940s, it was simply a syndrome noticed in most mental illnesses and did not receive any societal attention. In 1970, psychiatry demonstrated – with numbers to prove it – that depression was the most widespread illness in the world, while psychoanalysts noticed a net increase in depressive cases within their client base. Today, it captures the attention of psychoanalysts, just as psychosis did fifty years ago. And therein lies its medical success. Simultaneously, newspapers and magazines take it for a fashionable illness, perhaps even a kind of world weariness. Depression has become a tool to define much of our woe and, through various means, to lighten our load. Yet, given the sheer number of disorders they encompass, "anxiety," "malaise," and "neurosis" could have had just as much success as "depression." And therein lies depression's sociological success.

How and why has depression imposed itself as the major personal unhappiness of our time? How does this reveal the mutations of individuality during the second half of the twentieth century? These are the two questions that arise during this exploration of the depressive state.

Depression is a morbid state that gives us the ability to comprehend contemporary individuality and its dilemmas. Within psychiatry, depression is a crossroads for an excellent reason: yesterday, like today, psychiatrists did not know how to define it, and so they bestowed upon it a rare plasticity. The "choice" of depression over other categories is a result of a combination of internal elements of psychiatry and profound normative changes in our lifestyles. It is not, however, the first fashionable illness. Hysteria and neurasthenia knew analogous success towards the end of the nineteenth century. The history of depression is not without a link to these two pathologies. The nervous people of the twentieth century seem to be suffering from a pain as imperceptible as hysteria. Are we being toyed with again?

In 1898, in a work intended for the general public, a doctor could write: "Everyone knows today what the word neurasthenia means – it is, with the word bicycle, one of the most common terms of this era."[1] Because the same can be said of depression today is thanks, first and foremost, to a famous medication. We must approach the shores of the depressive question through the molecule known as Prozac.

In common terms, Prozac has come to stand for antidepressant in the way that Frigidaire stands for refrigerator or Kleenex for paper handkerchief.[2] How has a pill come to embody the hope – unreasonable certainly, but most understandable in these times – of instantaneously ridding oneself of psychological suffering? For a mental cure to hold such a fantasy, for it to produce a collusion between medication and social aspiration, the suffering at which it is aimed had to progressively acquire a central role in our societies. The language of the self has become integrated to such a point that each of us employs terms like "depression" and "Prozac" to say something about ourselves or our existence: they have become part of us.

Depression began its ascent when the disciplinary model for behaviours, the rules of authority and observance of taboos that gave social classes as well as both sexes a specific destiny, broke against norms that invited us to undertake personal initiative by enjoining us to be ourselves. These new norms brought with them a sense that the responsibility for our existence lies not only within us but also within the collective between-us. I try here to demonstrate that depression is the opposite of this paradigm. Depression presents itself as an *illness of responsibility* in which the dominant feeling is that of failure. The depressed individual is unable to measure up; he is tired of having to become himself.

But what does becoming oneself mean? The question is deceptively simple, while bringing to our attention serious issues of borders – between the allowed and the forbidden, the possible and the impossible, the normative and the pathological. Today, the private sphere is constructed by unstable relationships between guilt, responsibility, and mental pathology.

This inquiry is the third part of a trilogy that tries to draw an outline of the contemporary individual: the self that was established as we exited class-based societies, with their emphasis on political representation and the regulation of behaviours. The first part describes how the increased attention to the values of economic competition and sports rivalries in French society propelled the trajectory-individual to a conquest of her personal identity and an increase in her social status, commanding her to surpass herself in an entrepreneurial adventure. The second part describes how this achievement was accompanied by a new-found worry about psychological suffering. I examined two problems stemming from mass movements: (1) the self's being put on sale in reality television and (2) self-improvement through psychoactive drugs that modify behaviour and mood and increase individual abilities (e.g., through doping in sports).[3]

And this, the third part of the trilogy, is a study of the history of the psychiatric notion of depression. I chose this subject because the public debate now confuses psychoactive medication (which treats mental pathologies) and illegal drugs (which modify states of mind). The difference between these two classes of psychotropic drugs is not as clear as the medical world believed (with reason) during the 1950s, the period during which these medicines were discovered. We will have to get used to living with drugs that improve mood, increase control over the self, and soften the impact of existence: better to take the measure of the lifestyle they reveal.

The medical and sociological success of the notion of depression has not come about without issues, as is proven by the confusing and decisive controversy surrounding Prozac. Bliss on prescription is opposed by the chemistry of despair; the medicalization of angst is opposed by depression as an authentic illness; the publicity in praise of a miracle remedy is opposed by concern about toxicity or risk of addiction. The medicalization of life is a general phenomenon, but it seems to pose very particular problems in psychiatry.

The conflicting opinions on Prozac are not about the fact that, like all medication, Prozac can be both cure and poison: while a fatal dose of aspirin is quickly reached, a fatal dose of Prozac is another matter entirely. Yet we take aspirin to relieve pain even though it is much more dangerous than Prozac. Why should it be any different for an antidepressant as long as it is safe? By giving hope of overcoming all psychological suffering because it alleviates the mental state of those who are not "truly" depressed, the new class of comfortable antidepressants, of which Prozac is first in line, embodies, whether we like it or not, the unlimited possibility of restructuring our mental states to become more than the sum of our parts. The limit between healing ourselves and doping ourselves is suddenly blurred. In a society in which people permanently take psychoactive drugs that affect the central nervous system and modify behaviour, we would no longer be able to say *who we are* or even *who is normal.* "Who" becomes a key concept since it designates the presence of a subject. Has its reckoning come?

In fact, a sense of suspicion has taken over. Would an artificial sense of well-being be taking over from a cure? A series of unresolved questions flows from this. Is suffering useful? If so, what is its use? Are we moving towards a society of comfortable dependencies in which each person can take a daily psychotrope? Are we not mass-producing hypochondriacs? Can we still make the distinction between the unhappiness and frustrations of everyday life and pathological suffering? Is this distinction necessary? Sensitive questions, particularly since the latter presupposes a stable difference between "illness" and its absence. If medical ethics forces doctors to relieve suffering, even when they cannot cure the illness, why should this be any different when it comes to psychic problems?

Approached from this angle, the problem remains obscure. It is thus necessary to overcome the controversies associated with the treatment of depression through drugs by analyzing our problematic through a historical lens.

It is certain that an exploration of the institutionalization of the individual, which becomes clear as we follow the psychiatric representations of depression in the 1940s, the dawn of its contemporary period (with the introduction of electroshock therapy), will offer us some clarification. The transformations of the individual's avatar are a part of the history of democracy. They relate to its customs and morals, to what Montesquieu calls the general spirit of a society: "Laws are established, mores are inspired; the latter depend more on the general spirit, the former depend more on a particular institution."[4]

Two theories are put forward here: the first concerns the role played by depression in the normative changes that have come about in French society since the end of the Second World War; the second concerns the role played by depression in psychiatry, with regard to the mutations of the pathological individual, during the same period. These two theories follow an interpretive guide that I analyze later.

NOTHING IS TRULY FORBIDDEN, NOTHING IS TRULY POSSIBLE

The 1960s weakened the prejudices, traditions, walls, and bounds that structured our lives. The political debates and judicial disruption provoked by these changes were the signs of profound upheaval. We were emancipated in the proper sense: the modern political idea, that we are owners of ourselves, and not the docile serfs of the Prince, has widened to encompass all aspects of existence. The sovereign man who is only like himself, whom Nietzsche had imagined, has now become the norm.

It is precisely here that we are usually mistaken about the individual. Many are satisfied simply by bemoaning modern humanity's loss of reference points and the consequent weakening of the social realm, with the privatization of life and the decline of the public domain. These stereotypes bring us back to snivelling about the good old days. Retrospective illusions! Theological quarrels! Have we nothing to gain from this new-found liberty? We are much more likely to be affected by the confusion brought about by new reference points (e.g., new philosophies or religions, television programs destined to make sense of it all) than we are by their loss. Is not this increase in reference points a condition without which individual freedom simply could not exist? Rather than a decline of the public domain, what we are facing are transformations of our political references and modes of public action, which, in turn, allow for the discovery of a new identity within the context of mass individualism and the birth of globalization. Do we yearn to return to the disciplinary stranglehold? More important, how would we do it? Instead of pitying ourselves for the suffering that surrounds us, it is time to face, with some historical appreciation and good sense, the question of emancipation.

This new-found sovereignty does not make us all-powerful or free to do as we please, it does not bring about the rule of the private individual. Herein lies the individualist illusion, which does not want to "agree," as Claude Lefort says, "that the individual hides from himself by referring only to himself, that he is up against an unknown."[5] Two fundamental modifications, one on the importance of the law, the second on the importance of discipline, follow from this sovereignty.

The changes brought about by emancipation disrupted the intimacy of each and all: modern democracy – and this is its strength – has slowly made us persons without guides, progressively placing us in a situation in which we need to judge what surrounds us by ourselves and construct our own reference points. We have become individuals in the purest sense as no moral law or tradition can tell us who we must be and how we need to behave. The forbidden/allowed dichotomy, which had the force of law until the 1950-60s, has lost its pertinence. The overriding concern for the law – the need for new reference points and "limits-that-cannot-be-passed" – has declined. The right to live and the need to become ourselves place individuality within a feeling of restlessness. This leads to a rethinking of regulating limits within the self: the division between the allowed and the forbidden loses out to the division between the possible and the impossible. Individuality finds itself transformed.

And while the notion of the forbidden is put into perspective, the idea of discipline as a regulator of the relationship between individuals and society has become less important. Individuals resort less to disciplinary obedience than to personal decision and initiative. Instead of being acted *upon* by an external force (or complying to the law), persons base their actions on an internal drive or mental capacities. Notions like "projects," "motivation," and "communication" are now the norm. They have entered our social hierarchy and inhabit it from top to bottom; for better or worse, we have learned to adapt ourselves to them. Both the public sector and the private sector comprehend these notions; they are used as much in business management as in rehabilitation.

We must integrate these normative transformations into our thought processes. A failure to do so would prevent our understating how our perspective towards inequality, domination, and politics has changed. The measure of the ideal individual today has more to do with initiative than it does with docility. And here lies one of the decisive mutations of our lifestyles. This is because the modes of regulation are not a choice that each can make in a private way but, rather, a common rule valid for all,[6] social exclusion being the threat to possible offenders. These regulations are based on our societies' "general spirit": they are the *institutions of the self*.[7]

Hence a first hypothesis: depression teaches us about our current experience as an individual because it is the pathology of a society whose norm is no longer based on guilt and discipline but on responsibility and initiative. Yesterday, social rules demanded conformists, perhaps even automatons; today, initiative and mental capacities are required. The individual is confronted with a pathology of inadequacy more than with a pathology of the mistake, with the universe of dysfunction more than with the universe of law: the depressed individual is a person out of gas. The subordination of guilt to responsibility does not occur without clouding the relationship between the allowed and the forbidden.

In the workshop of societal ambivalences in which each person is her/his own sovereign, depression is instructive in that it makes visible the twin changes within the constraints that structure individuality: inwardly, these constraints no longer manifest themselves as guilt; outwardly, they no longer manifest themselves as discipline.

From the standpoint of the history of the individual, whether it designates a true illness or just social unease, depression is particular since it marks the helplessness of existence, be it expressed though sadness, asthenia (fatigue), inhibition, or the inability to initiate action (named "psychomotor slowing" by psychiatrists). The depressed individual, caught in a moment with no tomorrow, is left without drive, bogged down in a "nothing is possible." Tired and empty, restless and violent – in short, nervous – we feel the weight of our individual sovereignty. The decisive displacement of the difficult task of appearing healthy, is, according to Freud, the price the civilized person must pay.

DEPRESSION, OR THE DECLINE OF THE CONFLICT OF THE MIND

If psychiatry is to easily locate the displacement of guilt by responsibility, it must have an adequate interpretive guide. Before we turn to this, however, let us first formulate a second hypothesis.

In democracy, individualism has the peculiarity of resting on two phenomena: (1) being a person reliant upon one's own means (i.e., an individual) and (2) existing within a human group (i.e., a society) that finds in itself the signification of its existence. Gone are the days when we were guided by religious or secular leaders. Two notions have replaced them: inner nature and conflict.

In democratic societies, the mind, more than the body, is the centre of endless controversy. No matter the advances or discoveries of biological sciences, they cannot clear up the mind/body dispute. Just as in philosophy, so in neurobiology, we still lack agreement regarding the essence of the mind. These controversies intrude upon our fundamental beliefs. Instead of being expressed through the soul, which is wholly tied to sin, a person's inner self is now expressed through notions of the spirit, the mental, the psychological. In short, although hidden, our inner nature nonetheless signals its existence through various means. As sacred as the soul, our inner nature remains a taboo and cannot be manipulated without risk. Our inner nature is a fiction that we have created in order to explain what is happening within ourselves. But this fiction is also a truth: we believe in it as others believe in metempsychosis or in the mystical power of ancestors.

The institutionalization of conflict allows the free confrontation of contradictory interests and the achievement of acceptable compromise. It is the very condition of democracy insofar as it allows the representation of social division within a political arena. Equally as important, mental conflicts are the counterpart of the self-creation that defines modern individuality. The notion of conflict is what maintains the gap between what is possible and what is allowed. The modern individual wages war against the self: to be connected with herself, she has to be separated from herself. From the political to the private, conflict is the normative centre of democratic life.

The second hypothesis is that the success of depression lies in the *decline of conflict as a reference point* upon which the nineteenth-century notion of the self was founded. The identification of the notions of conflict and subject appeared with Freud's "Psychoneurosis of Defense," which explains that the history of psychiatry and depression is characterized by the difficulty of defining the self.[8]

Another difficulty with the self lies in a related field: addiction and dependence. Psychiatrists teach that addiction is a way of battling depression: it *abrades conflicts* through compulsive behaviour. Yet, since the 1970s, addiction and depression have been discussed together. Both are manifestations of a symbolic difficulty with the notions of law and conflict.

Addictions represent the impossibility of the self's controlling the self: the addict is a slave to herself, be she dependent on a product, an activity, or a person. Her capacity for self-achievement and for integrating herself within society (these two phenomena being similar) become impossible. She finds herself in an "impossible" situation with the law. The possibility of choosing morals and values (and hence the decline of the allowed/forbidden polarity) and overtaking the limits that nature has imposed on humanity (thanks to advances in biological sciences and pharmacology) make everything concretely possible. For this reason, today the addict wears the mask of the anti-subject. This is the same disguise the madman used to wear. If depression is the history of an undiscoverable self, then addiction is the nostalgia for a lost self.

In the same way that neurosis threatened the individual divided by his conflicts, torn between the allowed and the forbidden, depression threatens the individual apparently freed from his taboos but certainly torn between the possible and the impossible. If neurosis is the tragedy of guilt, depression is the tragedy of inadequacy. It is the familiar shadow of a person without a guide, tired of going forward to achieve the self and tempted to sustain himself through products and behaviours.

From neurosis to depression and addiction I explore the way in which we have moved from a collective to an individual experience of ourselves. I also try to follow a few mutations of subjectivity through changes in its pathologies.

"DEFICIENCY" AND "CONFLICT," AN INTERPRETIVE GUIDE TO A HISTORY OF DEPRESSION

The creation of the notion of neurosis towards the end of the nineteenth century offers us an interpretive guide to the movement from guilt to responsibility. Freud's guide is opposed by that of Pierre Janet, his famous rival. The following case is well known by historians of psychiatry and psychoanalysts. Freud and Janet modernized the old notion of nervousness by creating the notion of the mental: they made it acceptable to believe that the mind can be ill without a biological cause, and they "invented" psychotherapy by integrating the charlatan's use of hypnosis into medical science. Their contradictions are common knowledge, but I mention one in particular since it allows us, I believe, to interpret the metamorphoses of depression by joining them to those of individuality. Freud sees neurosis as originating in conflict, while Janet sees it as originating in lack or insufficiency. While with regard to conflict there is undoubtedly a subject (since the patient is considered to be an agent), this is rather less clear when it comes to depression.

I follow three main steps in this historical study of depression. The first step involves the subtle alliance between lack and conflict, which offered psychiatry the reference point it needed to treat the depression of the sick subject. This was the first paradigm of modern depression. The second step involves the breakup of this alliance during the 1970s, when neurosis began its decline. Depression emerged from the medical field without needing a pharmacological innovation as a vector for expansion (this was in a context in which emancipation led to a movement within the forbidden, while guilt remained hidden in the rise of responsibility). It became a fashionable illness well before the marketing of antidepressants like Prozac and even before the pessimistic turn of today. Depression appeared not as a pathology of unhappiness but more as a pathology of change, one in which a person yearned to become only herself: internal insecurity was the price of this "liberation." The third step, which occurred in the 1980s, involved depression's entering a paradigm in which inhibition dominated mental anguish, slowness, and anesthesia: the former sorrowful passion transformed itself into a failure to act, and this in a context in which individual action had become the measure of oneself. The notion of healing entered into a deepening crisis, and depression was redefined as a chronic illness much like diabetes. Yet, since the illness is of the mind, this chronicity led to a kind of identity questioning that did not exist during the 1960s: drug or medication? Depression and addiction are what trace the outline of the individual at the end of the twentieth century.

METHODOLOGICAL COMMENT

The key point of *The Weariness of the Self* is to shed light on the contradictory arguments that have forged both the scholarly and the popular image of depression. I do not hope to reach scientific truth so much as I hope to contribute to the public debate, and I try to comprehend more than to judge. To achieve a relevant societal critique we must be *realistic* in describing our world, *prescriptive* in evaluating livable worlds, and *political* in proposing intellectual steps that will enable appropriate action.

Depression, like all other mental pathologies, is not part of the classes of illnesses that are locatable in a specific part of the human body. Those who are interested in the history or anthropology of psychiatric categories and mental illnesses are faced with two issues: (1) a positivist tendency in the life sciences, which reduces these problems to biological imbalances, and (2) a relativist tendency in the social sciences, which does not take into account the biological dimension of human beings and that dissolves pathological realities within societal functions (e.g., labelling a deviance, managing certain disorders, or controlling behaviours). Sociologists too often settle for an approach that either medicalizes anxiety[9] or that analyzes a social problem through a psychiatric lens. These two tendencies are, without a doubt, a symptom of the difficulties involved in seeing the place that the *social* notion of the mental occupies in our societies.

How can we define suffering if we do not have the words to express it? Psychiatry, which is the only medical specialty that is expressly concentrated on the pathological individual, offers us this vocabulary. Although the mental can have an influence in dermatology or oncology, psychiatry is the only science whose object is the pathological individual. It is unique in that it observes how the relationships between the individual and society, along with their respective definitions, are simultaneously transformed. This is why *The Weariness of the Self* concentrates not on psychiatric practices but, rather, on psychiatric reasoning, by which I mean the type of experiences that a person perceives.

Psychiatry cannot read with certainty the characteristics of mental disorder – whether a feeling, an emotion, or a self-image – the way other branches of medicine read morbid signs in patients' bodies, blood or urine; rather, it focuses on emotion and/or the representation of the self. Throughout the history of psychiatry a question has remained unanswered: how does one objectivize the subjective? Psychiatry finds itself in quite a bind: when it discovers the cause of a mental pathology, as was the case with epilepsy, it was able to do so only because the illness was not a mental one. Psychiatry generally treats pathologies whose causes are not a matter of consensus.[10] The task of the clinician involves interpreting the symptoms and syndromes,[11] which she does not so much to distinguish the normal from the pathological as to achieve a diagnosis.[12] This distinction between the normal and the pathological haunts us today. One must not see this as a matter of insufficient clinical reflection so much as a practical consequence of the modern notion of interiority. The disagreements about the causes, definitions, and treatments of various pathologies and the uncertainties that accompany the history of psychiatric reasoning are especially revealing when we discuss the transformations of the individual.[13] We must then respect these difficulties by coherently reshaping them.

The Weariness of the Self tries to understand how psychiatrists formulate their questions and what type of solutions they bring to the table. One of depression's peculiarities is that, unlike monomania (Esquirol), hysteria (Charcot, Janet, and Freud), manic-depressive psychosis (Kraepelin), or schizophrenia (Bleuler), no famous clinician or great work is attached to it. I turned to a multifaceted corpus, which includes, among others, pharmacological, clinical, epidemiological, nosographical, and neurobiological aspects. Due to the lack of works available on the twentieth-century history of French psychiatry, a large number of the themes that I present are merely touched upon.

This book takes much of its information from a review of French psychiatric literature, beginning with works from the 1930s and 1940s, as well as Anglo-American works.[14] I also consulted *La revue du practicien,* a magazine that helped educate GPs from its first article on antidepressants in 1958, as well as two women's magazines (*Elle* and *Marie-Claire*) and a weekly (*L'Express*).[15] I was able to establish links between three different domains: (1) the internal debates of the psychiatric community; (2) strictly medical conundrums (and the help medicine can offer); and (3) the education received by the general public regarding an internal vocabulary that has guided social demand. This book does not deal with depression itself; rather, it deals with our notions of depression, our ways of reasoning about it, and our psychiatric models of it. I use this methodology in order to clarify a multitude of heterogeneous and contradictory phenomena that shape the notion of mental pathology. I hope *The Weariness of the Self* will help the reader both to grasp an overall view of the issues at hand and to respect the basic notions of psychiatry.

PART ONE

A Sick Self

Greek sculpture sought the logic of the body; Rodin sought the psychology of the body. The essence of modernity is psychologism, the fact of feeling the world and giving it meaning as an inner world, obeying the reactions of our inner self. It implies the dissolving of stable meaning in the flow of the soul, independent and pure of all substance, whose forms are but those of its movements.

> Georg Simmel, "Rodin" in *Michel-Ange et Rodin*, 1923 (102-3)

If, at one limit, narco-analysis is a psychological medication, that is, a chemical therapy, then at the other limit it is a psychological medication in Pierre Janet's meaning of the word – a psychotherapy.

> Jean Delay, *Études de psychologie médicale*, 1953 (227)

WHICH HISTORY OF DEPRESSION?

We have set our objective: to understand the mutations of the notion of the individual through the second half of the twentieth century. Which history of depression should we now study in order to reach our goal?

Let us begin by observing what was written on the history of depression in psychiatric treatises: first we find melancholia, whose long history originates in Greek antiquity. It was characterized by great pain, with its main manifestation being listlessness and torpor, once considered as one of the seven deadly sins (*acedia*). We then find delirium (*mania*), which Christianity believed to be the symptom of demonic possession, and in which, at the end of the eighteenth century, nascent alienists saw a loss of reason.

Then contemporary psychiatrists offered two views. The first
was that psychiatry in the first half of the nineteenth century
was intellectualist. Mental alienation was seen as an illness of
judgment or understanding since the madman was without
reason. This intellectualism could not conceive of delirium as
being the manifestation of profound emotional suffering, the
way in which the madman could speak out – albeit deliriously –
to interpret his pain.

The second view was that psychiatry in the first half of the
nineteenth century was nosographical: madness was seen as a
single illness composed of multiple symptoms. It was opposed by
reason. This concept was much too general to diagnose specific
illnesses: just as there is not a single sickness of the body, so it
is preposterous to propose a single illness of the mind. Alienists
undid this unity by expressing insanity through different mental
illnesses comprised of two main groups of psychoses. The first
was melancholia. Its definition stabilized during the 1830s,
becoming "partial delirium" and "moral anxiety." In France, as
of the 1850s-60s, the notion of circular or dual-formed madness,
characterized by phases of manic agitation and phases of depressive collapse, was expressed. Towards the end of the nineteenth
century, the German psychiatrist Emil Kraepelin defined this
form of dementia as manic-depressive psychosis, in which he
includes melancholia. The second group of psychoses, whose
most visible aspect is delirium and which results from the dissociation of the individual and his personality, was named "schizophrenia" by the Swiss psychiatrist Eugen Bleuler in 1911. During
the last third of the nineteenth century, various mental ailments
were defined by dementia. These ailments were both less serious
than melancholia or schizophrenia and were devoid of delirium.
They were named, depending on the case, neurasthenia, psychasthenia, irritable heart, and so on. These "neuroses" (the term
emerged at the end of the nineteenth century) included various
illnesses and were considered functional, meaning they had no
biological basis. Asthenic neurosis is seen as the second source
of depression after melancholia.

Psychiatric treatises note a certain stabilization of these morbid
groups between both world wars. They also make mention of
the shock techniques developed at that time and insist upon the
rudimentary nature of this therapeutic tool. They observe that

electroshock therapy has had some success treating melancholia. And here begins depression's stone age. Progress will only be made after the Second World War, with the discovery of medicine for the mind.

The crucial role played by the invention of neuroleptics (1952) in the transformation of clinical psychiatry and the beginning of neurobiological research has already been mentioned. Things became simpler: psychiatry gained the esteem of the medical community, which was working with the neurosciences that provided the bases for its clinical models. Psychoanalysis obtained this role during its short golden age from the end of the 1960s to the end of the 1970s. Neuroleptics would reduce the psychotic person's anxiety and keep her delirium at bay: they would put an end to the myth of incurability. The invention of antidepressants (1957) offered successful therapy for various disorders situated on the limits of psychiatry and whose sufferers had been filling the offices of general practitioners. This invention would allow the naming of an entire category of disorders, which was now referred to as "depression." Neurobiology would also see its task become simpler: the invention of these substances was a huge leap forward for research as it clarified, thanks to the discovery of neuronal receptors, the mechanisms that transmit information within the nervous system. Its major scientific consequence was the advancement of etiopathogenisis, the comprehension of mechanisms in which unknown causes trigger syndromes or illnesses. Both clinical psychiatry and biological research illustrate Hippocrates' aphorism: "It is the treatment that reveals the nature of the sickness." Since it efficiently treats morbid states, the treatment allows us to say, "This is a sickness." This is what medicine calls "the therapeutic test."

This historical reconstruction gives too large a role to technical innovation. Interpretation through therapeutic testing is not sufficient, and this for two reasons: (1) the status of anxiety and (2) the therapeutic support offered to mental pathologies.

The invention of modern anxiolytics (benzodiazepine in 1960) did not create an illness or a syndrome that we could have named, for example, "axiopathia" and that would now occupy a position similar to that of depression. If the expression "depressive illness" is widely used today (and challenged as well), the term "anxiety illness" is not. Except in a few cases, anxiety has remained closer to the notion of symptom than has depression. Thus, since 1980, the neurosis of anxiety has been split into two categories: panic attacks and generalized anxiety disorder. These two syndromes rapidly fell into the domain of depressive disorders since they are better treated, it is said, by antidepressants than by anxiolytics. Depression has also gained ground by absorbing various "anxiety disorders," to use the current terminology, thanks to the invention of new psychiatric categories: dysthymia and anxiodepression.[1] Today, anxiety is part of depression. In France, since the 1980s, anxiolytics have been the subject of many debates,[2] but psychiatrists have agreed to see them as medications acting upon symptoms. The picture is quite different for depression: innumerable articles have been written reminding us that it is a genuine illness, its gravity being tallied up not only in terms of its cost for social services but, especially, in terms of the risk of suicide it carries with it. This is why chemical treatment is now recommended for all types of depression no matter their degree of intensity – to the point where treatment is recommended for cases in which depression is considered subsyndromic.

The second reason that interpretation through therapeutic testing is not sufficient concerns the need to question the therapeutic support offered to mental pathologies. The progressive reduction of the toxicity of antidepressants, the comfort they offer patients, and their increasing simplicity of use would eventually lead to abuse, misappropriation of prescriptions, and so on; however, it was not possible to foresee this path at the time of the invention of antidepressants. From the 1940s to the 1970s, French psychiatrists would never consider healing a depressive individual without first wondering to what extent the illness stemmed from intrapsychic conflicts. The discovery of neuroleptics and antidepressants rapidly brought about a consensus: a chemical treatment can be effective as long as it is combined with a psychological one. This was an important credo in French psychiatry throughout the 1950 and 1960s, and it energized the development of both fields.

The preceding historical attitudes towards depression are not wrong, merely interpretively misplaced. Thus the opposition of chemical therapy and psychotherapy is much less important than are their respective composition and practices. Of course, melancholia, neurasthenia, and psychasthenia (listlessness and psychomotor slowing) are the main sources of depression, but it is not enough to say that depression comes from a combination of these factors. As of the 1940s, the history of depression became closely tied to the progress of pharmacology. But there is also the interpretive difference between the United States and France. The French metaphysical creature, the Subject, is absent in Anglo-American culture, and yet it is perfectly observable in the field we are studying.[3] We must combine a cultural and technical history of psychiatry, especially since it offers the biological means to treat pathologies.

Chapter 1 frames our thought processes, and by synthesizing the historical path that built a credible reputation for the idea of "mental" suffering during the nineteenth century, it casts the mould for the chapters to follow. We continue with the classical age of depression, the age of the "ill self" (chapter 2). A treatment with a terrible reputation starts the ball rolling: electroconvulsive therapy (ECT) (certainly not antidepressants, which only appear in 1957, twenty years later). ECT was the magic wand that broke the spell of melancholia. The impressive electrical discharges that shook the bodies of sick individuals undid their suffering and, miraculously, gave them a desire to live. But did it cure the asthenics, the doubters, the inhibited, the anxious, and all the other neurotic individuals whose symptoms resembled melancholia? Although this question shook psychiatry to its core, a consensus was never reached. ECT also brought about a new age in a more practical sense: it opened up nosographical, therapeutic, and diagnostic debates that continued on throughout the 1960s (chapter 3). These debates found their niche within the greater controversy surrounding the technique itself, while never concentrating on the issue at hand. But with the arrival of general medicine and the new-found attention to the self, they did succeed in socializing depression. The possibility of healing, a specific vocabulary of the self, industries that furnish molecules: all of these would bring about multifaceted and multiple demands from the public.

1

The Birth of the Psychic Self

As the first symposium on the depressives state in France opened at the Saint-Anne Hospital in November 1954, the speaker mentioned a specific name: Pierre Janet. "At the beginning of the century," declared Dr Julien Rouart, "there was much talk about certain neurotic depressions that have since disappeared, like neurasthenia, and Pierre Janet founded his entire psychasthenia theory on the notion of 'a lowering in psychological tension.' In fact … neurotic depressions are in contrast to the psychotic type as constitutional weakness is to illness."[4] Asthenia, lowering, weakness: the depressive mentality is built upon inadequacy. Freud, psychoanalysts have since pointed out, wrote very little on depression:[5] he preferred anxiety. Are anxiety and inadequacy opposed to one another? In fact, the border of their respective territories is guilt. Freud was guilt's protagonist, while Janet was deficiency's.

Questions brought forward by the study of mental illnesses have always been encumbered by timeless philosophical arguments over the status of the mind and the specificity of the ancient disciplinary disputes between biology and psychology and subject-specific antinomies. Beware of the self, say some, meaning the human being; do not forget the sick person, say others, meaning the body. Within the history of mental disorders there is an underlying tension between those who consider human beings in terms of animality and those who consider them in terms of personality (which is predicated upon their propensity for speech). This is an important opposition, and it brings about a series of conflicts regarding the source of illness, its definition, its treatments, and our concept of recovery. But the opposition remains tricky since we cannot imagine what the self

would be without a body. In which ways would it be "alive?"[6] Yet the
integration of animality and personality is the key to the subjectivity
that was handed down to us at the end of the nineteenth century.

If it is clear to our well-trained eyes that mental pathology is synonymous with psychological suffering, this has certainly not always
been the case. The contemporary individual can say: "I suffer" rather
than just "I suffer from…"[7]

To illustrate the genealogy of suffering with the self as the only
object, we analyze four different elements. The first is the discovery
that the insane individual suffers: this is the stage of melancholia.
The second involves the transformation from "I think" to "it thinks."
This undoing of traditional consciousness brings about a new concept of the individual: a stranger is at the helm of our conscience.[8]
Conscience leaves behind the mind, travels to the tip of the fingers,[9]
and the whole body begins to "speak" a language whose grammar
we must decipher. The third element involves the way in which the
connection to the self was opened and explored throughout the
twentieth century. This paves the way for individual worries and
identity questions, especially within the more well-to-do crowd.
Historians[10] have described in detail the increasing importance of
the dilemmas of individuals who have tried to make their way outside
of tradition and who now look at themselves from that perspective
(e.g., consider the democratization of the portrait, the circulation
of mirrors, the birth of photography) while simultaneously studying
themselves from the inside (e.g., consider the diary's monologue,
secret conversations with "mute interlocutors").[11] The fourth element of my analysis involves the creation of the notion of neurosis,
which opened up the possibility of a purely psychological injury (i.e.,
an injury that exists without being linked to a somatic disorder)
whose source is a traumatic event. This discovery reveals and energizes the socialization of the mind.

The history of the notion of suffering (although quite vague) is
less a progressive psychological rendering than a conflict-riddled
game that tries to cram biology, sociology, and psychology into the
mind. The progress of both the unconsciousness and the consciousness of the self, and a new-found sensitivity to interior upheavals
and shocks created by experiences, are this game's framework. In
the same way that Rodin tried to sculpt the "psychology of the body,"
psychiatry tries to define subtle movements, barely perceptible vibrations, interior upheavals, and anxiety.

This chapter shows the way in which psychiatry is a unique medical domain that, unlike other branches of medicine, is necessarily confronted with moral issues. Indeed, without confronting these issues it would never be able to treat those forms of suffering that are themselves moral. We then follow suffering through melancholia, through the decentring of consciousness embodied in the problem of reflexes, and through the reorganization of neurosis, in which neurasthenia enables the birth of functional illnesses. This dynamic opens the way for the study of the key notion of trauma, those exterior stimuli that result in mental disorders. Here we find two models of illness and two principle players, Freud and Janet, who structure the internal conflicts of mental health to this day.

HOW IS MENTAL ILLNESSES A PATHOLOGY OF FREEDOM?

Do mental illnesses result from an entity entering the body in the same way as would a virus?[12] Are they the result of heredity or a fragile psychology, affecting some but not others? Be it sickness or constitution, internal or external, when it comes to clinical work (e.g., defining the pathology, its causes and treatments), the issues are clear. Yet they are always connected to others, whether in science or in philosophy, since the mind can define how the individual perceives the internal and the external. This is the result of issues that were traditionally in the sphere of religion being displaced into the sphere of medicine.

In 1969, during a series of conferences devoted to Michel Foucault's *The History of Madness*, one of French psychiatry's most important postwar thinkers, Henri Ey, stated that madness had become an illness with "the arrival of the subject as the centre of an indetermination having its own organization. In this way, the notion of mental illness is a corollary of the idea of the individual."[13] His point is that alienation is the illness of a freedom that no longer finds its meaning and justification within an external divine presence. Without boundaries, this freedom is symbolically open to all possibilities. Psychiatry separates moral fault from the human being by transforming it into a medical object – a pathology of freedom or a life of relationships, to use Henri Ey's famous formulas. It is here, then, that we find the starting point of any thought processes regarding the relationship between psychiatry and individuality.

The birth of insanity supplied a solution, albeit an unstable one, to an emerging problem: how to differentiate between a moral question and a medical question within a context in which individual freedom had become political coinage, based in law, while, with the birth of the clinic, medicine evolved towards modernity. The medical domain would sit by the sickbed and lay a "knowing eye" on the body of the individual, which would, from that point on, be associated with illness.[14] To begin believing in a mental disorder where we previously saw only the Devil, we had to cleanse the body of its sacred image. With the notion of illness, the mind enters the domain of the body. As Freud wrote in 1923, the demons that once possessed our minds have become "psychological creatures" that we "regard ... as having arisen in the patient's internal life, where they have their abode."[15] If the mind is the soul, only secularized, then, if we are to decipher its grammar, it must have an equally secular physical body.

Here we see psychiatry's position between the medical and the moral: it transforms moral entities, for which the individual is responsible, into medical entities, by which the individual is affected. This situation leads to tensions within the individual. Sadness or delirium are no longer a sin against faith or an infraction against divine laws but, rather, an illness that prevents freedom. Not owned, but an owner of one's destiny, as specified in the United Nations Declaration of Human Rights.

Mental illness not only describes the irresponsibility of humanity's freedom but also functions as the non-attributable part of will or intention. Madness is a destructive player in the individual's mind, but there is an area in which medicine can help.[16] More than anything else, madness is reason's opposing concept.[17] The issue, writes Gladys Swain, is the "the deporting of madness from the human periphery to the centre of the being ... Within all, at the core there lies a conflictual instability that nullifies with a pre-emptive strike all attempts to define man as having a perfect balance within himself."[18] The modern psyche is defined by this conflict, and it is for this reason that it remains the individual's core. The psyche is the reasonable – and fragile – distance from oneself within oneself. It creates the modern self, making it receptive to a notion of law that is no longer guided and imposed by the divine.

When this distance is stretched to its breaking point, madness ensues. Inversely, this distance can be so small that it creates a fusion between the self and the self. The moderns referred to the victim of this fusion as a "drug user." In 1822, Thomas de Quincey explained that, unlike alcohol, opium is not associated with drunkenness because "it gives simply that sort of vital warmth which is approved by the judgment and which would probably always accompany a bodily constitution of primeval or antediluvian health." It allows "a healthy restoration to that state which the mind would naturally recover upon the removal of any deep-seated irritation of pain."[19] Drugs are a way of obtaining absolute health, but the price is high: a slavery to a different pathology of liberty. On one end of the spectrum we have the madman, on the other end we have the drug user: in both cases we find "the self's humanity flickering."[20] The madman and the drug user are the two symbols upon which modern societies rely to describe the dark side of the ideal individual. The first appears while democracy is born, the second appears two centuries later. Between them, we find the movement that drives some from alienation to neurosis, then from neurosis to depression.

MELANCHOLIA, FROM GREAT HEIGHTS TO HELPLESSNESS

The reason-alienation opposition does not fully describe the issues faced by mental illnesses; in particular, it does not breach the realm of suffering that is described by the happiness-unhappiness opposition. In order to consider alienation as suffering and not simply as a lack of reason, we need a cultural explanation.

The Age of Enlightenment is one of reason and happiness,[21] and these are the two main contributing factors to the secularization process that built modern societies. There appears a *personal life*, one that is developed at a time when a modern public sphere is being created in which, according to Habermas, personal thought processes are used in a public context. This personal life is independent from divine or royal authority and becomes the subject of much writing. The theme of happiness takes on a whole new dimension: it concentrates on "attention being paid to what is felt interiorly ... for the signs that are pleasure and displeasure allow man to become the agent of his destiny."[22] At the same time, the concept of "spleen" is developed: the contented consciousness and the anxious consciousness become connected. During a century in which a society that determines its own destiny is created (built on the fiction of a social contract between people who delegate the responsibility for governing them to a political power), lives can be justified by means other than religious ones, and happiness is one of those means. How can this be done? By sociability. Human beings are social animals, and their instinct brings them closer to others. During the eighteenth century, "Never was man less conceived of as a being alone ... Man's aptitude to understand his fellows and reveal himself to them goes without saying. We know no individual mysteries."[23] Those who desire solitude are misanthropes. The modern opposition between individual and society is one that lacks sense – and, according to Rousseau, if this opposition exists, it is because the society in question is built on shaky ground. But this happiness is faced with the issue of passions: they inflame the self, bring it beyond what is reasonable, and drive it to despondency, to melancholia.

Elation and despondency "lay the groundwork for art, and sow madness."[24] Melancholia has a twin destiny: artistry and illness. Its first destiny ensures that it is the mark of the inspired individual. As the romantic period begins, melancholia becomes one with the artist, that tragic and sublime figure whose genius is on the level with her suffering. Yet for the ordinary person, melancholia becomes an illness. But both these visions of melancholia are closely tied to the Western history of self-consciousness, in which it represents *exacerbation*.[25] And this to the point where Raymond Klibansky wrote that "to give an overall view [of melancholia] ... would be to write the history of contemporary man."[26] As the sixteenth century dawned, melancholia was "so well assimilated to self-awareness that there were no distinguished men who were free of melancholia, or who would admit as much, in their own eyes as in the eyes of others."[27] The melancholic individual does not flee her suffering, she prides herself on it. As Michelangelo said, "My joy is melancholia."[28] The pain and pleasure of being oneself: therein lies the theme of melancholia.

During the eighteenth century, as the brain began to occupy a central role in our actions, melancholia became defined as nervousness (in the sense that the nerves are irritated).[29] If the soul becomes corrupt, the brain tires, its forces become limited, and it requires rest and relaxation, music and sun. Humanity is predisposed to melancholia insofar as the nervous system is what ties us to the world. This state "is most often interpreted as the result of psychic shock or excessive tension due to external circumstances."[30]

In 1819, Esquirol defined melancholia as a monomania:[31] sadness, despondency, and a disgust with one's existence is often accompanied by a single-themed delirium (although reason is not absent). The melancholic individual is pursued by a single fixating thought that psychiatrists will later name *folie du doute,* or "guilt delirium." It is easily differentiated from general delirium, which is characterized by mania. Nonetheless, the idea of melancholia without delirium is born: "a sad and depressive passion" without signs of madness.[32] The absence of delirium reduces the role that reason plays in madness and allows the isolation of a specific pain in the burgeoning phenomenon that is alienation.

The main conceptual change began at the start of the nineteenth century, in the 1830s. Psychiatrist Michel Gourévitch compared Esquirol's description of a case of melancholia published in 1810 with one published in 1838. In 1810, the sick individual becomes delirious when bad news is mentioned; in 1838, the individual is "only" in despair.[33] This change in clinical analysis is remarkable.

From delirium to despair – the long decline of intellectual psychiatry had begun: "We can now, succumbing to the blows of fortune and the strength of one's passions, fall ill from sadness ... The status conferred by organic illness is extended to psychological phenomena, those once called moral."[34] It is here that the first hesitant steps are taken towards a definition of mental illness. Melancholia opened a way between the normal and the pathological:[35] instead of a difference of nature, we are now dealing with a difference of degree.

Furthermore, this illness "will make of suffering of the mind the very principle and element of disorder in the minds of the alienated."[36] An initial recasting is done by Joseph Guislain (1817-60) in Belgium, then by Wilhelm Griesinger (1817-68) in Germany.[37] It is based on two themes: (1) all madness begins with a change in temperament and (2) madness may appear without disorder in an individual's intelligence as only reason, emotion, and mood are affected. The notion of mood was imported by French thinkers in 1850, along with the idea of circular madness (an alternation between manic and melancholic states, separated by periods of lucidity). It was tied to melancholia towards the end of the nineteenth century. The psychiatrist Jules Séglas (1856-1939), who worked at the Salpêtrière hospital, defined the central point from which depression would evolve in the 1940s: "[with] melancholia without delirium or with consciousness," he declared in a class in 1894,[38] "*suffering is reduced to a feeling of impotence.* This moral suffering, this painful depression ... is the most striking symptom of melancholia; I would even say it is a characteristic."[39] The individual suffering from such an illness "is aware of the pathological nature of the phenomena he suffers from and against which he would like to, but cannot, react."[40] The fundamentals of psychiatry lie here: the distinction between mood and affect, between judgment and representation.

The transformation of an illness associated with the genius and his grand sentiments into a painful emotional affliction is no doubt linked to the social make-up of mental institutions. By the 1830s, the situation of the working class was the subject of multiple studies whose purpose was to explain the mental and material suffering of its members. The alienists saw here the source of the famous "moral causes." The disease's status disappears as we journey down the social ladder. Eugène Pelletan, a radical politician, went so far as to declare: "The illness is but decadence among the common, but among the great searchers for ideas, it is the natural predisposition to the sublime."[41]

REFLEX, OR CONSCIOUSNESS IN THE BONE MARROW

If in melancholia we find the birth of the division between affect and representation, in reflex we find one of the vectors associated with the decentring of consciousness. Reflex relates not only to sensation but also to movement. Movement has long interested science since, as Georges Canguilhem eloquently put it: "The essence of dignity is the power to order; it is the will. Hence, the attention given to setting out the boundaries between those movements that are simply animal (involuntary), and those expressly human, the fruit of will or of reason."[42] The attention given to the dignity attributed to humanity is reinforced by the fact that pain is not a medical object, it is not the illness itself. After all, didn't Magendie declare in 1847, during a symposium on pain held by the Académie des sciences: "Whether people suffer more or suffer less – should that interest the Académie des sciences?"[43]

Considering that, in the middle of the nineteenth century, there was not an issue with physical pain – there is but one language for sickness – why would there be one for mental pain? Physical pain is simply illness's companion,[44] at best a symptom, a helpful hint that a doctor may diagnose. Mental pain is mental alienation's barely perceptible companion.

Apparently we are very far from the question of the "self." Yet the secularization of the soul is also expressed by the physiology of reflex. Georges Canguilhem remarked upon this: "If the distinction between voluntary movement and involuntary has become a problem in physiology, it is above all because of its religious, moral and legal aspect. Before being a scientific problem, the question concerns the experience of guilt and responsibility."[45] The distinction between these movements is one of the battlegrounds that helps us understand the differences between the higher acts of humanity (courage, virtue, etc.) and simple reactions, mere reflexes, that are common to all mammals. Physiologists and alienists tried to explain physical activity based on a series of reflexes over which human beings have no control. This decentring involves establishing the relation between the brain and the body.

Today, the role of Darwinian biology in the birth of the Freudian unconscious and the research conducted on the reflex arc within a unified concept of nervous function is well known.[46] Yet the research conducted on reflexes has also opened the way for "a new model of subjective function,"[47] which culminates in the Freudian concept of the unconscious. We must not forget that Freud was a neurologist who had been taught by the best Austrian specialists: Ernst Brücke and his assistant Sigmund Exner.[48] Forgetting this would make it impossible to understand the multiple biological and physiological sources that not only attended the birth of the psychic unconscious but also allowed a new vision of humanity.

Sigmund Exner (1846-1926) "built ... a general theory of all psychic functions based on reflex, pushing the argument to the point of calling reflex what we would call a 'counter-*cogito*.' According to Exner we mustn't say I think, I feel, but rather, 'It thinks in me, it feels in me.'"[49] For this truth to appear, reflex had to be analyzed not only from the point of view of movement but also from the point of view of sensation (i.e., psychology). Involuntary movement becomes automatic action, an intelligence that would have no consciousness of itself.[50] Research conducted on the reflex arc situated the psyche "within the spinal cord."[51] By the middle of the century, researchers held the key to an integrated concept of nervous function that was

not limited to the encephalon.[52] They would be able to identify
within an individual a section both inferior and ancient, both animal
and involuntary, along with a section that was more voluntary and
less organized, a superior level that would be the last stage of
humanity's evolution. This disorganization removed the control over
the lower functions, and the result was mental illness. During the
twentieth century, a large part of organicist psychiatry found in this
theory its reference point (in France, one thinks especially of Henry
Ey). Later, brain biochemistry would remove its scientific basis.

Rightly or wrongly, the opposition between the self's suffering and
the pain of illness is a classic theme. So that suffering may matter
in and of itself, we must impose a language that allows the self not
only to be expressed but also to be understood. The public function
of the self, the common exchange, is the condition of the private
experience. The madwoman is a fellow creature, certainly, but a
fallen one, a degenerate. This is not only illness's essential issue, it
is of more importance than the sick individual herself. Treating the
mental suffering of the sick individual means identifying her as a
subject. It presupposes a step forward that cannot be achieved in
asylums, which are peopled by the poor and the homeless, but only
in liberal medicine, with its bourgeois clientele for whom mental
illnesses are largely disconnected from questions of public order.

NEURASTHENIA'S IMPACT, OR THE SOCIALIZATION OF THE SELF

Madness interests the public only through newspaper stories. Yet,
in the last twenty years of the nineteenth century, a new illness was
popularized: neurasthenia. We could call it the first fashionable illness, a sickness that interested not only scholars (Charcot, Freud,
Janet, Ribot, among others) but the press, public opinion, artists,
and writers. Neurasthenia was the starting point, through the birth
of functional disorders, for a new-found social attention to suffering.
The notion of the exogenous was born: something that originates
outside the individual creates a transformation within (i.e., a person's
pathological reaction). It renders moot the reference to heredity as
an answer to morbid behaviour or sensations. In the same breath,
the notion of the endogenous opened itself to psychic genesis and
so was rebuilt. This is what, in their different ways, Sigmund Freud
and Pierre Janet would explain.

THE NERVOUS VIBRATION

Besides asylums and hospitals, there existed in the nineteenth century a few private clinics,[53] led by alienists, in which a bourgeois clientele was treated through liberal medicine (neurology, gynaecology, ophthalmology, etc.) for a plethora of illnesses with colourful names: irritable heart, acute neuropathia, cerebro-cardiac neuropathia, hypochondria, and so on. During the 1860s, these illnesses were grouped under the banner of "neurosisms," or "nevrosisms," which described "people who, though they suffer from no organic disorder ... were nonetheless subject to mental torment."[54]

There is something modern about neurasthenia as opposed to melancholia. Its inventor, the American George Beard, described it as the illness of modern life as it springs from a trepidation associated with modern times, with industry and big cities. It represents the nervous dimension of industrial fatigue.

The notion of functional disorder allows us to leave behind the syndrome-lesion duality, which accounted for the traditional definition of illness.[55] If a syndrome can be a pathological reaction to an event, then the necessity of a lesion disappears. The importance of neurasthenia, then, is that is opens the way, through the notion of functional disorder, for a *social permeability of the mind*. It is the agent that brings about a whole new socialization of the mind.

Over the last twenty years of the nineteenth century, modern art imported nervousness, sensation, and instincts. "What is modern," wrote Hugo von Hofmannsthal in 1893, "consists of old furniture and young nervousness."[56] There was melancholic nostalgia for the stability of a world that was disappearing in a frightening race towards an ephemeral future. You had to be strong, as solid as a machine and as wise as a philosopher. Writers, poets, and painters simultaneously drew on modernity and nervousness. The speed of machines, the mystique of nerves, the cult of the unconscious, the theme of nervousness are all heard both in art and in medicine. The medical domain treated its patients, defined their sickness, and offered them hope of treatment, while art created a story describing what it was to be a soul that, if not torn asunder by its own will, was invaded by the most contradictory feelings.[57] Medicine offered treatment and culture that, by teaching the language of suffering, enabled the creation of a demand: the markets for inner peace announced their arrival.

In fact, neurasthenia appeared more as a form of nervous fatigue resulting from modern life than as a form of degeneration:[58] the social factor became etiology's first preoccupation. George Beard's 1869 work, *A Practical Treatise on Nervous Exhaustion,* became an international hit. Translated into French in 1895, it was already famous by the 1880s. A large amount of literature was sent out to medical doctors as well as to patients during the last twenty years of the century. The work of Gilbert Ballet and Adrien Proust, *L'hygiène du neurasthénique* (1897),[59] was hailed throughout Europe. In 1906, Ballet, a teacher of the clinical aspects of mental illness, created *L'Encéphale,* while Proust was better known as Marcel's father.

To what did the word "neurasthenia" refer? In truth, it encompassed everything. "If a patient," wrote Beard, "complains of general malaise, debility of all the functions, poor appetite, abiding weakness in the back and spine, fugitive neuralgic pains, hysteria, insomnia, hypochondriasis, disinclination for consecutive mental labor, severe and weakening attack of sick headache, and other analogous symptoms, and at the same time gives no evidence of anaemia or any organic disease, we have reason to suspect ... that we are dealing with a typical case of neurasthenia.[60]" A series of disparate disorders was classified according to this definition. According to Beard, these illnesses resulted from intense and repeated pressure on the nervous system and the cerebro-spinal arc. When we consider the uncertainty of diagnostics at the time, it is apparent that neurasthenia, hysteria, hypochondria, and melancholia came together unimpeded,[61] especially to the untrained eye.

The warm reception given Beard's book and the success of neurasthenia are not so much imputable to effective medication – none existed – as to one of the era's important issues: the physical fatigue of manual labourers as well as the exhaustion of young intellectuals, the middle and upper classes, and those occupying liberal professions in the big cities. Overworked individuals explained not only the degeneracy of the French population but also the defeat in the war of 1870. This degeneracy began to be studied in the 1880s. Fatigue was measured, and signs of overwork were discovered. Fatigue was an important issue as the century came to term, and it was seen as a main factor in the degeneracy of the nation. Insofar as its causes were social – they did not stem from some inescapable heredity – change was possible.[62]

Émile Durkheim, speaking of these "various anomalies that [were] commonly grouped under the term 'neurasthenia,'" added that "it [was] ... becoming more and more common."[63] Why? The explanations that have been brought forward by countless texts published from the late nineteenth century to the beginning of the twentieth century all observe a changing world, be it in the form of faster transportation and social mobility (e.g., the train), the spread of wealth and luxury (e.g., the birth of large shops and stores), the new role of the masses in politics, the decline of religion, alcohol as a poison of modern life, or a literature that explores the darkest depths of the human soul ("It offers the reader pathological cases, the problems of sexual psychopaths and revolutionaries").[64] Life in the big city, which was becoming "more refined and more agitated,"[65] brought sensual pleasure and aesthetic refinement to the bourgeoisie and middle class. It all came together without anyone's being able to distinguish modernity's criticism and pathology's diagnostics.

Much work has been done on the Ego's readjustment, which took place towards the end of the nineteenth century.[66] Scholars have suggested that artists painted personal dilemmas with the ambition of "making it." They wanted to uproot tradition and, as they stopped imitating nature, the brought forward questions of identity. They also provided tools for self-understanding and for enabling the bourgeoisie and the middle class to understand their world. Nerves made their appearance in culture and medicine: a picture of a humanity both more instinctual and more reflexive became the norm. In 1891, Herman Bahr spoke of "the solemn entry of a new life into inner spirituality" and called for "a mystique of the nerves."[67] In 1902, Willy Hellpach, in a book entitled *Nervosität und kultur* (*Nervousness and Culture*), tied the success of neurasthenia in the 1880s to the undoing of traditions: "It cannot simply be an accident that, around that date, we saw the eruption of the modernist movement – and it was no simple emergence, but a triumphant entry. Once launched, the modern era was mature enough to reflect on itself."[68]

In 1896, Otto Binswanger spoke of the "close connection between them [the symptoms of neurasthenia] and the modern way of life, the unbridled lust and haste for gold and possessions, those immense advances in technological spheres which have reduced to insignificance all limitations of time and space where communication is concerned."[69] In 1895, Krafft-Ebing evoked the transformation that had taken place over the preceding ten years in "civilized nations" and that had "abruptly transformed professional life, citizenship and property at the direct cost of the nervous system; this is then called upon to meet the increased social and domestic demands by a greater expenditure of energy, unredressed by any satisfactory forms of recuperation."[70] Wilhelm Erb conjured up the battle for life and luxury: "The demands on the ability of the individual in the struggle for existence have enormously increased, and he can meet them only by putting forth all his mental powers; at the same time, the needs of the individual, and the demand for enjoyment have increased in all circles; unprecedented luxury is displayed by classes hitherto wholly unaccustomed to any such doing."[71] Within this context, neurasthenia spread like wildfire. "It seemed to spread like an epidemic," wrote a psychiatrist in 1904: "The word neurasthenia is on all lips, truly a fashionable disease."[72]

We understand how Pierre Janet could write, in 1932, that "everyone was neurasthenic," while adding, "We were delighted to carry this weight." For what reason? As Janet commented, neurasthenia was "a weakening of the nerves, a weakening of the nervous function. That doesn't mean much." However, he then added charitably: "It's more interesting than it seems ... The nerves are not destroyed; they are weakened. That's more scientific than you might think, it was the beginning of the interpretation of functional disorders."[73] On the one hand, we have social reasons; on the other, we have functional disorders that allow for the perception that life in society can make us ill.

The nervous system is shaken, the mind's budget taxed, as Janet would say. These are the characteristics of neurasthenia. Functional disorders reorganized the partition between the voluntary and the involuntary. No longer simply indolence, fatigue is now the cause of the "illnesses of will." It holds the medical keys to moral weakness. Scientific psychology, which turns from introspection and moves towards materialism, carries the day in France and, with Ribot, "gives the illusory and the true alike the status of reality."[74]

Yet, the way in which these social causes operated to affect the nervous system remained vague. We could not base the idea of functional disorders on anything solid: the physiological or neurological elements that would establish the link between brain, mind, and society were lacking. It was difficult to give endogenous and exogenous causes following specific criteria. Charcot would tie it all together. He thought, contrary to the opinion of the times, that neurasthenia affected the working classes as much as it did the intellectual classes, and this for the simple reason that it could result from a series of *traumas*. So here we are, back to the notion of reaction.

REACTION: FROM THE RAILWAY TO AUTOSUGGESTION

Reaction first appears with Newton's physics before reappearing, as a medical term, at the dawn of the nineteenth century.[75] It kept its original physical sense of action/reaction, as we did not yet understand the physiological mechanisms that produced a reaction from an action. Nevertheless, reaction applied to living things because it was considered to be a form of resistance to a perilous situation. By the end of the nineteenth century, the term had been circulated and adopted so widely that Bernheim (an advocate of hypnosis) wrote in 1874: "it can no longer be defined, it does not carry any more specific meaning."[76] Perhaps it no longer carried a specific meaning, but it did carry a decisive consequence that would open mental disorder to the social world, rendering trauma psychological.[77]

This period's psychic trauma would involve train accidents. These were no simple mishaps as, during the nineteenth century, the train represented modernity, the *Bête humaine* whose imaginary effects on material and spiritual life were immense: "The railroad fixed the very idea of an accident with its modern meaning."[78] For the first time in human history, it was not only nature or war that caused catastrophe but also the human inventions of technology and industry. From this stems the issue of reparations and responsibility. Beyond the broken bodies, another phenomenon appears: uninjured people complain of headaches, backaches, partial paralysis, or amnesia. These injuries were not caused by lesions. John Erich Erichsen, a London doctor, in one of the first studies published on the subject in 1866 invented the term "railway spine" to name the "spinal shock" that caused such headaches. Another London doctor, Russell Reynolds, suggested that the symptoms of these disorders were comparable to those of hysteria and underscored that they were produced by ideas, though still far from the realm of madness.

During the 1870s, Charcot began working on hysteria and soon took over the territory. Among his patients we find men whom he considered hysteric. If hysteria is hereditary, it could also be brought upon by trauma caused by accidents, he thought, or consumption of alcohol and toxic substances. Further, he reckoned that female hysteria was caused by emotion while male hysteria was caused by accidents or toxic substances. We know that Charcot is one of the key players in defining modern hysteria: faced with patients who had suffered shock due to accidents, he demonstrated that the apparent neurological symptoms they had developed were actually symptoms of hysteria. Consequently, insofar as there were no lesions, which mechanisms could have caused these symptoms? Comparing this phenomenon to "the paralysis produced in hysteric individuals under hypnosis, through suggestion," he concludes that "these are traumatic self-suggestion phenomena, creating psychic or mental paralysis."[79] At the time, Charcot had on hand a concept of reaction that would be applicable to many situations. Amnesia, mystical ecstasy, or paralysis of a limb are the ways in which a subject may react (pathologically) to the shock received through autosuggestion. The marriage of hypnosis and reaction gave birth to the modern definition of neurosis: a mental disorder without an anatomical basis but with a reasonable cause.

Neurosis was born in a context in which mental alienation had been split into a series of various mental illnesses. Pinel had a single view of madness, characterized by many symptoms. Midway through the nineteenth century, there occurred a theoretical recasting that was due not to progress in psychiatry but, rather, to the anatomical and clinical concept that then reigned in medicine. It demanded a more precise semiology, of which the avowed goal was to "discover new illnesses through a differential effort, starting from several syndromes that could be subdivided" (hence the link between mania-melancholia and double-form or circular madness, which would later become manic-depression).[80] There was semiological progress when it came to illness being better differentiated diagnostically, and this made it acceptable to include psychiatry within medicine. Nevertheless, one issue still remained: the chronicity of most of these illnesses.

Yet, with regard to neurosis, there was not only an etiology but also, for the first time in the history of mental disorders, a successful therapy: hypnosis. The notion of reaction reduced the significance of the degenerative paradigm in favour of a new paradigm, that of personality disorder, an illness of which the mind is the cause and which was now the battleground and target of therapy. From this point on, we had a new criterion for defining an individual's inside and outside. Two legacies and two heirs emerge: Pierre Janet and Sigmund Freud.[81]

JANET AND FREUD: WEAKNESS OR GUILT?

Although Janet (1859-1947) did not receive as much glory as Freud, his contribution might well be more important with regard to our current subject. His illness model is an Ariadne's thread that wends its way through the history of depression.

Both Freud and Janet demonstrated that disorders of the mind are not what is left when we fail to discover an organic cause for a mental issue. They gave mental disorders their social and medical positivity. Neurosis was seen as a catch-all for any mental illness that did not have a physiological explanation. It concerned the mind through its negative image. In a book that, in 1909, presented itself as providing a synthesis of all neuroses, Janet wrote: "The intervention of the mind ... no longer has a purely negative character, a simple ignorance, as the absence of a lesion is to an autopsy, but has a positive, real and special character for illness."[82]

The main issue is both men's interpretation of anxiety. Freud saw it as tied to guilt while Janet saw it as a product of depression.[83] Further, Freud believed that "the sense of guilt" was "the greatest impediment to civilization."[84] Janet, a philosopher by training who became a doctor due to his interest in psychology, never offered a specific concept of humanity.

DEPRESSION AND THE SPLIT PERSONALITY OF THE ILL INDIVIDUAL

For Janet, neurosis is a functional illness, not a biological one, and it is located in the upper spheres of these functions,[85] "in their adaptation to current circumstances."[86] According to him, "Most neuropaths are depressed, exhausted, and have been since the start of their illness: their mental disorders find their origins in this very depression."[87] Both depression and exhaustion (a term that is synonymous with depression) are considered vectors of personality disorders, be it hysteria or disorders of the will, which Janet refers to as "psychasthenia."

His theory of hysteria breaks with Charcot's in that he demonstrates that the hysteric individual's bodily disorders are secondary to what he calls "moral symptoms": "The main one is a weakening in psychological synthesis, a narrowing of the field of consciousness … Hysteria is a form of mental disaggregation characterized by the tendency towards complete and permanent splitting of the personality."[88] The narrowing of the field of consciousness creates this scission. Hysteria is a personality disorder insofar as the functional aspect of the individual is no longer joined with her personal consciousness. This is the famous "splitting of consciousness": both personalities constitute two different individuals who do not know each other. The hysteric does not remember her second personality.

Of neurasthenia, Janet writes: "These patients who experience visceral disorders were also obsessive, prone to phobias, maniacal thoughts, doubters, and I have taken the liberty of summing up these disorders with a parallel term, the word psychasthenia … The weakness is not one of the nerves, but of the mind. This is not a medical or physiological issue."[89] He isolates asthenia from the plethora of functional disorders and specifies that it stems from Morel's "emotional delirium" (1866) – emotional as opposed to intellectual. The result is a particular emotion that is the very symptom of psychasthenia – obsession. It is characterized by indecision and doubt, an illness of reality. Obsession brings about pathological exhaustion "because of psycholepsia, a drop in psychological pressure."[90]

Janet has a static conception of psychic energy: he defines "psychological strength" as the quantity of energy that an individual possesses and "psychological pressure" the capacity to use this strength, from which stems his central theme of exhaustion. The "synthesis of the psyche" is undone in psychasthenia, and the patient is led towards automatic actions. This is the *psychic deficiency* that prevents synthesis.

Therapy consists, through hypnosis or other psychological medication, in increasing psychological strength and pressure. The goal is to solve the "the problem of economic administration of the forces of the mind."[91] Hypnosis, for example, allows direct action on the unconscious in the hope of treating the weakened personality by mending and bringing it back into action: the therapy, if successful, ends the pathological fatigue. For Janet, this equals recovery, as he concludes in his *Médications psychologiques*: "It is probable that one day we will learn how to establish the expenses and the income of a mind, just as we do so for commerce. Then the psychiatric doctor will be able to muster weakened resources while avoiding needless expenditures and direct efforts to a particular goal. Indeed, he will do better than that: he will teach his patients how to increase their resources and enrich their minds."[92]

Janet sees the doctor-patient relation as one between an active and a passive party. The doctor is the mechanic who repairs the patient's broken psychological motor – a patient in the literal sense of the word. Therapy consists of a "mental disinfection."[93] The doctor's "therapeutic capacity means he will give liberating but false information ... He must place [the patient] in the state of mind he inhabited during the event and relate it to him again in an improved version, thereby eliminating the intolerable and dangerous aspects of it."[94] Hypnosis is an out-and-out guiding of the mind: it aims to wipe clean the memory of the event that caused the illness. This forces us face the issue in the following way: the illness may be a personality disorder, but the therapy does not aim for the reason behind the illness; rather, it repairs a failure of the mind, a pathology that holds no truth for the patient (a truth that would belong to the subject). Janet, though he is a psychotherapist, adopts an animal model: he takes a patient exhausted by psychological exertion and disinfects his mind of anything that could hurt him by, in a way, making him forget his own story. Janet's hypnosis is a technique of forgetting. His model of illnesses is one of *deficiency,* and his therapeutic model is one of *repair.*

REPRESSION AND CONFLICT IN THE SUBJECT'S PERSONALITY

For Freud and Breuer, the hysteric individual's personality does not suffer from being split but, rather, from reminiscences.[95] The key to suffering resides in childhood. The predisposition must be sought for "in a surplus rather than in a deficit. The adolescents who later become hysterical are before their illness mostly vivacious, talented, and full of mental interests; their will power is often remarkable."[96] The cleavage of consciousness and the splitting of the personality are replaced by repressed conflict. As Freud bases his model of illness on it, let us return to neurasthenia as the starting point of our demonstration.

Freud proposes a counter-argument to those who would see the cause of neurasthenia in social pressure or exhaustion: "no one ever becomes neurotic through work or excitement alone."[97] Further, the etiology of neurosis does not lie in new-found permissiveness, as was believed by neurologists and alienists alike, since "our civilization is, generally speaking, founded on the suppression of instincts.[98]" He introduces a distinction between two types of neuroses. In the first type, toxic neurosis, "the phenomena are essentially the same as those due to excess or deficiency of certain nerve-poisons. These neuroses, usually designated collectively as 'neurasthenia,' can be induced by certain injurious influences in the sexual life, without any hereditary taint being necessarily present."[99] In the second type of neuroses, the psychoneuroses of defence, Freud argues that "A hereditary influence is more marked, and the causation less transparent. A peculiar method of investigation known as psychoanalysis has, however, enabled us to recognize that the symptoms of these disorders (hysteria, obsessional neurosis, etc.) are psychogenic, and depend upon the operation of unconscious (repressed) ideational complexes."[100] Here we find the essential displacement from heredity to filiation, conveyed by the notion of psychogenesis – essential because it distinguishes exogenesis from psychogenesis. One of Freud's most important contributions is his demonstration of the existence of the endogenesis of the psyche. This is important because, by distinguishing psychoneurosis from the rest of the neuroses, he invented an illness of conflict.

Jean Starobinski describes the respective spaces of the internal and the external: "Whereas trauma strikes the subject from 'without,' abreaction begins its movement from 'within' … The pairing of trauma-abreaction constitutes two notions that are symmetrical, inverse and correlative."[101] Neuroses with exogenous motives owe their existence to the external-trauma pairing. According to Freud, "defence psychoneuroses" are those that stem from internal-abreaction. He uses the term "psychoneuroses" because they result from unconscious repression due to intrapsychological conflict being played out by filiation. He uses the term "defence" because this repression causes symptoms (amnesia, paralysis, etc.) that allow the patient to defend herself from the anxiety and guilt produced by the intrapsychological conflict – for it is these that matter, not exhaustion.

Freud ends his *Studies in Hysteria* by describing the healing process: "I do not doubt that it would be easier for fate to take away your suffering than it would for me. But you will see for yourself that much has been gained if we succeed in turning your hysterical misery into common unhappiness. Having restored your inner life, you will be better able to arm yourself against that unhappiness."[102] Cure is less a return to a former state (repairing a malfunction by compensating for a deficit) than what psychoanalysts call "reshuffling," which makes facing oneself easier. It does not eliminate internal suffering, and it is not a return to a pre-disorder state; rather, it is a recomposition. More exactly, "Recovery often enough turns out to be merely an agreement to mutual toleration between the sick part of the patient and the healthy part."[103] A new patient appears on the scene as attention is now paid to the *subject of the illness*.

THE SUBJECT OF NEUROSIS, OR THE ANXIETY OF BEING ONESELF

Where Janet sees automatic reactions, what we could call an a-cogito in the sense that it refers to a weakness, a deficiency that needs to be compensated for by disinfecting the mind of its parasitic memories and thereby increasing its strength, Freud sees a counter-cogito: the patient's unconsciousness is intentional,[104] it does not stem from automatic reactions. In fact, there is no weakness associated with the neurotic individual but, rather, an unconscious desire that therapy tries to lift into consciousness. "Through my psychical work," Freud wrote, "I had to overcome a psychical force [and not a lack] in the patients that was opposed to the pathogenic ideas becoming conscious (being recollected)."[105] In defining the unconscious, Freud substitutes automatic reactions with intention, thus extending the conflict into the deepest reaches of our animality.

Freud does concentrate on the subject of illness, in the sense that the individual is both the agent and victim of a conflict (manifested by particular symptoms). It is this conflict, not exhaustion, that is the cause of illness. It is what must be treated since the illness itself is its (incorrect) solution. The individual, by definition, has a sense of the law, but the law within him does not let him gaze serenely at the starry skies above. His cage is named the "splitting of consciousness." For Freud, the symptom is not medical but, rather, a mnemonic trace created by repression, meaning that it must be understood as holding an important place in the patient's past – and it is this place that gives it significance.[106] The sick individual is not exhausted by her automatisms, she is anxious and tries to defend herself against anxiety through manifesting symptoms that are easier to bear. She is also the self of the oft-cited formula: to heal is to free oneself of the infantile fantasies we have about our parents, thus transforming neurosis into ordinary pain. She can then free herself from her therapist as well: theoretically, at least, it is possible for her to live by herself, to find her own way.

Conflict-history-separation; deficiency-ahistoricity-reparation. These are two ways of understanding and treating mental pathology. Even today, these two visions are stock references in the therapeutic arts.

But why is it such an arduous task to defeat interior pain? Freud answered this question more than once: "Experience teaches that for most people there is a limit beyond which their constitution cannot comply with the demands of civilization. All who wish to reach a higher standard than their constitution will allow fall victim to neurosis. It would have been better for them if they could have remained less 'perfect.'"[107] Neurosis is an illness (a medical entity) but it is also civilization's drive (a moral entity), the strange motor of the moderns' energy, the nobility of their life force. After all, did Breuer not mention the hysteric individual's vivacity, curiosity, and intelligence? Hysteria is the bodily cost of these qualities. It is an experience from which we must learn something. Durkheim's neurasthenia and Freud's psychoneurosis are both the terms and the consequences of civilization. For Janet, neurosis is a behavioural pathology caused by a "psychological depression that weakens the strength and tension of mental activity."[108]

Freud invented neither the unconscious nor neurosis;[109] rather, he discovered their target.

The conflict between Freud and Janet over the mentally ill individual is in no way a moral conflict. The controversy lies in the diagnosis, the etiology, and the therapeutic approach. Yet, Freud presented an ideal image of the self since he integrated the physiological and neurological teachings of the nineteenth century – the fact that we are mammals, made of instincts and desires – with a moral law. The individual keeps watch over himself "by setting up an agency within him to watch over it, like a garrison in a conquered city."[110] This image is ideal since it barely addresses morality. French psychoanalysis makes it its basis: from Angelo Hesnard (1886-1969), the first psychiatrist to write about Freud in 1913, to Jacques Lacan, neurosis is an illness of guilt.[111] As Freud writes, guilt "is the immediate expression of fear of the external authority."[112] Lacan, through the notion of "castration anxiety," places guilt at the top of his system. To emerge from the infantile and achieve maturity there is no other choice than to confront the forbidden, to feel its sting in order to differentiate the imaginary father (whom the child sees as all-powerful while she is nothing) from the father as incarnation of the law. Entering adulthood amounts to the *fear of becoming oneself*, it is inherent to the self's freedom. The self that is passed down to us from the end of the nineteenth century consists of the marriage of animality and guilt.

Between Janet and Freud, we find the tension between animal and human, which in no way parallels the opposition between psychotherapy and chemical therapy. This tension acts upon psychological therapies, as we have seen, as it will act upon chemical therapies, as we will see. Functional disorders of the personality are cast between two fault lines. The first consists of exogenous disorders, the internal resonance of an exterior shock. This damages a person who is treated first by psychotherapy, later by chemical therapy. Treatment is the *art of reparation*: we are in the closed system of illness, a specific medical paradigm. The second fault line consists of the psychogenic disorder, the revelation of a split consciousness that is the key to reaching the self. Here, treatment is the *art of separation*: we are in the open system of illness. According to the reparatory logic, there is nothing to learn from the illness since we are dealing neither with self nor experience but only with the pain from which the patient suffers, no matter the cause, lesion, or (in biological psychiatry's modern interpretation) difficulty in neurochemical transmission. According to the separatory logic, we rediscover melancholia's old lesson of the treatment found in the illness: "When the presence of pain and the correlative pursuit of a remedy disappear," writes Starobinski, "the vital energies are nearly exhausted. This serenity, this sense of peace, this apparent cure are the harbingers of death."[113]

After the Second World War, depression separates itself from melancholia. Depression travels between two versions of the difficult task of being well: (1) *anxiety*, which indicates that I am crossing into forbidden territory and am becoming divided, a pathology of guilt, an illness of conflict; and (2) *exhaustion*, which tires me out, empties me, and makes me incapable of action – a pathology of responsibility, an illness of inadequacy.

These two versions of wellness accompany the emergence of a new era for the self, who is no longer either the complete individual of the eighteenth century or the split individual of the end of the nineteenth century; rather, she is the emancipated individual. Becoming ourselves made us nervous, being ourselves makes us depressed. The anxiety of being oneself hides behind the weariness of the self.

At the beginning of the nineteenth century, the alienist focused on (un)reason; during the 1830s, he began to understand that involuntary actions can exist without delirium and observed the suffering of the madman. At the end of the twentieth century, psychiatry entirely reorganized itself around suffering, depression being the main vector of this reorganization. Originally, with madness, we had the question of representation (delirium); today, with depression, we have the question of affect (suffering). Between the two lies the culture of nervousness at the end of the nineteenth century. How do we resist exhaustion, which comes from modern life, with its emotional inadequacy? How do we overcome guilt, which comes from within and from the inscription of the individual within a specific filiation, to free himself from tradition? Through a triple dynamic of increased attention to the biological, psychological, and sociological aspects of the mind, neuroses created a language, uses, and habits for growing client groups – a language that allowed the definition and expression of the worries that hard pathologies, those of the abnormal person, had not previously been able to speak. What we can say, we can become. These are the pathologies of the normal person. If the end of the nineteenth century created the "chronic identity crisis,"[114] it did so only for the bourgeoisie. The proletariat had to wait until the second half of the twentieth century for the democratization of depression. Depression illustrates the tragic fate of the normal person when the notion of the forbidden is used as an instrument of domination. It then becomes as, according to Janet, neurasthenia was for Déjerine, "a crossroads from which all possible illnesses can flow."[115]

2

Electroconvulsive Therapy:
Technique, Mood, and Depression

"We no doubt meet all around us," Janet wrote in 1932, "many weakened individuals who are not at a normal level but who are treated more or less like normal individuals." He was apparently pointing out the lack of social and medical attention for these seemingly normal individuals who were, in fact, abnormal. He added, "If I am not mistaken, the analysis of this weakness, and its remedy, when it may come into existence, will become very important in the future."[1] Six years later, Freud referred to possible chemical substances: "The future," he said in his last book, "may teach us to exercise a direct influence, by means of particular chemical substances, on the amounts of energy and their distribution in the mental apparatus. It may be that there are other still undreamt-of possibilities of therapy. But for the moment we have nothing better at our disposal than the technique of psycho-analysis, and for that reason, in spite of its limitations, it should not be despised."[2]

Freud began working out his theories about the effects of these substances. Like psychotherapies, they would better distribute the quantities of energy in the "psychic mechanism," and the Ego would be freer in its movements. The conflict is costly for the neurotic individual since it acts negatively upon her energy. It can be interpreted as a deficiency (to be filled) or as a psychological issue (to be solved). Depending on the model to which we owe allegiance, the medication and the importance it is given in the treatment of pathology varies considerably. If the conflict is interpreted as a deficiency, the psychiatrist would think that chemical treatment would be effective in a plethora of cases, while if it is interpreted as a psychological issue, she would think that treatment would be effective only in limited cases and for a few pathologies. The question of a medication's specificity was the focus of discussion when biological therapies began after the First World War. These discussions continued up until the time of Prozac.

Biological therapies brought about durable progress with regard to the emotional aspects of mental illnesses: emotional syndromes gave way in a significant number of cases. Explaining this progress and its limits, eventually rethinking clinical classifications and modifying them, and one day even curing mental illness: this opens up an enormous laboratory. The old concept of moral suffering, that feeling of impotence that is everything in melancholia, as Séglas thought, would force intense discussion of the notion of *mood*, first within the realm of psychoses, then within the realm of neuroses. By the middle of the nineteenth century, Griesinger defined affect as "the feeling of oneself and one's moods,"[3] while Freud defined it as "the emotions of the Ego," even though he did not know, as he admitted in 1926, "what affect [was]."[4]

Whether we make reference to psychoanalysis or to organicism, affect is always more bodily, more animal, than reason. It is not only considered to be older in the history of our species but also to be unconscious in all senses of the word. It refers to the lower functions of human beings, to those they share with other mammals. Furthermore, emotional syndromes are the basis of many mental pathologies, from psychoneuroses of defence to schizophrenia.

Psychiatry refers to these syndromes as "mood disorders." Does the fact that these disorders are chemically treatable make them pathologies in the same way as are neuroses? Understanding mood is psychiatry's main point. To shed light on the role of technique in the changes of category and redefinition of pathologies, I look at the aetiological debates, diagnostics, and therapies that accompanied the use of electroconvulsive therapy (ECT).

ECT's invention in 1938 by Ugo Cerletti and his assistant Lucio Bini played a major role in the first controversies that contributed to the picture of depressive states. In 1954, during a colloquium on depressive states, a speaker announced, "If every psychiatrist is indebted to Freud for the ability to analyze his patients' personality, let us not forget that patients almost always owe the rapid curing of their attacks to Cerletti."[5] By placing himself between Freud and Janet, Cerletti marked the start of the technical phase in which the guilty person's and the inadequate person's stories were bound together. The concept of the ill self was built on a diagnostic question: to which underlying pathology must we tie the depressive syndrome? The answer requires us to concentrate on etiology and pathogenesis, on the motives of illness and its mechanisms.

From the end of the interwar period to the beginning of the 1950s, two factors characterize the situation of "depressive states." The first refers to the perception of psychological suffering in primary care medicine: multiple complaints are registered but are mostly ignored by general practitioners (if we are to believe psychiatrists). The second refers to the psychiatric field: the issue is to understand the role and position of affect in non melancholia-based depressions. The choice of therapeutic strategy depends on this. Can these depressions be treated with ECT? This is the key question. At stake is the meeting of the heterogeneous elements that define a *self sick from affect*.

GENERAL PRACTICE: IMAGINARY AILMENTS AND THERAPEUTIC IMPOTENCE

Spectacular demoniacal ailments were wrested from priests and gynaecologists only to enter the realm of neurologists and alienists; the nervous individual's silent or mournful exhaustion helped remove lack of will, laziness, and disobedience from morals and philosophy. An immense field of human suffering became visible through the decentring of consciousness and the fragmentation of the Ego, to which the term "neurosis" refers.

Yet, in the first twenty years of the twentieth century, neither hysteria nor neurasthenia commanded legions of people of letters, scholars, and journalists.[6] Works published during the interwar period as well as in the 1940s mention, without going into detail, the quantitative importance in general medicine of psychiatric disorders without delirium. "The problem of depressive states," wrote a psychiatrist in 1938, "appears in general medicine as much as in specialized psychiatry."[7] In most of these cases, doctors were faced with complaints in which obsession, doubt, and exhaustion reigned. When exhaustion stems from overwork, the term "neurasthenia" is still used.[8] Yet, when it stems from obsession, a constitutional weakness or depression is diagnosed. According to psychiatric literature, complaints abound in general practice. Nevertheless, three main difficulties seem to characterize these states and to prevent doctors from granting them sufficient consideration: (1) the recognition of psychiatric illnesses, (2) the patient's constitution, and (3) the haphazard use of medication.

Are They Really Sick?

The first difficulty was that doctors had real problems recognizing these illnesses, not only with regard to issuing a diagnosis but also with regard to determining that the patient was actually sick. The diagnostic is complex, since "we are not faced with one of these illnesses, a little too theoretical, with a shifting pathogenesis, or a well defined symptomology, and a fixed evolution." These patients, exhausted by their doubt and obsessions, must perform "an amount of work … without ceasing in struggle and effort."9 Since the patients showed no signs of delirium, doctors tended to believe they were imagining their ailments and being self-centred. They should be listened to patiently but also, from time to time, be given a good shake. How many hysterics, sleepwalkers, amnesiacs, spasmophiliacs, or individuals with multiple personalities were inventing their problems? Perhaps even shamming? Psychiatric articles and textbooks tried to convince general practitioners of the existence of these functional disorders, but what could they do about unfounded (at least biologically) complaints at a time when psychology had not yet become part of a broader cultural understanding that would have allowed the social comprehension of mental pathologies lacking in specific behavioural disorders or affects? Hence, the persistent mantra: "Neurasthenic allegations are sincere and real."10 Doctors needed lesions or pathogenic agents in order to be convinced of the existence of an illness.

Let us open the *Traité de thérapeutique clinique* by Paul Savy, published in 1948. The work remains interesting today because it is directed towards general practitioners and gives an indication of what was being said at the time outside of the psychiatric domain. Introducing the section devoted to illnesses of the encephalon, Savy writes with much optimism: "The spiritual has become material."11 Yet his text does not seem to provide general practitioners with an optimistic perception of psychopathological disorders. On the contrary, he notes "the extreme frequency of psychopathological states and the difficulty of their treatment."12 Doctors must differentiate these "states" from mental illnesses as they are functional disorders in which the exhaustion of the psyche apparently dominates, while the faculties of judgment and reason remain. The symptoms can be hidden behind gastric, muscular, cardiac, and genital ailments. Understanding the sick individual, not underestimating her pain, is equivalent to accepting the reality of mental anguish; it is the first step in helping the patient, while reassuring her as well as her family that she does not suffer from dementia or insanity.

Personality as Fate

A second difficulty stemmed from the patient's constitution. What if the patient's disposition or character were built in such a way that he had little capacity to enjoy his existence? "Modifying an inexorable predisposition to mood and psychological instability ... is an illusion for those who believe in the total irreducible nature of constitutions and who assign the fixed nature of a histological lesion to morbid behaviours."[13] What could be done about nature? Very little, although psychological analysis gave us the means to examine these fragile constitutions, the better to strengthen them. Medicine was easily impressed by nature's bulwark. When the constitutional state dominated, hopes for healing were slim. Doctors knew quite well how to diagnose anxiety neuroses that expressed themselves through short panic attacks, keeping the patient in a permanent state of fear of their return. If the diagnosis was easy, the therapeutic options were not, since "the basic predisposition that escapes the effects of medicine often gives sway to the occasional causes on which it is easier to act."[14] Besides, the prognosis was difficult to reach: we know patients who suffer from panic attacks for several months, with foreseeable relapses, and chronic forms sometimes last a lifetime. Psychiatry was unable to give general practitioners the necessary tools to address these complaints.

Haphazard Medication

A third difficulty was medication. During the 1930s, general medicine had various types of medication, and these were haphazardly used, to treat mental illness: remineralization; calcium therapy; tonics such as tea, coffee, cinchona, even strychnine; sedatives like barbiturates or opiates to treat emotionalism (the actual effects of treatment are highly controversial); faradisation (an electrotherapy with no connection to electroshock); physical exercise; and many more. Medical treatment "cannot be limited to the exclusive prescription of drugs and diets. Impressionability, the feeling of impotence, obsessive tendencies and pragmatic failure, the corollary of asthenia and spasm, demand moral medications. The medical treatment of constitutional depression demands patient and firm psychotherapy."[15]

Ten years later, treatment had barely evolved: "moral and physical rest [as well as] activity; calming as well as stimulating medication."[16] Thermal cures were quite useful, especially since the doctor was present for the duration of the treatment. Opium "exercise[d] an undeniable sedative effect, but barbiturates [were] easier to manipulate."[17] As for somatic symptoms, an in-depth examination "must serve as a basis for reassuring psychotherapy."[18] An attitude of comprehension and subtle direction, the importance of older medical psychological treatments was pointed out: the sick individual was not a madman, and his failing will could be replaced by his doctor's much stronger one: "Chemical treatment does not represent an essential, fundamental element in treating psychasthenia. However, *as an addition to psychotherapy*, and avoiding all forms of polypharmacology, the prescription of certain tonics can be useful ..., such as general sedative medicines to calm agitation and insomnia."[19] In any case, medication was rather eclectic. At the dawn of the discovery of medications of the mind, pharmacology had not advanced beyond the invention of barbiturates at the beginning of the twentieth century. Old-fashioned opium was still being prescribed, and discussions about its sedative and tonic properties continued for more than a century.[20]

No treatment had any strong evidence to back up its efficacy: there were no stable and reproducible effects. When illness was healed, doctors did not know whether they should thank the treatment or the natural evolution of the illness. There was no regularity associated with these medications, which might have allowed for the standardization of care.

Outside of insanity, psychological suffering remained shrouded in unknowns. Henry Ey mentioned this in 1947: "In general medicine ..., the domain of the 'psyche' is cast into the limits of epiphenomena or else the void."[21] There were no institutional connections that might have granted medical reality to functional disorders. Add to this a polarization of opinions in the constitution versus temperament debate, the haphazard use of medication, and the difficult prognostics of pathologies with polymorphous symptoms, and the problems faced by general medicine when attempting to deal with psychiatric disorders that did not display delirium are obvious. The social context did not give any attention to discreet mental disorders since, except in cases of insanity, privacy was of the upmost importance.

MANAGEABLE BODIES, HONOURABLE FAMILIES, MODEST AMBITIONS

Up until the 1960s, private disorders, including those of the mind, became public problems only when they threatened public safety or moral standards. Homosexuality was considered to be a social monstrosity (and was considered a perversion by clinical psychiatry and psychoanalysis alike), free love and freedom from moral standards were considered scandalous. *La Garçonne*, published by Victor Margueritte in 1922, tells the story of a young bourgeois woman who is determined to live her sexuality openly and freely, and it created a major scandal, followed immediately by commercial success. "So many autobiographical novels, memoirs, confessions … have enjoyed such great fashion over recent years," wrote Michel Leiris in 1939.[22] The increased awareness given to emotional experiences, be they sexual or auto-analytic in nature, is certainly not the domain only of literature, as is shown by the importance the bourgeoisie came to place on the diary.[23] Yet, the individual was still stuck in a normative configuration of social duty and conformity to taboos. Institutions (family, schools, business) were not only all-powerful but all-authoritative: discipline, obedience, subservience all guaranteed the well-being of social order. Bodies had to be manageable,[24] families honourable, and ambitions modest. In such a configuration, people either submit to discipline or revolt against it; they either observe taboos or break them. And, if they do break them and do not hide, then they create a scandal.

The life of the lower classes, played out in the factory or on the farm, was considered to be their social fate. The bourgeoisie, however, was organized by strict rules that promised something completely different. The great national dream of the interwar period was property:[25] it was the main goal of the French, who believed themselves to be a nation of landowners. In the rural sphere, the small family farm was the dominant organizational form. While farmers experienced a certain improvement in living standards, comfort was often lacking, and housing was often humble. As for lower-class workers, social progress was nonexistent: isolation and relegation was what shaped their world. The bourgeoisie, despite its heterogeneity, was united by its desire for social mobility and increase of capital. Its family model, with the father as the only figure of authority, was a reference point for the rest of society.

This society, in its private sphere, is built on notions of duty and destiny: the concept of the individual-societal relationship means protecting society from the excesses and defiance of the individual by keeping him or her within a strict framework. This relationship is a dichotomy. The self carries the conflict between the Superego and the created Ego, which, Freud tells us, is a "sense of guilt [that] expresses itself as a need for punishment."[26] The main function of social institutions is to maintain order and authority while conserving a balance between the rights and duties of all. Institutions are defined as being "the organizational means necessary for a group to meet its goals."[27] Individuality exists only when taken charge of by an exterior presence. The individual is never asked to adapt to or to transform new phenomena, never required to be motivated, only to fulfill a social role within a specific institution. The "bureaucratic phenomenon" described by Michel Crozier in a successful book published in 1963 caricatures this way of being. But could this system of rules have suddenly appeared absurd if French society had not already evolved from its authoritarian base and begun to transform its customs and lifestyles?

The political culture of this society may be described as consisting of a conflict between the individual and the State, weak intermediary bodies, and an active notion of citizenship. In the Republican structure, the citizen is the only authentic individual because he or she has chosen to refuse all private expenditure. The citizen is part of the public sphere, the space of liberty, equality, and universality; the individual is part of the private sphere, characterized by hierarchy and dependence. Family is the institution in which we best distinguish the public from the private, the domestic from the political. It "embodies, in opposition to citizenship, the aspect of our human condition that is not chosen, but bequeathed. Family is what defines the very meaning of the democratic contract by tying together what does not arise from the autonomy of wills."[28] Our homes are inhabited by both permanence *and* submission.

When individuality is bogged down in discipline, interdiction, and strict rules, privacy leaves the realm of the social and becomes a personal (or family) secret. Bourgeois families, of whom François Mauriac often wrote, cannot imagine their internal conflicts expressed outside of house and home, except through mental pathology or the courts. "The marriage bed," Breuer thought, "is among women the origin of most serious neuroses."[29] When the private realm becomes known through abnormal behaviour or suffering, it is because the patient has spoken of it to his or her doctor or priest. In such a context, both at the institutional and mental levels, it is impossible to consider private disorders as actual illnesses. Neurotic individuals are, for Freud, "psychical patients who clearly resemble the psychotics."[30] The notion of malaise can hardly function within this social configuration.

The problem for psychiatrists who are interested in the pathologies we have just mentioned involves extending the pathological domain, forcing other medical specialities to understand the severity of non-delirium mental illnesses. As of the end of the nineteenth century, more and more psychiatrists came around to the idea that what we consider to be normal is of the same nature as what we consider to be pathological. The notion of "illness" began to be challenged by a softer form – the syndrome.[31]

The road that leads to the sovereign individual, "like a man entering a promise, [who] could guarantee himself as a future," presupposes a slow maturing. It means, for Nietzsche, the marking of the body "with the help of the morality of customs and of social straitwaistcoats."[32] If the gap between the normal and the pathological was to become the centre of a moral debate, the notion of a disciplined and conforming individuality had to be questioned in favour of a new type of normative behaviour, one that would create a new relation between public and private spheres.[33] The lessening of disciplinary regulation and the sharing of what is allowed and forbidden, on the one hand, and the shifting of the normal-pathological problem towards a moral standpoint, on the other, are not two separate processes. Both occur simultaneously within the social and psychiatric sphere.

In psychiatry, this process included the invention of biological curative techniques. The first step involved the discovery of a method that was usually reserved for schizophrenics yet that soon revealed its uses for melancholics: electroconvulsive therapy. For other depressive states, no consensus existed as to its effectiveness. Depression was the first of ECT's avatars.

A Cure at Last?

After Henry Ey's 1947 initiative to create an international association of psychiatrists, the group's first meeting took place in Paris in 1950.[34] Jean Delay (1907-87), the holder of the chair of clinical psychiatry at Sainte-Anne Hospital, gave the opening speech (in place of Janet, who had died in 1947) at the Sorbonne's grand lecture hall: "If the word 'cure' is so important because of the hopes it conjures up, it must be pronounced only with great reservation, it is no longer forbidden to us. Mental medicine aims at treating today's patients; in that way it is like any other branch. Asylums have become hospitals, and just as the 1900 conference was placed under the sign of Assistance, the 1950 congress can be placed under the sign of *Therapeutics*."[35]

THE REASONS FOR THERAPEUTIC OPTIMISM

In retrospect, Delay's optimism seems doubly surprising. First, we would be hard pressed to say that asylums had become hospitals in the medical sense of the word. On the contrary, the committed populations essentially comprised chronically ill individuals, older people touched by senile dementia, "agitated" patients who were a burden for the asylum, and melancholic individuals whose suicide attempts unnerved the personnel. In 1952, the journal *Esprit* published a dossier, and its title perfectly sums up the then state of psychiatry: "The Miseries of Psychiatry." The concept of public order still dominated (with all the abuses associated with internment) in asylums, which were considered to be "the working class prerogative."[36] There was obviously a clear contrast between what psychiatrists described as the daily life of asylums,[37] on the one hand, and the modernist image that Jean Delay had painted a few years earlier, on the other.

Yet a modernist and therapeutic wind was blowing through the halls. The words "psychiatric revolution" lay on the tip of many psychiatrists' tongues. During the 1920s, the administrative side of psychiatric work conducted in asylums moved from the Ministry of the Interior to the newly created Ministry of Hygiene. Asylums became psychiatric hospitals, and, in 1937, their guards became nurses. But we would have to wait until 1958 before the word *aliéné*, or "insane person," was replaced with *malade mental*, or "mentally ill person."[38] Deinstitutionalizing the insane became the great working theme of psychiatrists.

A second theme explains our surprise over Delay's optimism. In the acts from the colloquium on biological therapies, we read only about the methods of shock therapy (ECT) discovered during the interwar period. The first neuroleptic, which saw the light of day in 1952 and whose success was so great that an international symposium in Paris in 1955 was dedicated to discussing it, was not even raised. The lack of different therapies is a recurrent theme in psychiatric literature whenever it speaks of medicines of the mind.[39] Is ECT not just a barbarous method that strikes fear into those who must submit to it? Ugo Cerletti concluded his speech at the 1950 conference as follows: "Yes, gentlemen, delivering man from electroshock was the first idea that came to me when I performed the first electroshock on man ... We are working in hopes of saying, one day, 'Gentlemen, electroshock is no longer practised.'"[40] This hope proved to be vain: ECT is still the most powerful treatment for melancholia, and it remains the last resort for depressions that resist antidepressants.

Psychiatry has at its disposal tools that today are considered rudimentary, a concept of public order that is authoritative, and hospitals that remain essentially asylums. Why would Delay's tone have been so upbeat? Was his optimism nothing but rhetoric? An attempt to please the psychiatric, neurological, and psychoanalytic schools from the forty-seven different countries that had sent more than two thousand participants?[41] Yet, ECT was considered, and rightly so, to be a revolution.[42]

Psychotherapies allowed us to act upon two types of pathologies: asthenia and hysteria. At the beginning of the twentieth century, French specialists agreed that there were many intermediate states between normality and insanity. For those most touched by illness, the psychiatric diagnosis could be nothing more than a prognosis. Two main categories of illnesses were defined during this period: manic-depressive psychosis and schizophrenia (or, rather, a group of schizophrenias).[43]

Manic-depressive psychosis, defined by the master of German psychiatry Emil Kraepelin (1856-1926), is characterized by the alternation between attacks of mania (which can reach frenetic delirium) and depressive lows, the lightest forms of which are characterized by an inhibition of the psyche and despondency. "Particularly striking," writes Kraepelin, "is the considerable *diminishment in the ability to act.* "[44] The reduction in the ability to act is, along with sadness and mental anguish, among the major manifestations of depression. In its most acute form, we observe that it becomes melancholia, with sensorial disorders and delirious ideas (delirium of guilt) leading to suicidal tendencies. Schizophrenia results from a change in a second group of psychoses, which Kraepelin defines as early dementia (early, since it begins in the patient's youth). It combines dysfunctions in the body's movements, emotions, and a hallucinatory thought pattern. The Swiss psychiatrist Eugen Bleuler (1857-1939) put forward a theory of psychic dissociation whose main symptom is a disorder in associations of ideas, which we call "delirium." It is this that defines schizophrenia.

But from Kraepelin to Bleuler, it is not only the definitions of two large groups of psychoses (i.e., manic-depressive psychosis and schizophrenia) that are stabilized. These two psychoses are certainly characterized by correlated symptoms and an evolution that is specific to each (Kraepelin), but they specifically correspond to two major psychic functions, personal initiative and detachment, absorbing "the whole manner of being of the sick person in relation to ambient reality."[45] Schizophrenia results in a loss of emotional contact, while manic-depressive psychosis leaves the patient intact between phases. Bleuler believed that there were two pathological aspects to the fundamental principles of human life: manic-depressive psychosis was seen as a pathology of "personal impulse," an impulse without which we could not live in the world; while schizophrenia was seen as a pathology of detachment from the world, a detachment without which a personality could not construct itself. The harmonious coexistence of the two underlying faculties, syntony and schizoidism, "seem[ed] to be responsible for the maximum of equilibrium, of felicity, of efficiency, to which we believe we have a right to aspire."[46] If Kraepelin's genius was his capacity to bring together the psychotic diversity in two types of psychoses, Bleuler's was his capacity to record them as a continuum with normality. Even if he did not explain psychoses,[47] he made understandable the types of subjectivity from which they arise.

As the biological means of acting on pathologies were taking their first hesitant steps, identity disintegration and affective distancing from the world were seen as the key features of the psychotic individual's territory. For Kraepelin, these features condemned the sick individual to incurability; for Bleuler, they forced the psychiatrist to make emotional contact in order to improve the patient's health.

The importance of shock therapy is that it paved the way for action. For the first time in therapeutic history, psychiatry could observe a *stable* relation between treatment and cure. These techniques established psychiatry as an integral part of medicine and allowed it to become part of scientific modernity – *that* is the meaning of Delay's speech. Acting *regularly* and with *durability,* these techniques allowed a definition of illnesses through "pharmacological dissection." Biological therapy became a fundamental element in psychiatric nosography and in the search for the causes and mechanisms that give birth to mental pathologies. Psychiatry now had access to a reliable witness: a patient's reaction to a specific treatment is a verifiable way of ensuring the accuracy of the diagnosis. Mental medicine had now entered the age of pharmacological dissection.

The question of mood became decisive since the interweaving of somatic and psychic aspects of mental illness was now done within a new context: shock therapy provided *experimental* foundations for understanding the aetiopathogenesis of mental disorders. Indeed, these methods confirmed, at the therapeutic level, the clinical thinking of the nineteenth century: diseased affect is the basis of insanity, while delirium and hallucinations are simply its consequences. Mood is to blame for the loss of reason, the fragmentation of thought, and the disintegration of the self's identity.

The Diseased Affect of the Self

Shock therapy, reserved first for schizophrenia, tried to produce coma or convulsion. Depending on the case, the goal was either sedation or stimulation. These methods included malariatherapy (for which Julius Wagner-Jauregg received the Nobel Prize for medicine in 1927), sleep cure assisted by barbiturates (narcosis supposedly being able to free schizophrenics from their automatisms), hypoglycemic shock with insulin, and convulsive therapy with cardiazol. But an epileptogenous technique, whose success was most striking, is what interests us at this juncture as it recast the problem of depression. Shock therapy came into general use in France (even outside Paris) during the Second World War.[48]

These techniques made it possible to test hypotheses regarding the pathogenesis of mental illnesses. Which mechanisms produced comas and convulsions? What were the reasons behind the therapeutic effect of shock treatment? And what was its nature? In short, what exactly were we treating?

THREE KEY FIGURES: HENRI CLAUDE, JEAN DELAY, HENRI EY

In France, most of the action took place at Saint-Anne's Hospital, under Henri Claude's (1869-1945) leadership. This neuropsychiatrist completely dominated French psychiatry between the wars.[49] Janet's friend, he came into the limelight at the beginning of the century for his work in endocrinology (the effect of adrenaline on the nervous system) and continued during the Great War in neurology (with Jean Lhermitte, he demonstrated the role of neurovegetative centres in metabolic and psychological regulation). Named to the research chair in clinical psychiatry in 1921, he set up the first open service at Saint-Anne and made a psychiatric internship obligatory for all medical students. He co-edited *L'Encéphale*, which was founded in 1906. Most of the postwar period's important names in psychiatry worked with Henri Claude, including Henri Ey, the director of the psychiatric clinic from 1931 to 1933 (during which time he developed a friendship with Jacques Lacan) and Henri Baruk, one of social psychiatry's main advocates, who made his name during the interwar period with his work in psychopharmacology and who established *Les Annales Moreau de Tours* in 1962. During the 1920s, Henri Claude welcomed into his service the founders of the future Société psychanalytique de Paris. Freud was barely known at this point and was hardly understood by doctors who saw him as a "German" Janet.

Henri Ey and Jean Delay belonged to the next generation. After the Second World War, they were among French psychiatry's most illustrious names. And both were, as was Claude, central players of their time.

Jean Delay was one of those rare psychiatrists who was also a professor and whose work received international acclaim. He headed the clinic of Professor Guillain, one of Charcot's successors at the Salpêtrière, "the Mecca of neurologists," and his first biographer. He undertook analysis (didactically, according to him) with Édouard Pichon, Janet's son-in-law, who would be among those to introduce psychoanalysis in France. Delay arrived at Saint-Anne, which is to psychiatry what the Salpêtrière is to neurology, towards the end of the 1930s. He was appointed to the chair of clinical psychiatry in 1946. Saint-Anne was, near the end of the nineteenth century, the centre for the "degeneration" school. Charcot's successes and those of his students at the Salpêtrière marked its decline towards the beginning of the twentieth century. Delay's interpretation of ECT, which became the word of law in the 1940s, and the first testing of neuroleptics in 1952 restored Sainte-Anne's prestige. Its reputation soon reached the same heights as those the Salpêtrière had known fifty years before. All of French psychiatry's currents would mingle and confront each other there: Paul Guiraud (France's incarnation of organicism and Ey's mentor) and George Daumézon (one of the main thinkers of Évolution psychiatrique) were department heads, and, in the 1950s, Lacan and Ey would hold seminars there.

Henri Ey's (1900-77) story is completely different from Delay's. He had Delay's prestige but not his influence. Head doctor of Bonneval Hospital and lacking a university career, he had no positions to offer. Yet, he remained an important figure for three reasons: first, throughout his career, he pitted psychiatry against psychoanalysis; second, from the outset, he participated in the Évolution psychiatrique group; and third, he contributed to the journal Évolution psychiatrique, which was first published in 1925 and edited by René Laforgue, a psychoanalyst. It was mainly through Évolution psychiatrique that the confrontation needed to bind psychoanalysis and psychiatry took place: the rapprochement would finally be reached towards the beginning of the 1960s. Some of L'Évolution psychiatrique's founders created, in 1926, the Société psychanalytique de Paris, which had its own journal, La Revue française de psychanalyse. In 1932, Henri Ey took over the editorship of L'Évolution psychiatrique, which he held until his death in 1977. For Ey, "psychoanalysis … provided a new understanding of the mechanisms of mental illness, and it [could] boast of impressive therapeutic results."[50] Meanwhile, he tried to open the journal up to neurologists. His life's work was to integrate psychoanalysis into psychiatry and psychiatry into medicine.

His institutional importance also stems from the fact that he was the main promoter of sector-based psychiatry and of the separation between neurology and psychiatry. He firmly believed in organicism, while retaining the idea that only through constant debate would psychiatry progress: imaginary consensus would not achieve this goal. The colloquia that he organized from the 1940s to the 1960s at Bonneval are still famous for the freedom of their content. Henri Ey is the second central player of French psychiatry.

FROM LESIONS TO FUNCTIONS

Henri Claude explained his psychiatric vision in his inaugural lesson in 1921: "In mental illness, most often we are faced with an inter-weaving of psychic and somatic factors whose study sheds light on the importance of the individual domain, a more precise and less strict concept than that of mental constitution. That is the objective of our teaching at Sainte-Anne, along with psychobiological meth-ods."[51] Psychiatric reasoning was changing from the ground up: theories on degeneration and hereditary fate were declining at the beginning of the century,[52] while psychopathological clinical tech-niques were coming into favour.[53] As of the 1930s, psychotherapeutic practices (institutional psychotherapy, occupational therapy, etc.) developed in conjunction with the introduction of shock therapy.[54] According to some accounts, they were often combined. The number of chronic psychoses were reduced, and patients were released from asylums.[55] The "therapeutic revolution" clearly preceded the inven-tion of the medication of the mind in the 1950s.

Biological treatments work, but how? The anatomical view, which looked for lesions, seemed vastly insufficient for a very simple reason: ECT does not repair lesions.[56] Mental illnesses had to be explained through different mechanisms. And many researchers began to describe the interweaving evoked by Claude not only at Sainte-Anne but also at Charenton and the Salpêtrière.

Shock therapy and the use of medication added experimental methods – specifically, those focused on humans – to clinical tech-niques. Nascent psychopharmacology contributed to an understand-ing of the effect of medication on the central nervous system: the origin of the disorder could not be found in a specific part of the brain but, rather, in a *dynamic* process attributable to certain areas of the brain. In other words, researchers were beginning to understand the *functions* of these areas (neurovegetative, diencephalon, etc.). These functions were seen as the biological basis of various pathologies. Some researchers tried to lift catatonic inhibition through prescribing cocaine, while others worked to produce schizophrenic states with the same substance but at very high doses. The first psychopharmaceutical laboratory was founded in Charenton (today called Esquirol) in 1930 thanks to the Rockefeller Foundation: hormones and chemical mediators (like adrenaline) were used in an attempt to understand pathology's mechanisms.[57] With Baruk, Claude published works on catatonia and, with Ey, works on hallucinatory psychoses. These showed that the affect is the basis of delirium, which results from a disorder of the thymia (a technical word for affect). Psychiatry could now exchange the anatomic viewpoint for a neurobiological one. In other words, *lesions gave way to functions*. It was believed that mental illness results, not from a lesion but, rather, from a functional deregulation that touches affect. It results from a dynamic state and is not static. Dynamics evoke change, perhaps even reversibility, and thus cure. As of the 1920s, analysis of a patient's personality, therapeutic experiments, and research on the central nervous system were combined to sweep away the anatomical view of psychoses and the inevitability of dementia (about which Kraepelin had theorized).[58]

Shock treatments demonstrated the existence of the biological mechanisms that underlie mental illness. They marginalized lesions and pathogenic agents. Combined with increasing laboratory research, these methods brought about precise hypotheses regarding the areas of the brain where chemical processes create emotional reactions.[59] In other words, they provided a way to empirically establish links between affect and representation: "The separation of the centres where intellectual acts occur from those that oversee instinctual reactions is not as absolute as some would have thought."[60] The aetiopathogenic mechanisms of delirium and rumination became experimentally comprehensible. What was the nature of these links between affect and representation?

SUPERIOR AND INFERIOR FUNCTIONS: THE GREAT CONSENSUS

The great doctrine of the interwar period and up through the 1940s was the hierarchy of functions. It refers to a model presented in 1884 by the neurologist John Hughlings Jackson. Mental illnesses are dissolutions of the superior functions of the brain, the last to be added during human evolution; they are more complex, more voluntary, and less organized than the inferior nervous functions. The disorganization of the superior functions undoes their control over the inferior ones. And this produces the mental automatisms that nascent scientific psychology would begin to study towards the end of the nineteenth century. These automatisms are of two different natures: positive and negative. Delirium and hallucination are the positive symptoms, while abulia, motor rigidity, and so on are the negative symptoms ("deficiencies," people would later call them). Jackson worked from a global, functional, evolutionist perspective, which was most emphatically not lesion-based. Mental illness appeared to him as a regression, as a "return to an ancestral or infantile state."[61] Jackson's theory was an important starting point, and it led to abandoning the idea that mental disorders were precise clinical entities – that is, illnesses.[62] French psychiatry (as seen in the work of Pierre Janet, Henri Claude, Henri Ey, Paul Guiraud, Jean Delay,[63] etc.) is essentially based on Jackson's theory of the unconscious.

ORGANICISM DEFENDS THE SELF

Henri Ey was taken with this doctrine: "It allows us to extend 'Janetism' to 'Freudism' while avoiding the errors and excesses of the latter."[64] In other words, there could be a psychogenesis of mental pathologies. According to Ey, a good Jacksonian, "Any lessening of superior mental forces brings about a liberation of energies designated by the terms 'unconscious' or 'instinctive.' Madness liberates animal tendencies."[65] This is where Janet and Ey meet: the illness is due to "an *energy deficiency*."[66] Inadequate psychological strength makes it impossible to control the body.

Only a "free and normal" psychic life comes from psychogenesis: "Psychic activity consists of integrating our history into the intentionality of the conscious." But this freedom "is rooted in organic life, it is nourished by it, it *integrates* it and consequently goes beyond it."[67] Freedom and psychic activity are two notions that completely overlap, the psyche being "the group of functions that allow[s] personal adaptation to reality."[68] This is why "mental illnesses are insults and constraints, they are not caused by free activity, that is, purely psychogenetic."[69] The link between the psyche and madness is one of exteriority. Madness does not hold any truth for humanity because it is the eclipse of the self, a disintegration of psychic activity: "No doubt we could correctly say of a hemiplegic person that he *is* paralyzed or *has* a paralysis, but we could not naturally say of a schizophrenic that he 'has' schizophrenia. We are touching on something real with these differences of language. I feel this so strongly that I could never write out a statement attesting that the patient is 'stricken with schizophrenia' or has 'chronic delirium,' but that he displays mental disorders that are characteristic of a certain structure."[70] The self is sick because the keystone of her freedom – her consciousness – is affected by hallucinations.

In 1950, Paul Guiraud (1882-1974), French organicism's other key personality, opened the chapter dedicated to psychoanalysis in his book *Psychiatrie générale* by writing: "One has to have lived through the period when psychoanalysis was revealed to psychiatrists to understand that it created a veritable revolution in our science."[71] Freud's contribution is, in his view, "to have found practical procedures for exploring the unconscious, and most of all to have shown that symptoms were the expression of an instinctive unconscious conflict."[72] Psychoanalysis pushed psychiatrists "into theorizing about the pathogenesis of deliria." It let them explain the patient's choice of delirium, while classic psychiatry was still wrestling with a "botanist" attitude. It helped them understand the patient's specificity and to search for the source of her delirium "closest to vegetative activity." The biological method learned from psychoanalysts that one "must enter the psychic region beneath the functions of the Ego." However, this method cannot reduce etiology to a purely sexual function since we must take into account all vital functions: "Emotional shocks, frustrations and conflicts, especially when they are repeated or accentuated, alter the function of the neurons as much as toxins and mechanical irritations."[73] Psychoanalysis gave us a means of making the patient specific, of understanding the illness through an individual's personal history. Combined with "the biological mind," it allowed psychiatry to become a medicine of the Self.

If Ey saw in madness the body's insult to human freedom, Lacan did not. For Lacan, "The question of truth conditions in its essence the phenomenon of madness … Man's being is wrapped up in it," and the intimate conflictuality of which he is made.[74] "Far from being an insult to freedom," Lacan replied head on to Ey at a Bonneval colloquium in 1947, "it is its most faithful companion, it follows its movement like a shadow. And man's being cannot be understood without madness, for he carries madness within him as a limit to his freedom."[75] From Ey to Lacan, the definition of the Self creates controversy. For the former, it is limited to normality; for the latter, madness is a "madness of the Self."

DELAY: A THEORY OF MOODS

In a book published in 1946, Jean Delay placed affect as the centre of psychosis: "It's through this particular angle, as mood disorders, that we consider the two psychoses [i.e., schizophrenia and manic-depressive psychosis]." Why focus on mood when a disturbed belief system is the major sign of psychosis? "The analysis of thymic disturbances has taken on special interest since the introduction of shock therapies into psychiatry ... These methods exert a truly remarkable effect on the thymic sphere, and therefore on psychoses where mood disorders constitute the primary disruption."[76] In both cases, we are faced with an illness of the affect – that is, a mood disorder. And this is the basis of hallucinations and delirium.

The ratio of durable successes in schizophrenia is, "according to our personal statistics[,] not more than 30 percent[,] whereas we have obtained 90 percent for melancholia."[77] There were no standardized statistical tools at the time, and Delay's count was inaccurate, even though the entire psychiatric literature confirmed that ECT was *the* treatment for melancholia.

Melancholia is described as a collapse of the life impulse manifested through moral anxiety: the feeling of incurability and delirium of guilt are such that the sick individual yearns for death and often commits suicide. "The collapse of the life instinct in melancholia," writes Delay, "comes with the absolute triumph of [a] moral consciousness that is all-powerful." Melancholia radicalizes the consciousness of the self under the sign of the illness of law: the influence of guilt is such that there is no room for the life impulse. Melancholia is like something found in Kafka: the law as pure punishment. In this case, writes Delay, "this sad consciousness, organized for and by pain, is transformed by *electroshock* that attacks its *thymic basis.*"[78] ECT regulates mood in a lasting fashion: it is a treatment that offers proof and helps distinguish, in a morbid entity, what part is syndrome (a clinical entity that relates to various illnesses) and what part is nosological (the pathology). When ECT temporarily releases the patient from a morbid form, the latter is usually only a symptom or syndrome; when it eliminates it permanently, it is an illness. Shock therapy is both a treatment and a tool for defining a pathology. As a treatment it provides proof and pharmacological dissection. If mood is the illness, writes Delay, "relapses rarely occur."[79]

Consciousness is thrown off centre, the Ego is fragmented; the "complete man," in his psychosomatic integrity, is the object of psychiatric reasoning. Janet-style psychological analysis, Freudian psychoanalysis, Jacksonian organicism, nascent psychopharmacology, and ECT mutually strengthen each other to draw a global configuration of the sick self. Mental disorder must be understood and treated on a double basis: (1) by acting on the centre of the lower functions (i.e., the thymia) and (2) by integrating the higher functions (as expressed in the patient's personal history). We could say that the sick self is affective: her emotional life is the meeting point of her thymic illness and her erroneous judgment. During the 1940s, a dynamic version of organicism brought together all the different schools.[80] Within this configuration, the debates raged.

Is This "Anxious," "Depressed," or "Asthenic" Individual
a Bit Melancholic?

Delay sees mood in the following way: "Mood is this fundamental affective disposition, rich with all the instinctive and emotional levels, that gives each of our states of mind a pleasant or unpleasant tone, oscillating between the two extreme poles of pleasure and pain. Insofar as we oppose, in mental life, a thymic sphere that includes affect and a noetic sphere that includes representation, mood is the most elementary and general thymic phenomenon."[81] During the 1940s, the effect of shock on the thymia became a common psychiatric standard of measurement. If unbalanced mood is at the centre of numerous pathologies, including neurotic ones, is mental distress and its corollary, a feeling of helplessness, enough to warrant the use of ECT? Or must we restrict its use to melancholia? In other words, have we discovered a treatment that can be used on all depressive states or only on specific entities?

The psychiatrist easily recognizes melancholia since the collapse of the patient's desire to live is observable in her attitude. She has "eyes that do not see," writes Delay.[82] She knows not from where her pain derives: "This collapse of the entire individual," wrote a young doctor in 1947 in his thesis in psychiatry, "in all his activities is primitive and apparently without etiology ... This suffering is without psychological cause: the patient feels it, suffers from it, but cannot explain it."[83] Lacking a psychological cause, and thus being endogenous, the unbalanced thymic source of melancholia can be broken by ECT.

Psychiatrists, at the time, considered depression to be associated with melancholia.[84] Should psychasthenia, "neurotic depression," reactive depression, and so on be treated by ECT? Although much less serious than melancholia, these phenomena possessed similar aspects (e.g., the loss of the life impulse and sadness).

This clinical reflection took place in psychiatric hospitals. In 1922, with the opening of the Henri Rouselle facility at Saint-Anne's – the first open service where non-psychotic patients could seek help – psychiatry's clientele increased.[85] Psychiatry welcomed, in part at least, patients who resembled those found in general practice. Should these individuals be categorized as melancholic? "In the minor melancholic state, we see patients who, when asked, recognize their sadness ... Expressing no suicidal ideas or delirium of self-accusation or humility, they appear to the doctor simply as fatigued individuals."[86] Minor melancholia or reactive melancholia: depression is still in its orbit. In the first case, depression is the entire illness; in the second, its place is much less clear.

IS ECT A SPECIFIC TREATMENT?

Depression's battle begins with discussions of the use of ECT outside of melancholia. It is a battle of definitions: should we characterize many different types of depression as functions of their etiology? Do these causes allow us to differentiate between defence psychoneuroses and traumatic neuroses? Must we consider depression as unitary? No one seems able to agree.

Jean Delay saw ECT as completely inefficient because "the sadness of the deep psychasthenic is of a completely other order than the pain of the melancholic person."[87] His concept of despondency is not linked to thymic disorder: the syndrome is due to a psychological conflict or trauma as only the higher functions are affected. Conversely, Georges Daumézon believed that we cannot distinguish between reactive and endogenous melancholies since both can be cured after a few rounds of ECT.[88] Meanwhile, as of 1943, Paul

Guiraud advocated its use in any depressive case.[89] At a 1950 conference, two Canadian psychiatrists stated that ECT "ha[d] shown itself
to be without a doubt effective and relatively harmless"[90] on more
than two thousand patients. Statistics on recovery and improvement,
as well as more precise information that accompanied them, were
all impressive in cases of hysteria, anxiety, reactive depressions, and
so on: "Clinically, the action of electroshock on psychoneuroses is
the same as on psychoses. Melancholic and anxious hyperthymia
is quickly calmed. Sleep and appetite become more regular. The
patient becomes more open to psychotherapy."[91] Disagreements
over the therapeutic effectiveness of ECT appeared when psychiatrists attempted to gain a consensus regarding the need to combine
psychotherapy and chemical therapy, which they did because – in
the Janet-Cerletti-Freud line – it was believed that "biological and
psychological therapies [were] not in opposition, but complete[d]
one another."[92]

The 1954 symposium, the first in France to be devoted to depressive states, provides us with a good idea of how the debate stood
after fifteen years of ECT. According to Julien Rouart, "Different
psychiatric schools ... have chosen [depressive states] as a battleground." He continued: "No doubt the universal character of depression as a lived experience makes it a perfect place to square off."[93]
What is the nature of this debate and what are its main arguments?

Jean Mallet saw the use of ECT in the case of neurotic depressions
as a negative thing as they were considered as partial melancholia
and therefore as less intense than other forms. Neurotic depressions
often resulted from an underlying neurosis and were "essentially
hysteria."[94] If depression was not the illness, then ECT would be
useless. Most often, depression was seen as a hysterical reaction to
a specific event – disappointment: "These events are experienced
as a loss of self-esteem or as a loss of external support that improves
self-esteem."[95] The notion of depression implies loss, decline, or
collapse of self-esteem. The depressed individual responds to disappointment by blaming herself and/or others. This everyday form of
depression differs from melancholia "for the neurotic patient tries
to hide it, though all the while it is expressing itself loudly in the
more or less delirious self-accusations of melancholia."[96] The neurotic depressive is ashamed, while the melancholic depressive has
lost the will to live. Yet self-esteem is, for psychoanalysis, linked to a
"particular pain," as Freud wrote, which is not anxiety, since it does

not signal danger, but, rather, a "reaction to the loss of the object
itself." This pain, which he names "narcissistic," "tends, as it were,
to empty the ego."[97] Narcissism and self-esteem comprised a marginal couple in this period, at least in French psychoanalysis. In the
1970s, they would become the main issue of psychoanalytic controversies over depression.

But if, like Ey, we do not accept the neuroses-psychoses distinction,
it would be logical to maintain that shock treatments work for all
types of depression. The clinical picture of the patient who is suffering from neurotic depression "gives the doctor the illusion of
being in the presence of a perfectly 'understandable' depressive
state."[98] This is an illusion because the doctor does not see that the
important issue does not lie in the distinction between melancholia
and other states but, rather, in the definition of the pathological:
ECT is useful in cases where we observe endogenicity.[99] To melancholia's "impossibility of being" comes "an insecurity of being,"
which is the permanent background in other cases.

Yet another problem arises. The distinction between neurotic
depression and melancholic depression is inadequate since there
are numerous atypical and transitional forms between these two
categories: "simple depressions, hysterical depressions, obsessive
depressions, melancholia of various types: agitated, variable, delirium-
based, schizophrenic, involving fantasy or states of stupor."[100] For
Laboucarie, the author of the preceding quote, this depressive
flowering can be mastered by ECT.

If there is no doubt as to therapeutic progress, the nosographical
question remains. Therapeutic proof does not seem to be the equal
of pharmacological dissection, and the general observation remains:
"Depressed patients resemble each other only on the surface."[101]
The term "depressive state" holds a negative practical value: it is a
way of identifying various disorders, giving them a certain similarity
by grouping them within the same entity – a "crossroads" – as
Dr Le Mappian wrote in 1949. All this seemed clear during the 1950
world conference and at the 1954 symposium of the Évolution psychiatrique. Here we see one of the issues within psychiatry that has
been constant since the invention of the first "effective" treatments:
we heal better and better, perhaps, but we cannot agree either about
what we are healing or about the effectiveness of the treatment.

What is at issue here is the interpretation of the role of the thymia
and endogenicity in neuroses. We can distinguish between two

models. The first is the ECT-melancholia model: the therapy must be applied to specific entities if it is to work, and these entities are not to be neurotic. The second is the non-specific model: only mood disorder is important, whether it stems from organic causes, as Ey believed,[102] or from an event that provoked it without affecting the lower functions (i.e., the thymic base). These two models help answer a question that is forced upon us by the invention of anti-depressants: can we distinguish between endogenous depression and exogenous depression?

As of the start of the 1940s, shock therapies were specifically used for melancholia, and they had important side effects. Psychiatrists working in hospitals used them widely for all sorts of mental illnesses, outside of any nosographical frame, at least when the symptoms became important enough to justify medical intervention. Certainly, ECT created risks for the patient (e.g., fractures) in its early use, but curare, a muscle relaxant and barbiturate-induced narcosis recommended by Delay in 1943 to calm the patient's anxiety before treatment, reduced these dangers. The use of ECT could then be extended. By the end of the decade, it was used for a plethora of mental illnesses, and its effectiveness seemed to decrease the closer we came to a normal state or, what amounts to the same thing, when the endogenous nature of the illness was not clear.[103] The same type of discussions and the same expansion of usage would be reproduced with antidepressants.

3

The Socialization of an Indefinable Pathology

The introduction of antidepressants and anxiolytics greatly amplified depression's medical and social ramifications. The prospect of using molecules to lift one's black moods led a growing number of psychiatrists to establish practices and allowed general practitioners to respond to complaints they had been hearing from their patients for some time. The generalists, however, had to contend with a number of uncertainties regarding their psychiatric tools.[1] The pharmaceutical industry had become an active player. As had the media: as of the late 1950s, magazines stressed over and over again that even those in the best of health could be liable to depression. The order of the day was to reassure: depression was neither a mental illness nor a matter of the imagination.[2] Suspicions of fakery and complaints about people having imaginary illnesses declined. Between 1965 and 1970, depression became an everyday aspect of general medicine.[3] Psychic life having emerged from its dark cloud, depression was now socially respectable.

Madness is mysterious and spectacular, while depression is subtle and discreet. Its presence is felt, but quietly, because depressed patients do not lose their reason. Psychiatry indiscriminately uses the word "depression" in the singular or plural and speaks of "depressive states." The depressed are alike only superficially because their illness is located at the crossroads of several pathological categories. How to recognize them? How to differentiate them in order to prescribe the proper treatment? Behind the doubts, the obsessions, and/or the fatigue, what pathology is at work within these patients? Are they suffering from a traumatic neurosis? A defensive psychoneurosis resulting from psychic conflict? Psychiatrists are forever asking themselves these questions.

However, depressions seem to present unique problems. First, intersecting, as they do, with other phenomena, they are extremely difficult to define. Second, as antidepressants are not equally effective for every emotional syndrome, the right distinctions must be made. Third, in uplifting mood, does one not alter perceptions, ways of viewing the world, one's self-image – indeed, everything that goes into making up a "personality"? Antidepressants create a whole new problem, that of the relationship between neurosis and depression. The need to differentiate between the mood that one *has* and the troubled personality that one *is* lies at the heart of the dilemma. Distinguishing between the person that one is and the illness that one has, while relating the one to the other, has been a constant challenge throughout the history of depression.

When the syndrome is removed has the personality been changed? And, if so, has it been altered in the same manner as it might have been had the person been subject to psychoanalysis? According to psychiatrists, if everyone can suffer from depression, then anyone can succumb to any kind of depression, though there are choices to be made with regard to the type. So who displays which pathology? The "choice" between varieties of depression is crucial to the debates we will be examining. For a period of twenty years, three separate notions were associated with the concept of "personality," and they dominated both nosography and diagnosis: (1) endogenous depression, (2) exogenous depression, and (3) psychogenic depression. This three-part division made credible a number of different relationships between self and affect. It should be stated that the boundaries between the two last categories tend to blur. Psychogenesis, increasingly, was equated with exogenesis.

AN IMPOSSIBLE DEFINITION

"Suffering is what does not deceive," wrote Jacques Lacan.[4] Depression, on the contrary, is deceptive. One fact soon strikes the researcher who consults psychiatric and medical literature: it is very hard to define depression.

In 1963, in the first special issue of the *Revue du praticien* devoted to depressive states, medical generalists were warned: "This illness is non-specific, because it is the common denominator of most psychiatric conditions."[5] Pierre Deniker, the "boss" of psychopharmacology at Sainte Anne, observed in 1966 that "the term 'depression' in common use today often refers to very disparate phenomena."[6] Depression's disparate nature has remained constant to the present day. In 1978, a specialist in the biochemistry of depression reminded us again: "The word depression is generic and vague, referring to a number of syndromes that one may classify according to their semiology, evolution, genetics, biochemistry and responsiveness to diverse therapies. Each of these groups can be subdivided without the resulting categories in any way matching those of the group following."[7] In 1985, it was acknowledged that "depression remains … a concept with blurred boundaries. What is known is that it is 'what antidepressants cure.'" Therefore, "the most common approach in treating depression is an empirical one."[8] In 1996, the same observation: "The concept of depression remains vague." What is more: "the adage according to which we know better and better how to treat it, but less and less what we are treating, remains valid."[9] But what do we treat better when we do not know what we are treating? What are the criteria for a cure? Some fifty years after the discovery of antidepressants, psychiatry, in the face of all that is vague and heterogeneous, is still struggling to produce a theory of depression.

In 1976, in "a review of contemporary confusion" dealing with the classification of depressions, Robert E. Kendell, a professor at Edinburgh University, judged that "over the last fifty years, and especially in the last twenty [i.e., since antidepressants were invented], countless classifications for depressive illness have been put forth. This is too well known to be repeated. However, conflicting statements and proposals as well as methodological issues are so overwhelming that those who are not intimately involved have increasing difficulty understanding what is happening … That nearly every type of classification logically possible has been defended by someone during the last twenty years attests to the complexity and absurdity of the present situation." The classifications of depression at the time ranged from a unitary type to nine different types. Kendall asserted that, if there was competition between the criteria of classification, it was because depressions "provide an opportune environment for disputes pertaining to the nature and classifications of mental illness taken on the whole."[10] Were we dealing with clear-cut illnesses or with extreme reactions to specific situations? With independent entities or arbitrary concepts? Should they be classified according to their symptoms, their etiology, or their pathogeny? There was no agreement even on the very substance of depression: "The boundaries between depression and sadness, between depressive illnesses and anxiety states, between affective psychosis and schizophrenia, and between recurrent depression and personality disorder are all arbitrary and ill defined."[11] This was a blunt summing up, by an internationally renowned British psychiatrist, of the perplexity that assails us whenever we try to get an intellectual grip on what we know as depression.

Since Kendall, the modes of classification, and the way in which mental illness is viewed, have been entirely rethought in light of work done in the United States. The goal of this work was to bring some semblance of order into the diagnostic confusion.[12] Herman van Praag, who has been called "Mister Biological Psychiatry" in Holland and who is one of the world leaders in the field of depression, wrote in 1990: "For 30 years, confusion has reigned where the classification of depression is concerned ... All things considered, the situation has in fact deteriorated. Once, psychiatrists at least acknowledged that diagnostic chaos was the norm. ... Today this chaos has been codified, and the confusion thereby masked."[13] These judgments are not the work of psychiatric outsiders.

Depressive states are thus lacking in all specificity, and their symptoms are astonishingly diverse. The term "depression" is vague, designating, if not a sad state of mind, at least an "abnormal" shift in mood for which there is no biological marker. All this results in the bizarre paradox that, although we do not know what we are treating, we are treating it better. What is depression? A shadowy phantom? An unlikely collective illusion? Simplistic answers are not good enough.

THE ONLY MENTAL DISORDER BOTH HETEROGENEOUS AND UNIVERSAL

Why this problem? Heterogeneity is far from being associated only with depression. For example, it also applies to hysteria, whose wealth of organic, psychological, and behavioural symptoms is

considerable. Indeed, has hysteria not been dubbed the "elusive illness?"[14] Yet it does not raise problems of definition and diagnosis:
its status as a sickness is unassailable.

There is a second trait proper to depression: universality. And this
it shares with only one other pathology – anxiety.[15] Contrary to
depression, anxiety is not particularly heterogeneous and is easily
diagnosed. To the degree that anxiety may be found in most pathologies, it, too, raises the question of pathological boundaries. Donald
Klein, one of our most eminent specialists in the field, reminds us
that anxiety is "an adaptive, and not a learned response to anticipated danger. Insofar as life teaches us to recognize a large number
of dangers, the appearance of unprecedented feelings of anxiety is
simply the product of an unusual experience of apprenticeship."[16]
As a consequence of this, some writers have criticized its medicalization – a position that Klein vigorously opposes.[17] It is easy to identify
the positive functions anxiety fulfills (i.e., as an alert to danger or
to the forbidden). But depression? Heinz Lehmann, who introduced
the first neuroleptic into North America in the early 1950s, asserts
that "anxiety is such an omnipresent phenomenon that it seems
futile to estimate its prevalence in the general population, other than
to discuss it in terms of the well-known slogan that we live in an age
of anxiety. Depression, on the other hand, makes a clearer cut-off
between the normal and the pathological. It is also more deadly
than anxiety."[18] We can see why anxiety, whose pathological limits
are hard to determine, and which does not lead to suicide, has
remained more closely associated with the status of a symptom than
has depression.

And so the reigning confusion surrounding depression derives
from a combination of *extreme heterogeneity*, as in hysteria, and *maximal
universality*, as in anxiety, a disorder so easy to recognize. Therein
lies the root cause for our difficulties in defining depression.

Depression and anxiety derive from feelings and emotions inherent
in being human, what Freud, let us remember, called "ego-feeling."
Part and parcel of our normal constitution,[19] they become pathological only at levels of high intensity, and this differentiates them from
hysteria and schizophrenia, which require no such calibration.

But is intensity of feeling enough to characterize a pathology?
Can antidepressants play a role in pharmacological dissection?

The work most often referred to in discussions concerning depression during the 1960s in France, *Méthodes chimiothérapeutiques en*

psychiatrie by Jean Delay and Pierre Deniker, can serve as our Ariadne's thread. Distinguishing two main categories of depression, "neurotic" (or simple) and "endogenous," the authors went on: "Our greatest diagnostic difficulty occurs when endogenous depression takes the form of a simple depression."[20] The cancer that was to eat away at the nosography and diagnostics of depression was anticipated four years after antidepressants were discovered. But during the period we are looking at, this cancer was "kept under control" by psychopathological thinking and a growing reference to psychoanalysis.

Introducing a long article in *L'Encéphale* in 1961, André Green presented psychoanalysis as the discipline that "casts light on the foundations of psychopathology, the pilot science of therapeutic psychiatry." "Only a few years ago," he added, "biological therapy and psychological therapy had almost no common ground. The introduction of chemical therapy soon raised a number of practical problems concerning their joint application."[21] What practical problems did the introduction of these treatments reveal? What psychopathology might resolve them?

TO CALM MANIC AGITATION, TO RELIEVE DEPRESSIVE MOODS

What does it mean to succumb to a mental disorder? Under what conditions can an abnormally troubled mind consider itself cured? To calm anxiety *without inducing sleep,* to stimulate *without inducing euphoria,* and, in each case, to do so with reduced risks of addiction, that was the "revolution" that neuroleptics and antidepressants made possible.[22] For the first time in the history of mental illness, true remedies were developed – molecules that restored to the individual enough freedom of thought, feeling, and bodily movement to bring her close to normal behaviour. Psychiatrists could not believe their eyes. Prior to the invention of neuroleptics, anxiolytics, and antidepressants, there were sedatives that calmed but put to sleep (e.g., barbiturates) and excitants that stimulated but rendered euphoric (e.g., amphetamines). Worse still, those substances carried with them serious risks of addiction.

Today, more than fifty years later, with psychotropic drugs (along with the language of psychic distress) playing an everyday role in our societies, we fear that these therapies may represent forces of social control in disguise. Our concern that the self is in danger of being lost has generated heated controversy. But this is the exact opposite of what was thought at the time – that is, that the molecule was a means of restoring the self. We must try to imagine how things were then and to understand psychiatrists' sense of wonder. The impact these remedies had is at the heart of the diagnostic, noso-graphic, and therapeutic debates that followed.

PEACE OF MIND

If electroconvulsive therapy (ECT) was the preferred treatment for melancholia, the manic behaviour and delirium associated with anxiety still had no cure. But anxious and dejected moods did not interest only psychiatrists, as the origins of the first neuroleptic show. Surgeons were also interested: the greater a patient's anxiety before an operation, the more anaesthesia one had to inject. That could trigger post-operative shock and, eventually, the patient's death. This is the problem that absorbed Henri Laborit, the military surgeon and anaesthetist.[23]

A team of researchers at Rhône-Poulenc tried to synthesize derivatives of a molecule called phenothiazine in order to develop a treatment for malaria. One of the derivatives stood out: it had greater side effects, both sedative and hypnogenetic, than the others. Rhône-Poulenc decided to seek out a molecule in which these features predominated. Henri Laborit included this derivative in a pre-operative anaesthetic because it enabled him to maximize effect while diminishing the quantity of anaesthesia used. Meanwhile, Paul Guiraud used the molecule with apparent success in treating twenty-four schizophrenics.[24]

This molecule (chlorpromazine) was synthesized in 1950. Animal experiments showed that it had the effect of "psychic deconditioning."[25] In June 1951, Rhône-Poulenc made the product available to Laborit, who published his results in February 1952: "It induces no loss of consciousness, *no psychic change*, but only a certain tendency to sleep *and above all a 'disinterest'* on the part of the patient as to what is happening around him … These facts point to possible psychiatric applications for the product."[26] Laborit did not simply note the possible uses for this molecule in psychiatry: he took the initiative of experimenting with it at Val-de-Grâce Hospital. On 19 January 1952, a twenty-four-year-old psychotic, who had already been committed on two occasions and subjected to two unsuccessful ECT treatments and some fifteen insulin comas, received a fifty milligram injection of chlorpromazine that calmed him immediately. He left the hospital after three weeks of treatment.[27] The head of the department presented an account of the case a few days later, and it was published in March. The patient was calm and did not lose consciousness. The sedative and hypnotic effects of chlorpromazine were thus separated, whereas they had been confused in the case of barbiturates (which both calmed and put to sleep). Jean Delay used the molecule in March. He administered repeated doses and obtained the same spectacular results.[28] The product did much more than calm excited states, it had a neuropsychic effect that Delay defined as follows: "The apparent indifference to or delay in responding to external stimulation, the lessening of initiative and of concern without any change in alertness or intellectual functions, this is what constitutes the psychic impact of the drug."[29]

What we had with chlorpromazine was tranquillity with no soporific effect or stupor.[30] The molecule produced peace of mind (ataraxia) and lessened the intensity of nervous agitation (hence its neuroleptic powers); consciousness was revitalized, and alertness, intelligence, and affect were no longer affected. It was truly a remedy that restored the mind's powers, rather than a drug. Many psychiatrists found it hard to believe because, up until that time, whereas the substances at their disposal (e.g., opium, barbiturates, and amphetamines) may have given comfort to the patient, they also altered his psyche. In other words, they did not restore the self in all its fullness. Heinz Lehmann, who conducted the first North American trials in 1953, recalled his astonishment: "Nothing like this ever happened with schizophrenia. I had never seen anything in any manual that made reference to such a possibility."[31] He added that, despite the medication's spectacular results and its tests on chronic schizophrenics, it took him two years to completely accept the idea that what he was seeing was not simply something that calmed anxiety but, rather, something that had an actual impact on schizophrenic syndromes.

If chlorpromazine's antimanic action was evident from the beginning, it took two years for its antidelirium effect to be accepted by the profession. Doubtless the tradition of sleep cures to calm the sick and the fact that chlorpromazine had first been discovered in the context of anaesthesia contributed to the impression that it was primarily a tranquillizer, a form of "artificial hibernation." The evaluation of the clinical results was very tentative. Delay first interpreted them as a "neuropsychic syndrome" and used the words "neurolepsy" and "psycholepsy" indiscriminately. The language wavered between references to the nervous system and to the psyche. "I was struck," wrote Pierre Deniker in 1975, "by the number of terms invented to account for what was new but difficult to define. Gangioplegic, potentializer, vegetative stabilizer, neurolytic, neuroplegic, psychoplegic, narcobiotic, ataraxic, and tranquillizers were each proposed in turn."[32] The word "neuroleptic" was adopted in France in 1954 by Delay and Deniker because it was the neurological activity that determined the remedy. "Though adopted with some reluctance," explained Deniker, "it entered the vocabulary of both pharmacologists and clinicians."[33] (In the United States the term "tranquillizer" was used when benzodiazepines made their appearance at the end of the decade.) Clearly, it was difficult to pin down the effects of a remedy for the mind when there was no tradition upon which such an evaluation could rely.[34] This point is crucial for mental pathology as it shows how difficult it is, when attempting to probe in detail the thinking of psychiatrists, to answer questions such as "what are we treating?" "how are we treating?"

In opening the 1955 International Conference on Neuroleptics in Paris, Delay acknowledged a debt: "Pierre Janet in his studies of psychological tension created the term 'psycholepsy' to indicate a drop in this tension. It is by analogy that we have proposed the term 'neurolepsy' in referring to that drop in nervous or neuro-vegetative tension which determines, in part, psychological tension, and corresponds to the clinical activity of remedies which produce, essentially, a relaxation."[35] The medication's action was consistent with a deficiency-oriented model of the illness (a drop in tension, in one's state of alarm). In closing the same conference, Delay stated: "From a therapeutic point of view, whatever the interest of these drugs, we should remember that in psychiatry such remedies represent only one moment in the treatment of a mental illness, and that the underlying treatment remains psychotherapy."[36] Note the crucial role reserved for psychotherapy. This statement was not a matter of form. Psychotherapy was not therapeutic by default – far from it – and the use of remedies for the mind did not reduce therapy to the ingestion of a molecule. The medicinal action was syndromic:[37] it modified the patient's personality but could not, on its own, cure a psychically ill individual.

MOOD LIFTERS OR PSYCHIC ENERGIZERS?

The Swiss Roland Kuhn and the American Nathan Kline both related the stories of their inventions in a 1970 collected volume devoted to discoveries in psychiatric biology. Kuhn discovered the antidepressive effects of imipramine, the most important member of a class called tricyclics; and Kline discovered those of iproniazide, the first antidepressant in the class called monoamine oxidase inhibitors (MAOIS). Both imipramine and iproniazide were at first called thymoanaleptics because their mood-lifting function seemed increasingly to constitute their main effect. Tricyclics were the most widely used antidepressants in the world. Their drop in popularity is recent and is the result of the appearance on the market of molecules called selective serotonin reuptake inhibitors (SSRIS), of which Prozac is the most prominent.

The juxtaposition of Kuhn's and Kline's respective texts shows that we are dealing with two very different conceptions of what constitutes depression. The controversy provoked by antidepressants in recent years was not inevitable.

Kuhn's point of departure was melancholia and the distinction between the endogenous-biological and the exogenous-psychogenetic. He drew on the phenomenological psychiatric tradition and brought to an understanding of melancholia a forceful conviction that "did not come from … biology or biochemistry, but, rather surprisingly, from philosophy." Karl Jaspers, and then Kurt Schneider, made a distinction between the patient's objective behaviour and her subjective experience, which, according to Kuhn, "could only be learned through self-description." The difference between what was endogenous and what was reactive was established "by distinguishing vital feeling – an experience that spreads through the patient's body with endogenous depression, without motive and psychotic – from 'emotional feeling' – a similar experience, but with a different nature – where depression has a cause and the cause is evident." According to Kuhn, the vital depressive disorder was characterized by "feelings of fatigue, lethargy, confinement, oppression and inhibition, accompanied by a slowing-down of thinking, acting and decision," while the emotional depressive disorder was characterized by "the inability to feel pleasure and maintain interest or even by loss of the ability to experience any emotion whatsoever."[38] The first was more corporal than the second; it resembled melancholia but lacked any sign of delirium.

Kuhn, like many scientists of the time, had decided to test phenothiazines on depressed patients. They had a calming effect when the patients were anxious but "no effect on the specific depressive symptoms."[39] In 1950, an official at the Swiss company Geigy suggested that he work on an antihistamine in order to test its hypnotic properties. The results were negative, but it seemed "the substance had some special 'antipsychotic' effects"[40] – special, but difficult to pin down. Geigy proposed another molecule, imipramine, whose chemical structure (tricyclic) was slightly different from that of chlorpromazine. He tested it for a year on various mental disorders and obtained results from three hundred patients.

In 1956, he decided to try the product out on cases of endogenous depression because he had come to the conclusion "that it must be possible to find a drug effective in endogenous depressions," a conviction, he notes, supported by the literature on depression at the time, by the results of electric shock treatment, and by psychotherapy.[41] Kuhn experimented with a specific diagnosis – melancholia-like depressions – not neuroses with depressive symptoms. In other words, the clinical action of the molecule was not tested at random. Furthermore, the testing was properly thought out with reference to the psychopathology. Kuhn presented his preliminary results (forty cases) at the Second World Congress of Psychiatry in Zurich on 6 September 1957 in front of an audience of – twelve people. "Our paper," said Kuhn, "was received with some interest, but with a great deal of scepticism. This was not surprising, in view of the almost completely negative history of the drug treatment of depression up to that time."[42] Kuhn's colleagues showed little interest in his results. Was this because the conference was entirely devoted to schizophrenia?[43]

The first published evaluation of imipramine indicated the following: "The substance is particularly effective in typical endogenous depressions provided there is a vital disturbance standing clearly in the foreground."[44] Imipramine could also be effective for neurotic depressions, but the preferred treatment remained, above all, "in the phenomenological study of the subjective *experience* of the patient, in the vital and emotional depressive disturbance."[45] Kuhn developed an approach distinguished by its specificity, in the ECT/melancholia tradition. Until the end of the 1970s, European psychiatry was convinced that antidepressants were most effective when applied to endogenous depressions, where affect was ailing.[46]

"What lessons does the Imipramine Story have for us?" Kuhn asked himself. The success of a specific treatment for depressive states depended on the clinical intuitions of the psychiatrist; he had to "recognize a particular pathological picture within which the drug is in fact successful ..., a picture only partly coinciding with the classical clinical idea of the depressive states."[47] In most cases, to succeed therapeutically one had to carefully select the patient through an extremely subtle analysis of his subjective experience; otherwise, the pharmacotherapy's effectiveness was greatly reduced. Of course, luck played a role, but one had to be "able to 'invent' something completely new, something hitherto unknown, namely *a new disease.*"[48] This was a creative act and not a miraculous effect involving some vague nosographic entity, which is why Kuhn claimed to "have achieved a *specific* treatment of depressive states."[49] All Kuhn's thinking addressed what it was to be psychically ill. For him, what was required was a subtle understanding of human experience. This discovery was not, according to Kuhn, a matter either of chance or of science. He found philosophical bases for his psychiatric and pharmacological thought in the work of Heidegger and Binswanger.

But imipramine had yet another lesson to teach: Kuhn had noted that it was antidepressive, not euphoriant. This meant that it differed from a drug. What is more, it was a sedative and not a stimulant. Now, endogenous depressions were almost always accompanied by lethargy. Alan Broadhurst, at the time Geigy's director of medical research, recently declared: "Everyone was expecting that an antidepressant, if it ever saw the light of day, would be a stimulant."[50] Sedation was counter-intuitive. In fact, amphetamines were being used to treat melancholia and depression, but they were shown to be both ineffective and dangerous. Kuhn's clinical breakthrough was to invent a mood elevator that was also a sedative. Jean Guyotat, one of the rare French psychiatrists with an international reputation during the 1960s (apart from the big names at Sainte-Anne), wrote in 1963 that imipramine had an anti-obsessional effect: it made it easier to deal with frustration, which "doubtless explains as well what Kuhn observed, the absence of addiction to imipramine."[51]

What Nathan Kline took from the MAOI story ran exactly contrary to Kuhn:[52] what he saw was not just a remedy specifically designed for endogenous depression but one applicable to all depressions –

one that was not just a mood elevator but a euphoriant. Assigned in 1953 to do a comparative study of Rauwolfia serpentina, otherwise known as reserpine (one of the alkaloids that Ciba had just isolated), and a placebo, he launched a study of 710 patients. And, in 1954, he was the first American to confirm the antimanic properties of reserpine, the second neuroleptic. He abandoned his work after a few years as he found he was inducing serious depressions in psychotics. Nevertheless, his clinical insight was the starting point for biochemical hypotheses dealing with mental disorders.

The 1953 study led Kline to postulate "the existence of drugs that would function as antidepressants (or *psychic energizers*, as I subsequently designated them)."[53] In April 1956, a colleague told him about an animal experiment in which a molecule called iproniazide (an antitubercular) had been administered and had made the animals "hyperalert and hyperactive." In Kline's words, this "led me to speculate whether this was the psychic energizer for which we had all been looking."[54] Several studies had already been conducted on this molecule, but their aim had been to make a comparison with the tranquillizing effects of chlorpromazine. The data did indicate that iproniazide had secondary euphoriant effects on patients who were being treated for tuberculosis, but this antidepressant effect had not been noticed by the researchers. In May 1956, Kline's team was visited by the medical director of Hoffman-La Roche, who was "much impressed with the antidepressant action of opiates and had been working on the possibility of developing a nonaddicting opiate with such antidepressant action."[55] He was, however, "singularly unimpressed by their idea."[56] Kline tried to convince Hoffman-La Roche to help them. The laboratory was not interested: "Here indeed was a fairly unique situation! A group of clinical investigators were trying to convince a pharmaceutical house that they had a valuable product."[57] In November 1956, he began a study of some hospitalized patients with premature dementia and then sought out depressed patients who were being treated in private practice. He found nine, and began the study in May and June 1957. After that, the antitubercular treatment was recommended for depressions.

For Nathan Kline, the MAOI story "is not only the secret of treating depression but the key to its cause and prevention. This door is beginning to open, and behind it we find even now evidence that the mechanisms of schizophrenia and perhaps of some neuroses will become visible and treatable."[58] Kline staked all his hopes on a

biology of ⬚⬚⬚⬚⬚⬚⬚⬚⬚⬚⬚⬚⬚⬚⬚⬚ nent for
a specific ⬚⬚⬚⬚⬚⬚⬚⬚⬚⬚⬚⬚⬚⬚⬚⬚ le Kline
discovere⬚ ⬚⬚⬚⬚⬚⬚⬚⬚⬚⬚⬚⬚⬚⬚⬚⬚ ant. Did
he not w⬚ ⬚⬚⬚⬚⬚⬚⬚⬚⬚⬚⬚⬚ ?"[59] The
remark c⬚ ⬚⬚⬚⬚⬚⬚⬚⬚⬚⬚ AOIS, as
stimulants, to create dependency.

On the one hand, we had a psychopathology based on clinical experience and, on the other, a malfunctioning of the nervous system that was interpreted biologically. Two visions presented themselves: the first sought to chart, as far as possible, the pathology underlying syndromes (this was the melancholia–ECT model), while the second sought the biological causes of those syndromes.[60] Kuhn thought he had discovered a specific; Kline thought he had discovered a non-specific. We were back to the debates over ECT but within a totally different scientific context. The future would confirm the "victory" of Kline over Kuhn, with depressive syndromes being cut loose from any underlying pathology, the diagnosis of which was no longer considered a precondition for treatment. Further, antidepressants today act upon such a wide variety of syndromes that even the term "antidepressant" is being questioned by psychiatrists and pharmacists.[61] In the wake of all that, psychiatry has abandoned its probing of the relationship between the self and sickness. Kline's victory over Kuhn also meant the posthumous revenge of Janet on Freud. Today's pathological human is different from that of 1960, but then so is today's normality.

In the years that followed the introduction of these medicines of the mind, the two points of view, at least in France, supported one another when it came to responding to one question: can a molecule, on its own, cure?

BETWEEN THE PERSONALITY THAT ONE IS AND THE MOOD THAT ONE HAS

As of 1955, the pharmaceutical race was under way: there was an abundance of psychopharmacological and neurobiological research, a whole plethora of psychopharmacological conferences and societies.[62] The term "psychopharmacology" was a sort of "hook that functioned as a centre of attraction for disparate groups of clinicians, statisticians, specialists in animal psychology, and other professions brought together to evaluate the therapeutic possibilities of new remedies."[63] The development of a series of pharmacological tests on animals made possible an analysis of the effects of molecules that had been synthesized by chemists. A work published in 1959, a pharmacologist notes, "boasted 240 pages of reference material just for the period of 1952-1957."[64] These publications described the effects of psychotropic drugs, comparing pharmacological, bio-chemical, and metabolic studies, among others. A dozen conferences on "psychotropic drugs" were organized between 1955 and 1960, and they "generated a literature that would overwhelm the most devoted researcher were he capable of reading them."[65] Between 1952 and 1965, a hundred molecules saw the light of day – of which only a few made their way to the market. This was something with which the medical community had to come to terms.

The consequence of these discoveries was the mobilization of a number of professional bodies.[66] "Psychopharmacology," declared Delay on opening the conference of the International Neuropsycho-pharmacology College in 1966, "interests in different ways the chemist and the pharmacologist, the physiologist and the doctor, the psychologist and the sociologist. Given that its very nature is to modify behaviour with chemical substances, it finds itself at the crossroads of biological science and ethics."[67] Delay's interest here was not one of philosophical inquiry. There were two reasons for his position. The first was that neuroleptics acted only on syndromes and that the action of antidepressants was "essentially *suspensive*, which is to say it must be maintained for as long as the attack con-tinues or becomes a chronic condition."[68] In other words, the chemical action altered the mechanisms but did not eliminate the causes; it was pathogenic but not etiological.

The second reason for Delay's position derived from the fact that antidepressants affected not only endogenous depressions but also neuroses, often called "simple" or "exogenous" depressions. This, for Delay and Deniker, "[was] one of the most interesting and least known discoveries." Compared to neuroleptics, which greatly enhanced the possibility of treating well-known illnesses, antidepres-sants were deeply innovative; it seemed, our two authors continued, "that there was a future for antidepressants' treating neuroses that were *constitutional in nature*."[69] And so the Janet-type neuroses were treatable, and the molecules seemed equally effective for certain defence psychoneuroses. Jean Guyotat, in 1963, gave the example of an individual who had been suffering from an obsessive neurosis for seven years. Imipramine brought an end to this. "We cannot in this case," commented Guyotat, "talk about symptoms in the classic sense of the word."[70] Something more was happening on the frontier between the personality that one *is* and the symptom that one *has*. The antidepressants were modifying the "personality." "It is striking," Guyotat continued, "to observe that there are many common elements shared by psychotherapy and chemical therapy. We must insist on the fact that the sick person does not react to a psychotropic drug as to an explosive, he does not vanish into thin air. The observed changes lead us back always ... to his overall personality." And so we must "avoid the dichotomy that would make psychotherapy part of the natural order and associate the chemical therapies with one that is artificial."[71]

The new treatments, unlike ECT treatments, were of long duration. In that respect they resembled psychoanalysis, with its extended time span during the course of which a personality slowly altered and resolved its conflicts. The patient was transformed incrementally. A few shocks were not, from this point of view, in any way comparable to the slow impregnation of the molecule. Nuanced reactions could emerge over time, as in a talking cure. The pathological shifts in emotion and thought associated with antidepressants were such that, in 1972, a psychiatrist could declare: "All those who in 1957 were privy to the first publications, the first conference reports concerning the use of imipramine for depression, and who tried it on their own patients, likely felt, as I did, that modesty was the best policy when talking about depression and psychotherapy."[72]

It was important to understand, as Delay and Deniker recommended, "the psychodynamics of chemical action."[73] Pierre A. Lambert and Jean Guyotat targeted this problem. They sought, for example, to reveal the mechanisms through which an antidepressive molecule could enable an obsessive individual, as in psychoanalysis, to create a distance between herself and her compulsive rituals. The chemical action had to be understood and interpreted in terms of "the global personality" of the patient. They analyzed the antidepressive action of the molecule using Freud's model for melancholia as a starting point: the patient was sick from not being able to mourn the object in which she was emotionally invested. She internalized the object and turned her aggression against herself. The antidepressant re-established the relationship with the object and enabled psychotherapy to resolve psychic conflicts with which, earlier, it had been unable to deal.[74] Thus their goal: "To be able to prescribe a chemical therapy, not on the basis of symptoms in the ordinary sense of the word, but based on the structure of the patient."[75] This goal would not be achieved.

A STRONG AND CONFUSED IDEA

These clinical debates were accompanied by heated metaphysical discussions concerning the nature of the global influence of antidepressants on personality. "The 'psychiatric field,'" Claude Blanc declared in 1965, "ranges from the metabolism of serotonin to the philosophical implications of our psychopathological knowledge about humanity."[76] Incomplete hypotheses concerning the functioning of the central nervous system were no longer enough for neurobiology. Antidepressants "force the psychiatrist to think physiologically," as Delay said.[77] They began, in concrete terms, to encroach on philosophy's territory and, in psychiatry, on that of phenomenology and psychoanalysis. The medications were restoring personal powers. In his report presented to the Bonneval conference on the unconscious in 1960, Claude Blanc made clear the anthropological consequences of pharmacological progress: "[it] reintroduce[s] the idea of the self into the study of how the brain functions."[78] What psychopathology could incorporate the new pharmacological data? That is what was at stake.

In fact, "the notions of sedation, drowsiness, excitation and euphoria are totally inadequate because they are too crude, and the experience of patients eludes such categories."[79] These concepts came closer to describing what animals experienced, to a "veterinary psychiatry," as André Green termed it.[80] They allowed us to account for changes in affect but not for changes in the inner life of a human being (especially since molecules successfully tested on animals had no effect on humans). What was needed was a psychopathology that would account for medication in such a way that psychopharmacology would not "strip away that meaningfulness which is our human prerogative."[81] So that it would not reduce what was human to a kind of life that is a simple projection of the nervous system: "One of the most instructive lessons we have received from these new [neurophysiological] discoveries is how central meaning is to the observed phenomena. The preselection of signals requires that a distinction be made between the signifier and the non-signifier when our attention is being focussed in a particular way."[82] Serge Lebovici and René Diatkine reminded us that the unconscious was an expression of the biological and the psychic, that the model of the reflex was fundamental to Freud's conception of an economical division of energy.[83] Other psychoanalysts emphasized that it was wrong to condemn "psychoanalysis for practising pure psychogenesis" as organogenetic factors were never ruled out.[84]

But these arguments remained theoretical. The psychopathological question was important, above all, because the molecules had one practical limitation: the patient's resistance to their effectiveness. In certain cases the pathology was resistant: the product worked on a patient at one point and then stopped working. How to explain this? How to relate the impact on one's mood to that on the personality? What took place between affect and thought, "body" and "mind?" To answer those questions would be to define the illness.

In 1966, Delay again cautioned, with consensual enthusiasm, that "psychiatry cannot be reduced to chemistry"[85] because, in a medicine of the mind, there had to be a relationship. But Ey was more specific in discussing the clinical and professional problems posed by the new molecules. What did it mean for a psychiatrist to think physiologically? And what kind of psychiatrist would this be? "Almost always," Ey wrote, "... a confused but strong idea makes itself felt when one resorts to biological methods: they pave the way for and favour psychotherapeutic action."[86] Strong, because the medication was not considered mechanistically but as part of a relationship: a medicinal relationship and a doctor-patient relationship; confused, because the nature of this dual relationship was constantly being questioned by the profession on one point in particular – when was the medication the principle cause of change and when was it but one part of a therapeutic system?

REALIZING THE POTENTIAL OF PSYCHOTHERAPY

A substance's impact could not truly be appreciated independently of a series of contexts: the treatment environment, the patient's history, his relationship with one or more doctors, and so on. What is more, the pharmacological contact and the human contact were like the two arms of one body. Chemical treatment, whether it consisted of old narcotics or new molecules, was "a chemical psychoanalysis":[87] it brought inner conflicts to the surface, and it made it possible to purge them. The profession was in agreement that molecules acted on the personality as a whole because a psychic disorder was, as a close collaborator of Baruk wrote, "a global threat to the personality, which is disturbed, not only where the patient's mood is concerned, but also from an intellectual and instinctive point of view."[88] But this action could not provide a cure all by itself. That much was clear.

A mental disorder was not cured by treating the brain; a medication for the mind was not the same as a somatic medication. This argument was particularly widespread in psychiatry at the time. We find it in the Évolution psychiatrique group,[89] in the École de Sainte Anne,[90] in the Lyon school (Lambert, Guyotat), and among the supporters of Henri Baruk.[91] Only the believers in psychic causality viewed the medication as sedatives. The medications were relational substances as they allowed the patients to face up to their conflicts, while the doctor *was* the medicine.

This argument was already basic to the idea that some shock treatments made the patient more amenable to psychotherapy; the impact on the patient's state of mind, which was utterly ravaged before the treatment, allowed the patient to renew her contact with reality. The fact that she was surrounded by others during the treatment represented "a psychotherapeutic gesture."[92] Ergotherapy, institutional therapy, and shock treatments facilitated a new connection between doctor and patient, put the accent on their renewed relationship, and gave a therapeutic role to the nurse, encouraging dialogue between her and the psychiatrist.[93] The therapy was global.[94] "Biological and psychological therapies, far from being in conflict, complement each other," declared Delay at the 1950 conference.[95] Thanks to shock treatments, the patient could see beyond her symptoms, and the psychiatrist could initiate a therapeutic relationship.

And so the terrain had been prepared, and psychotropic medications fit naturally into this model. If the neuroleptics "'realized the potential' of anything, it was psychotherapy," declared Le Guillant at the 1955 conference.[96] Psychiatrists soon realized that the effectiveness of chemical therapy varied greatly and that the overall context of its delivery played a major role. It was, in fact, the only plausible explanation for a significant proportion of failures and the extremely varied degrees of its success. The medication was incorporated into a therapeutic dynamic that was largely present before its advent, and it was promoted as a modernizing element in psychiatry. The addition of laboratories, the psychiatrist's training in related disciplines, and so on all gave psychiatry an air of medical modernity.[97]

Psychotropic medication was truly advantageous. It allowed one to diversify the therapeutic arsenal and to maximize the potential of the various therapeutic techniques by playing one off against the other. Everything seemed to anticipate a solid marriage between the two types of therapy. It only had to be determined how exactly they would interconnect. During the Lyon conference, "La relation médecin-malade au cours des chimiothérapies psychiatriques" in 1964, all agreed that there was "one positive phenomenon to be underlined ...: it is the recognition on all sides that as of now psychotherapy is a resource for all psychiatrists. We are all aware of this fact. Let us generously acknowledge that this is a recent development, and that it is good to see it given pride of place today."[98]

What other branch of medicine could boast a sophistication enabling it to manage the complex procedures involved in biological and psychological techniques, leading to remissions and often cures of such a wide range of pathologies whose causes, to boot, were unknown? Pathological humanity could be treated in its entirety. And that is what, in large part, lent psychiatry its excellent medical legitimacy. Before as after the discovery of medication for the mind, the true treatment was psychotherapy. Medication laid the groundwork, or so ran the psychiatric gospel. It was repeated over and over by all psychiatric schools at the 1950 and 1955 world conferences. It was at the core of the 1964 conference organized in Lyon on the doctor-patient relationship within a chemotherapeutic setting, as it was at that on the relationship between psychopharmacology and psychotherapies organized by the Évolution psychiatrique group the same year in Paris.

After a short period of optimism suggesting that a cure for madness had at last been found, psychiatry found itself dealing with a chronic issue. Most schizophrenics had to take their molecule for the rest of their lives in order to remain more or less stable, but these molecules had significant side effects (in particular, late-onset dyskinisia, or bodily stiffness, failing intellectual capacities, etc.). Psychiatric hospitals gradually emptied, especially after the 1968 introduction of delayed neuroleptics, which only required an injection once or twice a month. Patients were treated medically as outpatients, were supposed to see their personal physician on a regular basis in an outpatient clinic, were to receive psychotherapeutic support, and, thanks to social assistance, were to be able to live (or at least survive) outside an institution. No one questioned the fact that psychoses were genuine illnesses; this was not so with depression.

With regard to the "psychic disorders of a sane individual,"[99] the endogenous, exogenous, psychogenetic trio were what provided access to the relationship between the patient and the illness. Did pharmacology not show that it was impossible to talk about a patient without making reference to biology? On the other hand, did not efforts to explain why a molecule did or did not act on one patient or another lead doctors to get interested in the personality, in a "structure" that would account for pharmacological vagaries? Antidepressants, it was then thought, were more effective when the life force was touched by the illness, when the depression was an endogenous disorder resembling melancholia. However, this criterion was purely theoretical. How to distinguish in practise the three types of depression? How to get one's bearings when they could resemble each other, as Delay and Deniker emphasized? On what could doctors rely to make a successful diagnosis and prescribe an effective therapy? These were crucial questions for general practitioners, who were on the front lines in dealing with these disorders.

GENERAL MEDICINE: DIAGNOSTIC CHAOS

Depression is a deceptive illness. Psychoses certainly present significant diagnostic problems, but what is unique about depression is that it is both heterogeneous and universal. It is a delicate matter to assess the impact of medication on depressive states whose surface symptoms are more complex than delirium, hallucination, or agitation, and whose sufferers, who are from all walks of life, run the gamut of the asthenic, the anxious, the demoralized, the doubting, the hysterical, the obsessive, and so on. All these people come to consult a general practitioner.

If it was difficult to accurately describe the effects of neuroleptics, it was even more difficult to describe the effects of antidepressants. First, it was not clear that the medication was responsible for the remission. Often, the judgment was made in a manner described by the Swiss Paul Kielholz in 1962: "A depression, although it was not cured by electroshock or by medication X, finally lifted on the administration of medication Y, from which one may erroneously deduce that the last medication was the most active,"[100] In fact, it could have been a simple synchronicity between the end of a depressive episode and the taking of an antidepressant. Charles Brisset, in a 1965 overview of evaluation methods, judged that an evaluation involving the isolation of one aspect of behaviour "is accurate enough for general behaviour (agitation, for example)" but less adequate for more complex symptoms such as "a depressive tendency."[101] In 1970, Jonathan Cole, who, during the 1960s, was director of the pharmaceutical division at the National Institute of Mental Health and one of the most prominent American scientists in the field, was particularly harsh: "In my judgment, both the anti-anxiety agents and the antidepressant agents suffer from overpromotions. [...] On the other hand, a lot of depressions, particularly neurotic depressions, get better anyway, and severe retarded endogenous depressions did well with electric shock therapy before the antidepressant drugs ever came along. [...] On average, the superiority of these drugs over placebo is not impressive, particularly in the case of hospitalized patients with depressive illnesses."[102] If neuroleptics did not exist, he went on, they would be missed from the therapeutic arsenal; on the other hand, antidepressants could be replaced by ECT and some carefully selected barbiturates. The vagaries involved in the evaluation of pharmacological treatment soon confused depression's nosographic status. Five years after Kline's and Kuhn's communications, Kielholz painted a catastrophic picture: "At the present time the conditions surrounding pharmacological treatment are close to chaotic. The literature's data regarding improvement and cure vacillate, for imipramine for example, between 25% and 50%. For certain monoamine oxidase inhibitors, they range, even, from 0% to 65%."[103]

How to bring order into this chaos? One had to select a therapeutic strategy, prescribe the "right" antidepressant, and perhaps recommend psychotherapy or psychoanalysis. To educate the medical community meant clearly recognizing the type of depression and distinguishing it from the pathologies it resembled. The heart of psychiatric reasoning was etiological. It meant asking the following question: what is the pathology underlying the observed symptoms?

AN INCREASING DEMAND, AN EVOLVING MEDICAL FRAMEWORK

In 1960, a CREDOC (*Centre de recherche pour l'étude et l'observation des conditions de vie*) study noted that, after seasonal complaints (colds etc.) and digestive troubles, "the most important category is ... made up of a group of disorders which can seem quite unlike each other.

They include psychic disturbances, insomnia, migraines, headaches, neuralgias, and pains with no obvious cause."[104] Functional disorders accounted for 11.8 percent of pharmaceutical consumption. The authors emphasized that their methods did not allow them to distinguish between autonomous psychic disorders and those with organic origins, but they pointed out that this difficulty was also due to "the very status of medical concepts, and the diagnostic possibilities."[105]

In 1963, in the foreword to the first special issue of *La Revue du praticien*, which was devoted to depressive syndromes, Dr Laplane noted that "depressive states play an important role in medical practice, given their frequency, the risks entailed in their not being recognized, and the effectiveness of the therapies that can be proposed for them." He emphasized as well, as did all the literature of the time, that they "certainly represent a significant proportion of a general practitioner's clientele."[106] A 1965 study of private practices estimated that 80 percent of the clientele of general practitioners was made up of individuals with "functional disorders."[107] In 1966, Claude Blanc confirmed that the "vast collection of depressions and neuroses [were] treated in private practice."[108]

Private requests for treatment of psychological problems increased significantly during the 1960s. All sources are clear on this. In 1967, there were 1,600 psychiatrists in private practice: "We only know that no one is idle and that the arrival of new clientele in a doctor's office or clinic translates into rapid success."[109]

The doctors had to know at least something about clinical psychology and to possess a minimum of psychiatric knowledge. "Much remains to do," Ey asserted in 1965, "but the introduction of psychobiology into medical schools is a development of major importance."[110] Three years later, Jean Guyotat had a similar message: "As of this date, we can say that what increasingly characterizes the psychiatric movement is the ongoing infiltration of the social environment by psychiatry and psychiatric institutions."[111] He was referring, of course, to his own sector, but he was also referring to general medicine as "more than 30%" of the clientele was afflicted with problems demanding psychiatric knowledge. Psychopathological training was therefore essential. Many conferences had this question on their agenda: the 1966 World Conference of Psychiatry in Madrid, the 1967 French Language Conference of Psychiatry and Neurology in Dijon, the Symposium on Psychosomatic Medicine in Paris in

1967, the conference held by the Society of Medical Psychology in Rennes in 1968, and so on. But the lack of psychiatric training among generalists was a recurring theme; they could not get beyond their functions as "dispensers of medication," and they over-pre-scribed the tonics and stimulants that they habitually equated with tranquillizers.[112] In a study on the practice of psychiatry in France, the great majority of psychiatrists questioned insisted on the need for close collaboration with general practitioners, "but there were serious complaints concerning the generalists,"[113] who either diag-nosed neurosis too quickly and sent the patient, who had had asked for nothing and was now frightened, off to a psychiatrist, or they focused on the symptoms.

If chemical therapies made psychotherapeutic treatments neces-sary, who was to design them? Their definition "was as general as it [was] imprecise," it "range[d] from simply listening, offering good advice and an understanding attitude, to an attempt to know and master the relationship between patient and doctor."[114] What is more, the term referred to a number of different techniques whose command required training: this included not only Freudian psy-choanalysis but also Jungian analysis, waking dreams, autogenic training, relaxation, group therapy, and so on. Did general practi-tioners have to learn about all that? And, if so, how were they to do it? Because "we know that psychiatry is, in the teaching of medicine, but a minor adjunct to neurology."[115]

As of the late 1950s, hospital psychiatrists became more and more interested in psychotherapy and, above all, in psychoanalysis,[116] which began to take on greater importance in psychiatry. The impact on the psychiatric community of the 1960 Bonneval Conference on the Unconscious organized by Henri Ey, the proceedings of which were published in 1966, enhanced the appeal of psychoanalysis.[117] In 1960, no psychiatric department heads in the Paris region had analytic training; in 1965, ten out of thirty-three had this training.[118] One-third of the neuropsychiatrists in the Seine *département* were psychoanalysts: compared with the rest of France, this proportion was unique.[119] Psychoanalytical trends were "becoming more and more powerful," confirmed Ey in 1965, while group and psychoso-matic psychotherapy made parallel progress.[120] The first interna-tional conference on the training of doctors was organized by the Tavistock Clinic in London in 1962, and the second took place in Paris in 1964. According to Ey, "[they gave] us the opportunity to

widely discuss all the problems presented by the psychological training essential to doctors."[121] Pierre Pichot was elected to the first
chair of medical psychology at the Paris Faculty of Medicine. Manuals
aimed at medical students and doctors were published,[122] and they
demonstrated a variety of techniques (hypnosis, autogenic training,
etc.). The first Balint groups appeared in 1959, and the Medical
Society of Balint Groups was founded in 1967. These groups coached
doctors in establishing therapeutic relationships in daily practice.[123]
But the impact of these groups remained marginal. "Ten years ago,"
Dr Kammerer declared, "at a time when very few of us had been
analyzed, many of our most advanced colleagues had no idea what
psychotherapy was. Not the slightest idea."[124] By the end of the
1960s, psychoanalysis was a force in psychiatry, many interns were
being psychoanalyzed, and some would become leading lights of
French psychiatry.

DIFFICULT DIAGNOSIS, DELICATE THERAPY, OR A GENERALIST'S EDUCATION

The first article in *La Revue du praticien* that raised the subject of
antidepressants dates from 1958: "Psychotropic substances have
continued ... to dominate the news where therapy is concerned."
According to this article, Imipramine, which was not yet commer-
cially available in France, "acts on depressive states. However, it
neither sedates nor renders euphoric."[125] There was an astonished
reaction to the specifics of antidepressants. The medical literature
was already considerable but so was "the perplexity of clinicians."[126]
This was because articles on the therapeutic indications were rare.
But managing the diagnosis and medical prescriptions was an essential role of generalists, all the more so in that, as *La Revue du praticien*
never tired of saying, those in need constituted a large segment of
their day-to-day clientele. The key task was to properly diagnose the
underlying pathology of those "patients poorly adapted to the circumstances (professional, familial) affecting their lives."[127] According
to Perrault, the use of a molecule "must *under no circumstances* be
divorced from psychotherapy; we must *never* lose sight of the fact
that its symptomatic action on anxiety, emotional tension, or insomnia
are palliative only, and that the deeper biological or psychological
causes must be carefully researched and treated."[128] Distinguishing
the symptoms from the illness was a constant in the journal's articles.

But how to diagnose a pathology with many clinical signs and an unknown etiology, for which there would soon exist "an increasing number of drugs, as a psychiatrist already indicated in 1962, all of which [would] claim to be superior to their predecessors, with fewer and fewer toxic effects on the organism as a whole?"[129]

In fact, depression was "a diagnosis made both too often and too rarely." Too often, because general practitioners diagnosed periods of anxiety, hysterical crises, and episodes of delirium as depressive states; too rarely, because depressive states, including "the most typical, [were] described as asthenia or overwork, and the period of rest in the countryside that [was] then prescribed, disorienting the patient inappropriately, [could] lead to a tragic end."[130] And so the chaos described by Kielholz was very real, and, beginning in the 1960s, depression started to infringe upon a whole series of minor mental pathologies. Indeed, it redefined them.

The existence of an effective chemical therapy was considered "an event of considerable consequence … It [was] now widely accepted and ha[d] been … from the beginning, with a simplicity of use and record of success that satisf[ied] the most sceptical and persuade[d] the most reticent."[131] Antidepressants showed up in the category of stimulants, as new products taking their place side by side with amphetamines.[132] About ten molecules were on the market in the mid-1960s, and new substances continued to be made available. What criteria could doctors use to make their choices? Especially as they tended to confuse different types of psychotropic drugs and to have a poor grasp of the treatment methods associated with antidepressants. What might be the physical reactions to procedures, modes of application, and properties that were so varied? The doctor had to take into consideration a multiplicity of factors (social, psychological, and organic), which elicited a variety of pathological responses (anxiety, asthenia, etc.).

She should not take the place of a psychiatrist because therapy was simple only in appearance: "the symptoms [were] so personal and the traps so common."[133] The frequent occurrence of these pathologies in general medicine and the variety of symptoms, which rendered diagnosis difficult and therapy delicate – these were recurring themes. To do no harm is, let us remind ourselves, medicine's prime ethical principle. Doctors had to distinguish "melancholic depression, [which was] the classic type,"[134] and which was hereditary and recurring, from simple and/or neurotic depressions, which were reactive. A strict watch had to be kept on treatment not only because the progress of a deceptive series of symptoms had to be traced but also because the risks of suicide were great for those who were melancholic or suffering from endogenous depression.[135] The major fear of doctors was suicide because the lifting of inhibitions preceded improvements in mood. Doses had "to be carefully weighed: in serious cases, the delay in action plus some inconveniences inherent to antidepressants [could] lead them to prefer other therapies, notably electroshock treatment; in mild cases, it [was] best not to have the patient run risks not justified by the state of his health."[136] The treatment had to be administered for at least one or two months after symptoms were relieved so that the remission could be well established.

Symptoms of sadness and mental pain were at the heart of the depressive mood. "Inhibition and helplessness ... [that] amount to an overall sensation of sadness"[137] were the common denominator, "without which it [was] impossible to speak of depression."[138] These produced "a feeling that one's self [was] being devalued, which cast a shadow over all other aspects of life, with a weakening and slowing of one's train of thought and ability to act."[139] Sadness was at the root of the slowing, which, in the final analysis, was produced by it. The sadness was not to be confused with a state of anxiety, especially since the distinction between antidepressants and anxiolytics was not always understood in general medicine.[140]

When the doctor diagnosed a depressive syndrome, she had to specify what type of depression she was dealing with: melancholic-endogenous, neurotic, reactive, or symptomatic (i.e., of an organic illness).[141] Neurotic depression itself could take many forms. The only sure thing was that it was not a psychiatric entity but, rather, a "syndrome observable as much in the mentally ill, recognized or not, as in the patient who [was] normal on the surface."[142] The relationship between anxiety and depression was especially tricky to define: even if depression was not the same thing as anxiety, anxious depressions did exist. Luckily, the molecules put on the market brought into focus one distinction: some acted on anxiety in particular, while others were stimulants. By 1967, this division seemed well established.[143]

Another problem complicated the approach even more. To the degree that, thanks to psychotropic medications, the mentally ill no longer evolved naturally in two different ways (i.e., towards either chronicity or cure), a key question arose: did the medications alter one's conception of mental illness or did they modify the clinical picture to which psychiatrists had subscribed since before their invention? The symptomology shifted rapidly under the impact of the treatment,[144] and the symptoms presented often increased the confusion. The problem had arisen before, with ECT, but not at all to the same extent; there were many different medications, and not all were equally effective even within the same class. According to Delay, the "morbid examples ... seem[ed] heterogeneous."[145] How to even things out?

The use of antidepressants remained limited because prescribing them was a delicate matter. They were slow to act, and there were side effects (dryness of the mouth, memory problems, constipation, trembling, weight gain) and toxic consequences (cardio-vascular problems, sometimes fatal). Their management was complex because their dosages had to vary depending on the patient. If the medication persisted in having no effect, one had to start over with another. It is not surprising that antidepressants were little used. Between 1965 and 1970, the medical consumption of psychotropic drugs moved from ninth to fifth place thanks to the prescription of hypnotics and anxiolytics.[146]

In such a context, the medications aroused very few suspicions. A 1970 publication intended for the general public explained that, in our well-off societies, "we move from medication for the sick to medication for normal people in difficulty, then to medication that makes life easier for people in a state of normality."[147] The reader was informed of research that was trying to develop "chemical compositions free of toxicity ... [that would] be tomorrow's true medication for good living."[148] There was no questioning of whether one should be treating a weariness with life. This allusion to future remedies free of toxicity appeared just as chlorpromazine was being introduced. "My friend Henri Ey," declared Delay in 1955, "has quite properly criticized this notion of 'psychiatric aspirins,' but let me just say that aspirin is a great medicine, and that we would very much like to have available to us in psychiatry a few 'aspirins.'"[149] From a perspective that encouraged patients to take an interest in their psychic conflicts, a harmless medication that would contribute to their inner peace was good news; no one wondered if they were dealing with real illnesses. On the contrary, people were being given authorization to be psychically ill. This was one of the ways inner life entered the everyday world.

The idea of modern life was part of the same trend. It turned up in 1958, in the first article *La Revue des praticiens* devoted to antidepressants. Modern humans have "too many ambitions and they are contradictory; Western civilization is not all blessings, and even these take their toll," especially given "our states of neuropsychic discomfort." The role "of psychotropic drugs" was "to give these patients back their zest for life, which modern living and technical progress [were] constantly threatening."[150] "Modern life" did not raise any doubts in the doctor's mind as to the existence of certain pathologies. On the contrary. "Do we not see patients every day who, with or without an organic syndrome, see their lives dominated by their psychic condition?" asked a doctor at a 1962 symposium. "Depression seems to be at the helm of modern man's entire life. That fact is disturbing."[151]

The accumulation of difficulties hardly gave the generalists a chance to develop a coherent and standardized practice. To distinguish anxiety from depression; to separate out the types of depression; to link them, if need be, with a neurotic underpinning or to another psychiatric category – all that amounted to an impossible task. Endogenous depression was modelled on melancholia; the signs were the absence of an exogenous cause, a family or personal history (whether manic or depressive), a death wish manifesting itself, for example, in the feeling that one is a useless burden to others. In exogenous depressions, which were the majority, the cases were differentiated according to the presence or absence of a connection between the personality and a triggering event. When the depressive episode was linked to a triggering event, it was not a defensive psychoneurosis. Things were different when the event played an insignificant role as this meant that the cause was of psychogenic origin and that the depression was a symptom of unconscious psychic conflicts.

Between failed psychotherapies (good only for exclusively thymic disorders) and pharmacotherapies (effective for all neuroses) did not the nosographic chaos make diagnosis impossible? The magic formula for resolving this uncertainty became a therapeutic test: "In practice, it is most often the success of antidepressive therapy that will confirm doubtful cases."[152] In the end, the main consequence of antidepressants was that they showed doctors that depression was not an imaginary illness. According to Louis Bertagna, who had been responsible for the "Psychiatry" section in *La Revue du praticien* since the 1950s, "depressive illness ... ha[d] now shown its true face as a genuine illness linked to a physiological disorder and differing from other types of medical conditions only by its psychological expression."[153] In 1970, 9 million cases of neurosis and personality disorder were diagnosed.[154]

PHARMACOLOGY: AN INTEREST IN ONE'S INNER LIFE

If anyone could suffer from any kind of depression, the nuances, approximations, and contradictions were such that it was impossible to correlate one type of personality with one type of depression. From this, we draw a minimal consensus: by acting chemically on the thymic syndrome, the medication prepared the patient to face up to his psychic conflicts and thus made him the therapeutic agent for his own illness. Amidst such chaos, affective shortfall and psychic conflict mutually reinforced each other: despite the many difficulties of which we have spoken, they guaranteed that symptoms and syndromes would continue to be regarded as a set of problems associated with a sick individual. The advent of the biology of mood, and then the discovery of neuroleptics, anxiolytics, and antidepressants, was the driving force behind the new attention doctors paid to affect, feelings, and emotional life.

Depression was part of general medicine's landscape during the second half of the 1960s. During the regional medical conferences in 1972, which were devoted to depressive states, several speakers called attention to the increase in the use of the term "depression." This increase occurred for two reasons: (1) to broaden the diagnosis itself and (2) to reassure the patient's family, to avoid stigmatizing the psychotic patient with medical certificates destined for her employer, and/or to avoid confronting her too brutally with a diagnosis of schizophrenia. As Porot commented: "The public, the doctors and, their hands forced, the psychiatrists [were] being led to name as depressions an excessive number of psychic disturbances, the majority of which [did] not fall into the category of depressive states."[155] Depression was a socially acceptable disorder; however, in being so, it lost its medical meaning.[156] It became a semantic attractor.

During the 1960s, there emerged a language that facilitated the formulation of an appeal for care. Mass-market magazines and books of popular psychology, as we shall see, spread the word. They created

a social environment within which was inculcated a popular phrase-
ology that each individual could appropriate at his or her leisure:
just how the individual appropriated it was another problem. These
magazines and books attached *commonly held* descriptions to what
each individual was liable personally, indistinctly, to feel within herself. This carved out a social space for inner life, creating a language
proper to the psyche. To heal, including with the help of a molecule,
the patient had to cultivate an interest in her inner self. She could
not be reduced to her illness; rather, she had to be the subject of
her conflicts.

The difficulty in associating depression with one category or
another was at the core of the diagnostic uncertainty. Depression's
deceptive nature, resulting from a combination of heterogeneity
and universality, was what allowed it to thrive. The impossibility of
defining it led to the piling on of depressive syndromes, to disman-
tling the old to add on the new. This sea change in psychology would
have considerable practical consequences, reshaping the idea of the
individual – a process already begun, quietly, with the concept of
well-being, with mass consumption and social mobility. By introducing modern life's vicissitudes into medical care and making medicine
cognizant of them, we initiated a process that, in the end, produced
a social language expressly designed to translate inner life. It contributed to the socialization of the psyche. At the same time, it trig-
gered the "psychologizing" of society. The disciplinary frameworks
and taboos that had provided a structure for the individual began
to crumble.

PART TWO

The Twilight of Neurosis

I could no longer submit to Fate. My wish was not to be good, in the way of our tradition but to make good. But how? What did I have to offer? ... This anxiety began to eat away at me.

V.S. Naipaul, *A Bend in the River*, 1989.

Sexual liberation has replaced the fear of sin with a desire for normality.

Augustin Jeanneau, "Les risques d'une époque ou le narcissisme du dehors," 1986

THE CRISIS OF NEUROTIC DEPRESSION: A SHIFT IN THE ROLE OF THE SELF

We could, at the end of the 1960s, reasonably divide depression into three groups: endogenous depression, neurotic depression,[1] and reactive depression (which is necessarily exogenous). Endogenous depression had deep somatic roots and its mechanisms were biological in that they affected sensations, feelings, and emotions (i.e., subjective and psychic experience). Neurotic depression was the most involved with the idea of personality, and it was the one that came closest to being a *psycho*pathological disorder. Reactive depression emphasized the influence of external circumstances, and it could affect the healthiest and the most stable among us.

If the role of antidepressants in treatment remained controversial, there was no doubt, during the period at which we have been looking, that psychotherapy was the preferred therapeutic choice. Whatever its limits, the categories of neuroses and of melancholia

set the standard for depressive syndromes. Delay referred to Janet
when he identified the types of effects induced by psychotropic
medications; Freud, because he also furnished insights into
the psychogenesis of psychoses, was the authority when people,
from Lacan to Guiraud, attempted to define psychotherapies.
However, there was such difference of opinion over what types
of depression to include and what were to be their nosological
boundaries that the result was an impasse – an impasse that was
reflected in classificatory disarray and in what was actually being
prescribed by general practitioners.

Depression was a crossover entity: all the professionals agreed
on this, whatever their orientation. In 1980, during the final
address at a European conference on depression, Pierre Pichot,
who was, with Pierre Deniker, Sainte-Anne's most prestigious
representative, declared: "We find ourselves facing the question
of the possible subdivisions for a class that is both unique, given
its shared bases, and multiple, given the ways in which it mani-
fests itself, the conditions for its appearance, and its mechanisms."[2] We have just seen that it was difficult to establish criteria
that clearly differentiated, on the one hand, endogenous from
exogenous depressions, and, on the other hand, the different
types of exogenous depression. Was there any way out of this
diagnostic chaos that general practitioners had to navigate as
best they could?

In the discussions on etiology, diagnosis, and the therapeutic
effectiveness of a particular approach or product, the weakest
and the most diagnosed group was neurotic depression. Neurosis
was the key word here: the intrapsychic conflict manifested itself
through depressive symptoms, and it was that conflict that the
therapy aimed to treat. In this pathological class, the notions of
self and conflict overlapped to the point where they were one
and the same: a self was the self of its conflicts.

Psychiatry came up with two important classificatory solutions
to make diagnoses a bit more coherent. Each one contributed in
a totally different way to the decline of neurosis as an expression
of psychic conflict.

The first solution was proposed by psychiatrists with a psychoanalytic bias. They emphasized the idea of a depressive personality. For them, the depressive syndrome was neither psychotic nor
neurotic; rather, it was a "borderline state." The neurotic was a

conflicted individual, for she was "the one who manifest[ed] the unconscious conflict."3 The "depressive personality," on the other hand, was unable to bring her conflicts to light, to give them form; she felt empty, fragile, and had a hard time dealing with frustrations. This led her to addictive behaviours and to seek out sensations. In psychoanalytic language, we could say that the personality in question found itself less in a conflictual state than in what we might call a split state, characterized by a sort of inner tearing apart, where the elements were neither in conflict with nor in relation to one another. The individual was overwhelmed by a feeling of inadequacy. Here we had a shift in the self's representation: the private rift became an inner gulf.

Thanks to a "neo-Kraepelinian" model, the second classificatory solution did away with the idea of personality and the clinical competence of the psychiatrist. Since psychiatrists could not agree on causes, and therefore on the illnesses underlying syndromes, they just had to remove symptomatology from the etiological problem. That is, they had to remove it from the question: what underlying pathology is associated with a series of symptoms? Technically, the procedure involved the development of *standardized* diagnostic criteria that clearly described the syndromes and, thereby, acted as reliable guides for diagnosis. This solution was developed in the United States, where the face of psychiatry was largely transformed with the release of a document representing the second psychiatric revolution: the third edition of the *Diagnostic and Statistical Manual of Mental Disorders*. In professional jargon, this document is referred to as the DSM-III. The biological, the psychic, and the social formed a key triad in the new psychiatric mainstream that emerged in the course of the 1970s. We had entered the age that psychiatry refers to as "biopsychosocio."

These two solutions confirmed the divorce between the deficit model and the conflict model. In medical terms, the individual experiencing a deficit was first and foremost the object of his illness, in the sense that he was defined by his suffering from something (never mind if it was a lack of mother love going back to early childhood or an insufficient level of serotonin). The depressed individual hardly needed to face his conflicts because he had a pathology from which he could be freed, thanks to the doctor who is the agent in Janet's medical model.

In psychoanalytic terms, he was not capable of being the agent of his conflicts, of being an active agent who could picture his conflicts and so be better armed to recover "the freedom to decide this or that,"4 as Freud said in talking of a cure. Part 2 traces the decline in references to conflict and guilt in favour of figures who focused on references to deficit and well-being.

This transformation of the idea of depression took place in the context of a normative change that became obvious during the 1960s. In fact, the traditional guidelines for structuring individual behaviour were no longer accepted, and the right to choose the life one wanted to live began, if not to be the norm for the relationship between the individual and society, at least to become part of everyday life. The relationship between public and private changed drastically; the former became an extension of the latter. In place of discipline and obedience, there was the shoring up of the self; instead of imposed limits and a destiny to which one must adapt, there was the idea that everything was possible; instead of traditional bourgeois guilt and the struggle to free oneself from the law of the father (Oedipus), there was the fear of not measuring up and its ensuing emptiness and impotence (Narcissus). The portrait of the self was considerably altered; it now meant being fully oneself, Nietzsche's sovereign individual. From the moment *everything was possible*, illnesses of inadequacy provoked ruptures in the individual to remind her that *not everything was allowed*.

At the crossroads between psychopathological discussions and these normative changes, depression positioned itself as the obverse of a certain self-image. It associated classic melancholia with the egalitarian passion of democratic times, when, in the notorious words of Andy Warhol, everyone would be famous for fifteen minutes. Depression was the drama of a new normality that was at the same time a new prescriptivism (chapter 4).

On the medical front (chapter 5), data now pointed to the increased insistence that a range of personal problems be addressed by general medicine. At the same time, the psychiatric expertise on which this medicine might rely was offering practical solutions to deal with the diagnostic chaos. This expertise emphasized the effectiveness of the deficit model. Depression abandoned all attempts to unearth an underlying pathology. Why force patients to face up to their conflicts when medical

assistance can compensate for feelings of inadequacy? The crossroads phenomenon became a catch-all. At the same time, the
therapeutic status of psychotropic medications began to be questioned: were we drugging people or really treating them? The
disconnect between the two models of illness, along with the
erosion of the regulating functions of the forbidden, led to a
questioning of the boundary between the normal and the pathological. The land of the permissible would be subordinated to
the land of the possible.

4

The Psychological Front:
Guilt without an Instruction Manual

During an international conference on depression held in October 1970 in New York, Heinz Lehmann proposed a percentage and a number that would be picked up and repeated for a long time to come: the prevalence of depression at any one moment represented 3 percent of the western population, meaning 100 million people were suffering from it.[5] It had become the most widespread mental pathology on the planet.[6] The Swiss Paul Kielholz, director of the psychiatric clinic in Bâle, after having organized two conferences at Saint-Moritz in 1972 and 1973, respectively, founded, in 1975, the International Committee for the Treatment and Prevention of Depression, with the aim of training general practitioners. The medical press widely referred to depression as a fad. According to Reigner: "The visibility granted by non-medical media to the 'depressive phenomenon,' the relative ease with which patients talk about 'their depression' or that of someone close to them, leaves the impression that we are dealing with a fad ... The arguments advanced to make its case throw stardom, overextension, drug taking (and sometimes depression wrongly considered as a consequence thereof) all in together, more often than not on the front pages. There can be no doubt that the word depression itself is being bandied about irresponsibly."[7] The idea had taken off. It cropped up as much in psychiatric publications as in general medicine. "And so civilization is particularly depressing," wrote Dr Ragot in 1977, in the most venerable French psychiatric journal, the *Annales médicopsychologiques*.[8] The psychoanalytic journals also picked up on the depressive theme: "If depression has attained the status of the illness of the day," pointed out the psychiatrist-psychoanalyst Jean Bergeret in 1976, "we must recognize that it is in part the consequence of a collective consensus to devalue Oedipus."[9]

PSYCHIC LIBERATION AND IDENTITY INSECURITY

Depression "may be found along the entire length of a trajectory running from medical folklore to death. At one end ... depression 'of all flavours,' confounding the unpleasant with the depressing, and swallowing whole the myth of the depressed individual whom we must reinflate like an old tire. At the other end, the event that lends meaning to a man's life; in other words, death."[10] That is an excellent summing up, by a psychiatrist in 1973, of the astonishing situation in which depression found itself at that time. With its multiple guises, from the truth at the core of human existence to a minor, everyday despondency, depression seemed to cover a spectrum wider even than that covered by neurasthenia a century earlier.

How was it that depression assumed all these flavours? What was this devaluation of Oedipus that favoured the explosion of depressive disorders? Why was civilization depressing? Did the times no longer find optimism appealing? Had not the conditions bearing on private life and intimacy improved over the years? Had not the right to live the life one chose begun to receive the respect it deserved?

The dawning age boasted a dynamic whose two faces were *psychic liberation* and *identity insecurity*. Centre stage, the emancipation of the masses was in full swing; the media, as of the 1960s, lavished enormous attention on private lives, while the techniques that, in 1966, American sociologist Philip Rieff called "therapies of liberation,"[11] claimed to offer every individual the practical tools to fashion his or her identity, free of all constraints. In the wings (those of psychopathology), new controversies cropped up in France; they pointed to a newly emerging, widespread insecurity vis-à-vis one's identity. The most frequent clinical manifestation of this was a depressive void compensated for by addiction. Did the passion for being oneself, encouraged by the new norms, have as its dark side a marriage between addiction and depression? Between the two poles of apathy and stimulation two large pathological territories were emerging.

Neither Mad Nor Lazy: Inner Life Is Not Psychology's Business

Just as depression was infiltrating general medicine and everyday life, French society was undergoing a radical transformation: it was freeing itself from the world of notables and peasants and of an unalterable destiny imposed by class. Economic growth; the development of social programs; reforms in the educational system (the end of the separation between primary and secondary paving the way, in principle, for children from the working class to pursue their education to the end of high school); new opportunities to rise in the social scale; changes in the family; housing and recreational policies that lessened crowding and allowed more space for one's private life – all this contributed to a shift in how the relationship between the individual and society was viewed. Improvements in living conditions made well-being not just a distant aspiration but, rather, something within reach of the working class. If, in the past, comfort was something to be achieved, perhaps, at the end of one's life, "young couples ... [could] start out with a guaranteed economic status that it took their parents an entire lifetime to attain."[12] There was a democratization of the idea that anyone could make her way; mass humanity was on the move. The result was a different set of confusions.

EPIDEMIOLOGY: A PATHOLOGY OF CHANGE

Epidemiology teaches us that depression insinuated its way into our societies as a pathology of change and not as a pathology of economic and social difficulty; it accompanied the transformations affecting most of our institutions after the Second World War. It was the child of abundance, not an economic crisis. Depression took wing during the thirty years of prosperity following the war, during a period of economic progress, of growing well-being, and widespread optimism. Its prevalence, its scope, and its effect on the population's state of health turned it into a public health problem.

In 1967, an expert from the World Health Organization estimated, based on the first studies conducted on the general population, that the frequency rate of mental disorders had almost doubled in fifteen years.[13] An epidemiological synthesis published in 1975 by the head of the mental illness division of the same organization adopted the figure of 100 million and asserted that it would get larger for four reasons: (1) the increase in life expectancy would make for more depressions (given the illnesses associated with aging); (2) the constant change in the psychosocial environment would cause stress that could result in depression (e.g., disintegration of the family, solitude, etc.); (3) cardiovascular, cerebrovascular, and/or gastrointestinal diseases, themselves on the increase, bring on depressive reactions in one case out of five; and (4) the number of medications that generate depressions was growing (hypotensors, hormones, and/or oral contraceptives).[14]

According to the American Medical Association, which in 1989 published a synthesis of epidemiological studies based on representative samples of the general population,[15] the increased risk of undergoing a depression among people born after the Second World War was indisputable. Not only were all age ranges affected, the frequency being somewhat greater for men than for women,[16] but adolescents and young adults, relatively untouched up to that point, were now vulnerable as well. Correlations were established with alcoholism and drug abuse; a rise in the rate of suicide, especially where young whites were concerned; and homicides, especially involving young blacks. This despite the fact that individuals born after 1945 not only enjoyed the best physical health in modern history but also were raised in a period of unprecedented prosperity. Urbanization, geographical mobility (with its consequent emotional ruptures), the increase in social anomie, changes in family structure, and the weakening of traditional sexual roles all contributed to the rising incidence of depression in our societies. Following this 1989 synthesis, working groups were set up in order to minimize bias and to check the compatibility of the various studies undertaken in several countries. Their conclusions matched. They confirmed the assessments made of depression's incidence since the Second World War and "found a threefold increase in the rate of first-onset major depression in the most recent birth cohort (<40 years of age) as compared with older birth cohorts."[17]

Do such figures suggest an increased occurrence of this pathology? A tendency to consult a doctor more frequently for a psychological problem? A change in diagnostic practices? The most constant factor in these epidemiological analyses and statistics was the emphasis on social change.

THE LANGUAGE OF A NEW SELF-AWARENESS

Two simultaneous developments accompanied the postwar improvement in living conditions: (1) social opportunities for the poor and
(2) a new awareness of self, with language derived from magazines
and books devoted to popular psychology. This new self-awareness
evolved because the hierarchical conception of life was fading away,
especially in the family, where institutional roles (being a mother, a
spouse, etc.) were being replaced by a desire for individual fulfillment and new roles, especially among children. The compulsion to
obey moral or religious principles was weakening steadily and was
being supplanted by models offering interpretive tools for resolving
or surmounting personal problems. The media absolved their readers of any guilt (you have the right to feel psychologically bad) and
facilitated the emergence of a demand by providing the words to
formulate it. They created a public space that gave shape to psychic
reality, and they devised a style for mass psychology. For the inner
life was not in the heads of people who invented its language on
their own; rather, it was in the world and in us at the same time. It
required individuals who formulated shared concepts that everyone
could understand and make their own and that would express what
they felt inside. Without institutions dedicated to the inner life there
would not, socially speaking, *be* an inner life. The inner life was the
product of an act of collective creation, which provided a social
context within which it might reside. There was a change in the
perception of what was personal. It had become not only the domain
of what was secret, of one's self-sufficiency or freedom of conscience,
but also that which allowed one to *free oneself from one's destiny* and
to choose one's own life. Conformity to a single norm gradually gave
way to a range of values and different ways of life.

If depression appeared in psychiatric literature and in general
medical literature in the guise of sadness and mental distress, with
other symptoms flowing from these,[18] it appeared in the large circulation magazines in the guise of anxiety, insomnia, and overwork.
Fatigue, in its two-pronged relationship with modern life and the
individual's psychological difficulties, was a popular topic for the
opinion media. And it was through them that the language of
depression made its way into French society.

There existed a venerable tradition of advice-giving in the popular
almanacs and the feminine press. It had three main features: (1) its

language was authoritative (a guide to good behaviour knew what it had to teach to an ignorant reader); (2) its style was prescriptive (here is your problem and this is what you have to do); and (3) it presented a vision of life that posited a collective destiny to which one had to adapt whatever happened (i.e., the reader was asked to play an institutional role [e.g., to be a good mother, a good wife, etc.] and not to throw it over if the wish to do so should arise). This ordering of private life did not encourage the individual to ask questions; what was important was to preserve the stability of family life for it was through doing one's duty that one found happiness. The times still called for discipline in the household.

Marcelle Auclair, the columnist for *Marie Claire*, wielded this rhetoric masterfully. In a February 1963 article on "the abuse of tranquillizers," she wrote: "These days, 'to listen to oneself' is no longer a flaw, it is not even a foible. We delight in listening to ourselves, and ... the least of our revulsions, like the least of our enthusiasms, is sacrosanct ... The idea of 'getting a hold on ourselves' rather than 'listening to ourselves' occurs to us no more than if we were canaries or monkeys, rather than thinking individuals." This cast of mind led straight to the consumption of tranquillizers, which represented, "and I weigh my words carefully, cowardice vis-à-vis oneself and life."[19] Here we had a moral issue involving error and guilt; it was less a question of understanding what was happening within oneself in order to resolve one's difficulties than of getting a hold of oneself and moving on. In October 1963, in an article devoted to seaside cures to help deal with "modern life[,] which is weighing us down," she did recognize that, on occasion, "however we may 'take things upon ourselves,' we need help from the outside." But this consisted primarily in halting work for a short time, in avoiding being overtaxed in order to find oneself: "One must not throw oneself into the arms of psychiatrists; before taking such a radical step, one must ... tap all the resources that nature offers us."[20] This traditional view of succor for the soul left little room for attending to one's inner life.

In 1970, in the same magazine, Menie Grégoire used very different language. She explained to her readership that a woman's equilibrium derived from "the good relations she maintains with herself and her surroundings." Not only psychoanalysis but also psychodrama and group therapy allowed an individual to relive the situations that first structured her relations with herself and others:

"One then discovers, as though seen from outside, one's own reactions along with those of others. One emerges little by little from oneself and one's secret prisons. By trial and error one establishes other relations, and one sees one's life change."[21] The rhetoric of destiny, already very marginal in *Elle* at the beginning of the 1960s, declined visibly over the decade; a discourse of inner life, in which everything was a relationship between self and self or the self and another, and that invited the reader to question his or her psychic conflicts, gradually gained the upper hand. By creating a public space that gave form and meaning to the difficulties of private life, the media contributed to the socialization of the psyche.

A POPULAR GRAMMAR FOR THE INNER LIFE

Dr O.P. wrote the column "Docteur, répondez-moi" ("Doctor, Answer Me") in *Elle*.[22] " Doctors have only recently acknowledged the crucial role of the 'psychic,' and have admitted ... that it is important to pay attention to the patient's life, to his past, his personality, his activities, his concerns, his difficulties."[23] Because the psychic life was everywhere, it caused innumerable organic problems (gynaecological, dermatological, etc.). Depression, "the price to be paid for a hectic life," appeared a little later, in 1957, but it "ha[d] nothing in common with mental illness" and it was "curable." It could strike "the healthiest and the most balanced of individuals." Nor did it derive from weakness of character ("Depression is not an illness of the lazy").[24] However, if they were to be treated, the depressed still had to admit they were ill.[25]

In 1960, Marianne Kohler, a journalist, took over the column, and the number of articles increased significantly. Six issues were devoted to a large-scale investigation of anxiety,[26] an investigation that was to "answer[] all the questions [people were] asking [themselves] about this strange illness, this 'cancer of the soul.'" The author told the story of her journey through the tunnel, her ruminations, her insomnia, her consultations with doctors, her consumption of stimulants and tranquillizers. A medical psychoanalyst diagnosed hysteria ("that rather annoyed me") and taught her what was most important: "the cure is in yourself." "To overcome this solitary suffering, each of those who are afflicted by it can draw on the experience of all the others." The articles on self-control, physical exercise to combat depression, and ways of recovering in the wake of violent emotion were followed by a long succession of practical suggestions for insomniacs, the depressed, and the "ultra-nervous."[27]

The first "in-depth" article on depression was published in *Elle* in 1965:[28] "Nervous depression attacks all segments of society, the industrious, the lazy, the poor, the rich." Fatigue was *the* initial sign of depression: it made one irritable or drove one to shrink into oneself, and one could not recognize it on one's own. It could take hold from one day to the other or arrive "on the tips of its toes"; the depressed person had, above all, to listen to her doctor ("someone who speaks her language and who, manouevring gently, weans her from her obsessions"). "The ideal would be to pay a visit twice a year to one's psychiatrist, as one has become accustomed to doing with one's dentist." The language was doubly reassuring: psychic suffering was not mental illness; fatigue was neither laziness nor weakness of character but an illness. As of 1966, the articles multiplied.[29] Most important, however, in February and March of that same year, the magazine devoted five weeks to a pre-publication presentation of Pierre Daninos's *Le 36ᵉ dessous*. Its immense success owed much to the author's status as a famous humorist ("Nervous depression as recounted by our number one humorist writer"). After suffering many tribulations, he was so helped by an antidepressant that he ended up feeling like the master of the world. "A constant stream of letters from the depressed" arrived at *L'Express* to ask Daninos' advice. Doctors also wrote to the magazine: "Psychiatrists are recommending the book's purchase to their patients, and are going so far as to advocate their reimbursement by the National Health."[30] A few years later, in 1972, Jacqueline Michel had a big commercial success with *La Déprime*. After seven years of bouncing from doctor to doctor, she regained her appetite for life thanks to an antidepressant: "It is happiness, upper case, vibrant, permanent. Your work! [She is in conversation with her psychiatrist.] Needless to say, I am spreading the gospel of the blue pill."[31] *Elle* spoke of antidepressants for the first time in 1965, but the portrait it painted encouraged no one to request them.[32]

A collective volume on the relationship between stress, fatigue, and depression was published in 1974. It gave a panoramic view of the many connections between these three evils of modern humanity.[33] The authors noted that asthenia was present both in current neuroses and in defensive psychoneuroses. In this second category, "neurosis is not an expression of psychological weakness, but of the strength of one's urges and their conflicts."[34] Alvin Toffler's *Future Shock*, published in the United States in 1970 and in France one year later, was a global success. It portrays a society in which malleability, the feeling that everything is temporary, and a surplus of choices would risk inducing an overall fatigue whose principal consequence would be depression.[35] There was a constant reference to themes of individual performance and continual change. Several writers raised the subject of change, as much at the regional meetings on depression in 1972 as at the international conference on masked depression organized by Paul Kielholz in 1973.[36] In January 1981, *L'Express* devoted its cover to stress. In the magazine, a doctor who had just published a book in collaboration with the concept's inventor, Hans Selye, declared: "The increasingly rapid pace of change requires us to constantly accelerate this adaptive process. To survive, twentieth-century man must adapt to a society in a permanent state of flux, where everything is changing before his eyes … Out of ten patients who come to see me, seven show symptoms that are the direct consequence of this plague … Stress is of psychological origin."[37] And depression, of course, was one of its primary manifestations, resulting from the weakening of the immune system's defences.

According to a 1965 issue of *Elle*, fatigue was "our response to things." This was a recurring theme: four years later, in *L'Express*, a doctor responsible for fatigue counselling at Sainte-Anne declared, "Fatigue is a refusal to see inside oneself."[38] "The problem of fatigue is also a personal problem," added *Marie-Claire* in 1976. That is why the magazine advised taking one's life into one's own hands.[39] In 1969, *L'Express* published a series of reports on modern life. Pierre Deniker commented laconically: "The bar has been raised."[40] Overall, magazines were very cautious where medication was concerned and, for the most part, advised their readers to take an interest in their personal lives and to reflect on their psychic conflicts.[41] Magazines tended to absolve their readers of guilt where their private problems were concerned by emphasizing that these difficulties were to be expected in a hectic society. If there was no question of either madness or weakness, then what could be more legitimate than to take an interest in what was going on inside oneself, especially since many everyday evils (fatigue, back pains) could be explained by mental processes? Being able to detect the early signs of depression in oneself and one's intimates, and taking an interest in one's psychic conflicts: these were the two main thrusts of the media's teachings. Bodily pain appeared more and more to be an extension of inner disorders whose source was in the psyche.

Translations of American books shot through with psychotherapy, a sea change in the rhetoric of advice columns, increased attention to these questions on the radio: all of this created public space for a language attuned to the inner life.[42] Menie Grégoire's program on Radio Télévision Luxembourg in 1967, *Chère Ménie*, was the first notable example (followed closely by Dr X, with Françoise Dolto, a well known psychoanalyst, on Europe 1). The media introduced the questions pertaining to the inner life into everyone's daily lives. The extraordinary impact of *Chère Menie* and the polemics that followed in its wake, along with the profusion of competitors and the adoption of a similar style in the written media and on the radio, brought into play, from one day to the next, a new type of intimate language: you are not alone with your private problem (whether it be insomnia or a personal relationship) as it is shared by all.

In traditional advice literature, the question imagined by the reader was, "What should I do?" The answer never changed: "Live up to your obligations and you will achieve happiness." The new rhetoric opened the door to other questions. You could no longer reply to the question, "What should I do?" without asking, "Who am I?" The answer now took on a different complexion: conform to your desires and you will achieve happiness. Self-esteem was the clear goal of this advice, and a grammar of the inner life was now within reach of the masses. This grammar provided a housewife, however ignorant she may have been of the unconscious, with introspective tools that equipped her to take an interest in her private life. And she allowed herself to do so because people like her were expressing themselves openly. The media lessened the shame or guilt that one might feel in talking about one's personal problems (depression can strike those in the best of health). It bestowed social legitimacy, and people felt reassured.[43] We were witnessing the increasing prevalence of a type of self for which the right to a freely chosen private life was considered normal. The crux of this was one's relation to oneself (do not shrink from confronting your conflicts, the remedy is in you, etc.) or to another. Inner peace became the mainstay of an immense, eclectic marketplace, and self-esteem gave rise to a relational service industry with its own language (advice to the careworn); its own technologies (medicinal, psychological); its professions (sexologists, group therapists); and its own literature.

And so a large number of everyday vicissitudes gained admittance to the terrain of psychiatry and clinical psychology. Mental disorder was no longer associated primarily with madness but, rather, included a variety of more commonplace problems. Medicine, like the media, encouraged people to seek treatment ("One had to take seriously an illness that caused so much damage").[44] The widening view of what was pathological facilitated the incursion of private life into public space and heralded the beginning of its institutionalization: the intimate zone was no longer a private affair.

CHOOSING ONE'S LIFE

The 1970s was a transitional period during the course of which the idea that every individual was responsible for her own life began sociologically to make its mark. Mass humanity was becoming its own sovereign. Its horizon was each individual's self-management of her/his own life. The notion of taboo was in decline. The normative changes introduced in the 1960s were making their way into everyday life.[45] We were witnessing a retreat from the picture that set the individual up against her society, that depicted the individual as someone who had to be hemmed in by disciplinary norms in order to socialize her and to protect society from her excesses. In France, May 1968 was a symbolic reference point. It accelerated the moral dynamic at work in French society and brought it into the political debate. It became the focus of conflicts in the public arena through social movements whose demands had serious implications for moral standards: equal rights for men and women, the right to abortion, divorce by mutual consent, the acknowledgment of common law relationships, the right to contraception. The Neuwirth law on the "pill" was passed in 1967. One demanded, in the streets if necessary, individual freedoms that became the focal point for clashes between left and right and that were debated in Parliament (before being exposed to public view a few years later on television shows). There entered into the controversy and into the political arguments a way of looking at one's private-sphere rights in terms of individual choice. On the left, the very idea of law was likened to a kind of domination from which it was crucial to free oneself.[46]

Neitzsche's sovereign man, his own man, was becoming a mass phenomenon: there was nothing above him that could tell him who he ought to be because he was the sole owner of himself. Moral pluralism with no compliance to a single norm, the freedom to make one's own rules rather than having them imposed: the development of one's self became, collectively, a personal affair that society had to endorse. A type of self, less disciplined and conforming than "psychic," and enjoined to figure itself out on its own, was now legion.

"Psychological Culture": A Way of Fighting against Depression?

A new therapeutic style, of American origin, spread into France and seemed rich with promise; it promoted inner well-being through the lessening of external constraints and linked the idea of taboo to social repression. In 1976, a psychiatrist noted: "Perhaps discussions that tend to *deny* the unhealthy nature of certain psychic states are nourished by the desire no longer to speak of 'pathology' and individual deficiencies, but to shift the responsibility onto society."[47] All this found expression in the popularization of therapies designed to free the individual from these constraints. The overwhelming question was: how does one find a cure for social constraints and become wholly oneself?

In 1966, the American sociologist Philip Rieff, in a book that caused something of a sensation, identified this phenomenon as the triumph of therapy. He proclaimed the coming of "psychological man," who was characterized by a decline in renunciation. The great disciples of Freud, Jung, and Reich, in particular, promoted a "releasing" therapy. The post-Freudian therapeutic era proclaimed "the cultural defeat of the Superego,"[48] the garrison installed in every psyche to instill, as Freud contended, a feeling of guilt. For Rieff, the post-Freudian age embodied the "revolt of the private man against all doctrinal traditions urging the salvation of self through identification with the purposes of community."[49] "Anxious to increase ... psychological capital,"[50] post-Freudian therapies brought to light a massive process of deconversion in our societies, which were "now committed, culturally as well as economically, to the gospel of self-fulfillment."[51] The 1980s literature on individualism was content to recycle this dual motif of the privatization of existence and the personal realization for which it became the dogma, the authors differing only in their positive or negative appreciation of these changes.

The social mission of therapy was to embed in its practices the idea that society was a means to pursuing individual ends. The leading lights of these practices stood behind their emancipatory views: there was nothing to be expected or learned from psychic conflict. It was not a matter of negotiating a quid pro quo within the realm of what was forbidden but, rather, of freeing oneself from it in real terms: how was one to live a full life? The new therapies provided, via group relationships, normative substitutions.[52] The idea was to live, on the one hand, on one's own terms and, on the other, through the ongoing quest for the approval of others.

THE GOSPELS OF RELATIONSHIP

During the 1970s, the world of psychotherapy was being turned upside down. First, the American group therapy techniques spread far and wide, most prominently Arthur Janov's primal scream, Alexander Lowen's bioenergetics, and the human potential movements. By the 1980s, the New Age groups were carrying the flame. Their goals? To achieve an inner well-being that would facilitate relations with others. Then religious revival, both Protestant and Roman Catholic, began to take hold. The old tradition of healing through religion was revived, including in its fold the psychological difficulties of modern humanity. Its aims? To achieve personal fulfillment by imbuing God and religion with the psychotherapeutic. Now religion answered to earthly demands and God was the end point of self-realization, with a psychotherapeutic Jesus as mediator. In both instances the technique for healing relied on a goal that was diametrically opposed to the idea of a conflicted self: how to multiply the capacities for well-being of individuals who, if they were not finding life difficult, were at least seeking to lead lives of more "authentic" fullness. This constituted a logistics for the emancipated individual as its aim was not to make tolerable what was forbidden at a reduced psychic cost but, rather, to do away with all suffering. A guilt-inducing education, allied with society's repression of feeling, was what underlay pathologies. Therapy targeted one's emotions via a therapeutic treatment of the body; it was in rediscovering the animal sensations that reside in humanity that the individual discovered herself to be truly human. The essential took place in a realm beyond words – in feeling, in culture, in the body's return to nature. In other words, this psychotherapeutic paradigm was based on a conception of the human being as an animal. Its affinities were with the biological psychiatry that was coming into its own at the same time.[53]

The Primal Scream was published in 1970 in the United States, where it had an enormous success, and was translated into French in 1975.[54] For Janov, the pain of neurosis was pathological rather than a product of civilization. It resulted from social repression, which prevented individuals from adequately fulfilling themselves. It burdened them with all sorts of taboos that prevented them from discovering their "true selves." The cure took place in a group setting, and its method consisted in reliving primitive experiences through techniques that enabled patients to regress and to express themselves – that is, to express their (suppressed) hatred for their parents, their despair, or their frustrations. To go back to the beginning not through words but through the body, to release buried emotions: this was how to purge the pain, to bring to the surface those energies stifled by education and social taboos, and to profit fully (i.e., with no restrictions) from life. The three curative steps were: (1) to vent the negative, (2) to affirm the positive, and (3) to demand or impose what the true self desired. In 1973, a medical psychiatrist who had converted to Janov's method explained to *Elle* that, "for Janov, every frustration counts, from the first bottle our mother refused us, from the first day we cried so she would take us in her arms." This therapy propagated a message of love: "When we discover within ourselves the possibility of freely expressing this love, we can take pleasure in ourselves and others. We regain our zest for life. We are cured. We have nothing to seek beyond that."[55] The Christian message was rendered entirely secular. It was emptied of all theology and replaced by a gospel of relationships.

Alexander Lowen, the promoter of bioenergetics, was a disciple of Wilhelm Reich. He published a book on depression and the body, which was translated into French in 1975.[56] Bioenergetics, like primal scream, was a group technique that acted on feelings and the body. It was designed to help the individual to better express her emotions and sensations; a discharge of energy, stifled by civilization, was the focus of the therapy. For Lowen, as for Janov, everything passed through feeling and the body for it was there, and not in the realm of reason, that authentic human spirituality resided:

"True spirituality has a physical or biological basis ... Faith is rooted in the deep biological processes of the body." This approach sought the roots of spirituality in our bodily nature; it was a kind of mystic biology.57 The goal of the cure was to help individuals to rediscover a faith in themselves that was analogous to that which a Christian found in God. It was, essentially, a process of secularization. Faith in oneself, confidence vis-à-vis others and a newly meaningful life – this is what each person could find within herself. "People don't get depressed when they are the loving ones," Lowen went on: "Through love you express yourself and affirm your being and identity."58

The birth of the Charismatic Renewal Movement in France at the beginning of the 1970s was part of the same dynamic. However diverse its groups and their options – more religious and primarily concerned with the salvation of souls or more secular and primarily concerned with the healing of its members – their psychotherapeutic dimension was always important and sometimes central. For example, beginning in 1977, the Béatitudes community proposed "psycho-spiritual gatherings" in a monastery where techniques such as Binswanger's existential psychiatry, or neuro-linguistic programming, were used "in an approach that is both therapeutic (healing) and religious (salvation)."59 In these groups, the religious was constantly being penetrated by the therapeutic.60 One of the Charismatic Renewal Movement's touchstones, as with the New Age therapies, was that transformation of the individual was a vehicle for the transformation of society.

What were these groups' clienteles seeking? According to a study conducted at the end of the 1970s on bioenergetics sessions, "one of the major elements involved in the participants' demands is related to the present; a present made up of experiences and emotions, of the investment of feelings on a 'relational' level, independent of social roles ... Above all, it is a matter of becoming independent of the constraints weighing on personal relationships, so as to experience these in an authentic manner."61 The author of the preceding quote shows that the group, as such, attracted a clientele that felt psychologically alone and that it "offer[ed] an experimental framework with no taboos; they [could] try things out, put their desires to the test, live relationships in keeping with their emotional investments."62 It is through the group that each person could discover his own individuality – his "true self." The group provided the practical support of the validation of oneself by others. It showed one how to proceed.

This therapeutic religiosity was centred on the body, propagated a message of love, and saw healing as a faith. Such were the principal ingredients. Its conception of pathology perhaps gave the impression of being new, but it in fact only recast the old deficit model of dysfunction. Except that instead of repairing a failure of the mind, it sought to enhance the power of the ego. If the aim of psychoanalysis was to render manageable the forbidden, and if it presented itself as an art of creating distance, these techniques, by embracing the goal of smoothing over every conflict, situated themselves in the line of those arts that put things back together. Psychic conflict made no sense to them, it was one of the rotten fruits of civilization. The therapist had to compensate for the frustrations life imposed on her patients and free them from the artificial structures that prevented them from being themselves. And behind the technical focus on feeling and the references to deficit, there was no opposition between psychotherapy and chemical therapy. The conflict and deficit models could be applied to all therapies, and there were as many illusions and fantasies on one side as there were on the other. In fact, the pertinent opposition, let us repeat, was not between psychotherapy and chemical therapy but, rather, between deficit and conflict.

A NEW IMPERSONAL RULE: PERSONALIZATION

The success of this therapeutic style had its origins in a shift in the normative context: the insistence on conformity or submission to a single and preexisting norm had lessened. A new tolerance for "the right to be different" – an expression that would grow in popularity – was making inroads. From now on, all people could be normal, whatever their differences. What was important was not only to be able to express these differences (the opportunities to do so would multiply) but also to assume them (the practical means of doing so would also multiply). This pluralization, enabling every individual to choose her life without fear of being stigmatized, resulted from the fact that that joyful era saw the development, sociologically, of the pure individual, a type of person who was her own sovereign. This individual was by definition uncertain of herself since there was no longer anything outside herself that told her how to behave, and she had to make up her own rules. These were not, for all that, a personal cobbling together as it was their social context that had changed. The norms of the day encouraged people to become

themselves, just as those of the past demanded that they be disciplined and accept their condition. And nothing allows us to claim
that there was less subjective experience in disciplinary constraint
than in personal flowering. "Personal" was a normative artifice; it
was, like every norm, perfectly impersonal.

The new therapies revealed a radical rethinking of what was
normal and what was pathological.[63] They were the clinical reflection of a set of standards that had abandoned its ties to guilt and
discipline. In the social realm one could make up one's own rules,
while clinically, the measures taken served less to encourage a state
of equilibrium for the individual than to remove his inhibitions and
enable him to widen the scope of his own possibilities.

According to Philip Rieff, what the new therapeutic age had to
offer was the collective determination "not to pay the high personal
costs of social organization."[64] Not to pay? This glorious innerness
went hand in hand with different ways of expressing our private
anxieties. Mental pathologies where intrapsychic conflict was not
present but where, on the other hand, a sense of one's valuelessness
prevailed were an object of concern that did not exist in France
during the 1960s. A lowering of self-esteem, feelings of inferiority:
these bore a strong resemblance to deficit. If conflict was linked to
guilt, deficit was bound to narcissism. This was the great lesson that
depression would impose on the individual who thought he could
set himself up as his own legislator.

THE GREAT DEBATE: NEUROSIS OR DEPRESSION?

In their books Janov and Lowen outlined a number of pathological
cases, chiefly concerning depression. Behind the appearance of a
therapeutic treatment transcending the pathological there emerged,
rather, an *identification* of well-being with healing that resulted in
the *separation* of the conflict model and the deficit model. If there
had been an absolute point of consensus among psychoanalysts, it
was that a cure "begins after one no longer sees oneself as in a state
of well-being."[65] Now the deficit model, isolated from its old rival
and ally, had well-being as its exclusive goal. It no longer acknowledged the limits reality imposed on all lives, whose recognition had
been a requirement for any cure. The new psychological culture
seemed like a posture of defence against that depression whose terms
it was at the same time prolonging. "Therapeutic gregariousness,"

thought Jean Bergeret, "constitutes an ... example of reactive anti-depressive training."[66] It gave support, said the psychoanalysts, to the individual's narcissism; however, it did so like a drug nourishing an insatiable Ego, with no limits imposed. The techniques for bettering the self did away with the individual's inhibitions but did not afford the means for her to structure herself. A new way of viewing depression spread through the analytic community. It defined a mode of despair that previous generations had not known.

PSYCHOANALYSIS FACE TO FACE WITH MOOD

As of the 1970s, French psychoanalytic literature paid particular attention to a clientele that, it seemed, was growing rapidly. A new kind of patient was stretching out on the psychoanalysts' couches. These patients presented a daunting challenge because, unlike neurotics, they were not able to recognize their conflicts, to picture them. They lacked the basic underpinning without which it was difficult to achieve a cure: guilt. Sometimes distressed, these patients above all felt chronically empty; they had great difficulty coping with their painful emotions because they did not intellectualize them. Their representations were poor, they were not able to give symbolic form to their suffering: they were prisoners of their mood. This new species had a name: borderline personalities.[67] Depression dominated the clinical picture.

The basis for an analytic cure, let us remember, was to enable unconscious psychic conflicts to emerge because these were at the root of all symptomatology. Depressive symptoms, like all symptoms, had first to find their meaning; they were not themselves the target of the cure. A depressive episode could, in fact, represent a crucial stage in the healing process. The patient divested himself of imaginary identifications that accorded him secondary benefits;[68] having lost the objects he held to, he became depressed. More generally, the "depressive position" was an indispensable step in the development of the child because it was the source of personal maturation. Depression was part of the process that structured the individual. At the pathological level, it manifested itself as "a state that could not be more elusive for psychoanalysis, and criticism of the theory of depression is certainly not new."[69] In short, mood was of little interest to the psychoanalyst. The preface to a 1985 issue of the *Nouvelle Revue de psychanalyse*, which was devoted to this subject, made the point: "Mood," it declared, "is not a psychoanalytic concept" because the psychoanalyst "sees there the corporal impact of representations that have not achieved consciousness, or the confused, deformed indices of repressed, cornered feelings."[70] In fact, "becoming conscious" was central to analytic healing.

Now, suddenly, mood began to interest French psychoanalysts. During the 1970s, neurotic depression was the source of intense debates in the community. A number of clinicians noted the new prominence of depression as an issue. In 1970, in the *Encyclopédie médicochirurgicale,* Jean Bergeret was the first Frenchman to devote an article to borderline personalities.[71] Two years later, in an article aimed at general practitioners, he estimated that systematic studies in consultation services had concluded that 20 percent of patients had a neurotic structure, 30 percent a psychotic structure (which would manifest itself in very few cases), and 50 percent an intermediate structure whose primary symptom was "essentially depressive."[72]

All analysts noted, whatever the nosological status it was accorded, the quantitative importance of the work devoted to "depressivity"[73] or to "a return to the subject of depression in current psychoanalysis."[74] The thirty-sixth Congress of French Language Psychoanalysts, held in June 1976, was devoted to depression. It gave rise to two special issues of the *Revue française de psychanalyse,* which presented two very thick reports by André Haynal and Jean Bergeret as well as the many discussions that followed. Roland Kuhn evoked, rather wearily, "the inexhaustible subjects of neurosis and depression."[75] Neurosis and depression do seem to have presented a delicate diagnostic problem concerning the status of mood in an analytic cure. Psychoanalysis did, in fact, bring to the fore a certain type of humoral depression.

DEPRESSION BETWEEN THE PATHOLOGY OF IDENTIFICATION AND THE PATHOLOGY OF IDENTITY

Before we can understand the reasons for this new attention to emotional disorders and their diagnostic issues, we must remember where, historically, psychoanalytic tradition situated depression and, more precisely, what its relationship was with anxiety.[76] When patients presented depressive symptoms, the psychoanalyst had first and foremost to investigate their psychogenesis in order to understand why they reacted in this way. We saw this general problem being raised in the previous chapter: what type of personality was subject to one or another type of depression? In analytic language, this was translated into a diagnosis of how these patients' Egos were organized, whatever the reasons for the depression or the nosographic situation (melancholic psychosis, neurosis with depressive manifestations, etc.).

Psychoanalysts distinguished, as we noted, two large categories of emotion that Freud referred to as "displeasure": anxiety and depression. These two emotions were not the same. Anxiety was always provoked by a danger or by the violation of a taboo, while depression was brought about by a loss. Freud based his clinical approach to melancholia on mourning. He wrote that, in mourning, the external world had grown empty and deficient, while in melancholia the Ego itself did so: "The patient represents his Ego to us as worthless, incapable of any achievement and morally despicable." He was afflicted, Freud went on, with "an extraordinary diminution in his self-regard."[77] The loss of the beloved object provoked a "peculiar painfulness" of which "so little is known."[78] This painfulness was designated in German by the word *Hilflosigkeit*, which was translated, depending on the circumstances, as distress or impotence.[79] It was a matter, Freud explained, of an inner pain that we could compare with bodily pain: "When there is physical pain, a high degree of what may be termed narcissistic cathexis of the painful place occurs. This cathexis continues to increase and tends, as it were, to empty the Ego."[80] The melancholic individual had lost her self-respect. Her Ego was split in that one part of it systematically devalued the other.

Beyond melancholia, two situations could present themselves. In the first, sadness and helplessness were neurotic symptoms in the same sense as were obsession or hysterical paralysis. But there was a second type of depressive emotion more difficult for psychoanalysis to classify: it was not a symptom but, rather, a pathological system characterized by the loss of an object, and it was much more tenuously related to the idea of the forbidden. In this case the conflicts were pre-Oedipean. That indicated that these patients had stalled at a stage preceding their identification with parental images, which were the first objects presented to them. The patient had remained at a phase where he was still one with the mother. If neurosis was a *pathology of identification*, then the borderline condition, because the individual had not been able to develop relationships with objects, was a *pathology of identity*. Indeed, he had great difficulty identifying himself. He was, one might say, his own impotent sovereign – which was the source of the "extraordinary diminution in his self-regard: his delusion of inferiority."

Depression, then, was not a neurotic symptom because the personality structure associated with it was different from that associated with the neurotic. Psychoanalysts called it "the depressive personality." "The depressive personality," wrote André Haynal, "seems unable to free itself from the problem of loss, unlike various neuroses that will bring to bear defensive strategies in order to control the negative inner states it creates ... With neurotics, depression is the indicator of a particular loss ...; but depressive structures live chronically in the shadow of an unresolved problem of constant loss, of being always the loser, the disappointed."[81] The borderline condition was not a vague catch-all, it was a structure with the same legitimacy as neurosis, psychosis, or perversion. The great difference between a neurosis with depressive symptoms and this pathological system was that, in the first instance, the individual managed to construct stable defences, while in the second, her identity crisis was permanent and often manifested itself in chronic depression.

And so psychoanalysis found itself face to face with a depression that was not melancholic and that did not play itself out in the one realm where this therapy had the most success – neurosis – leaving it with an impassable conflict that made the individual ill. This type of patient attracted the attention of British psychoanalysts in the 1930s and became the focus of much attention in North America in the 1950s and 1960s. These patients first turned up in psychiatry at the end of the nineteenth century, at a time when the boundary between psychosis and neurosis was being established. They had character disorders stemming from their constitution but did not suffer the implacable destiny that led to dementia. Twentieth-century French psychiatry was very familiar with such patients. Henri Claude talked of schizomania; Eugène Minkowski of a schizophrenic character with no habitual dissolution of identity, as in schizophrenia; Henri Ey of schizo-neurosis. The patients lived in a state of permanent psychic disequilibrium.

These pathologies were called "narcissistic."[82] This narcissism was not that love of self that was one of the products of joie de vivre but, rather, the experience of being captive to a self-image so idealized that it led to impotence and paralyzed the individual, who had a constant need to be reassured by others and could easily become dependent on them. One can see how group therapies might compensate for this fragility. The psychoanalysts had a tool to define their pathology, which was the Ego Ideal. The phenomenon was defined variously in Freud's thought, but we could say schematically that it was linked to narcissism just as the Superego was linked to the forbidden; the feeling of inferiority was to the first what the feeling of guilt was to the second.[83] In fact, if the Superego told one not to do, the Ego Ideal urged one to do.[84]

In narcissistic pathologies, the Ego was so invested that any frustration was hard to endure. The patient never derived any satisfaction from her impulses; she felt empty and reacted aggressively, impulsively, or by acting out. If the neurotic was defined by her psychic conflict, the borderline personality was not able to enter into conflict: she was empty. This type of patient posed very special problems for a cure because it was difficult not only for her to work through her psychic conflicts but also to negotiate a transference with the analyst, which was a precondition for successful healing. She was not open to analytical "influence" because the identifying processes had not been instilled in early childhood. The prognosis for these depressions was poor.[85]

Many analysts confirmed this: "We are facing more and more frequently the problem of depressive personalities ... It is *banal* to say that the clinical pictures we are facing today are not exactly the same as in Freud's time."[86] Were there fewer classic neuroses by comparison with the new pathologies? The psychoanalysts did not all agree on this distinction between depressive and neurotic structures. For Lucien Israël, the depressed were above all hysterics: "The complaints that arise in these states are for the most part none other than hysterical complaints: pain of various kinds, dizziness, feelings of weakness and exhaustion."[87] It was known that hysteria drew its symptoms from what society had to offer, and so it was possible that these varied in accordance with social norms: ecstasies in a culture that was still religious, depression in a culture with a highly refined self-consciousness. Now, depression became a fashionable illness just as these norms were coming into their own. "We have observed, in our day, fewer great hysterical syndromes," remarked another analyst, "and concomitantly, an increase in depressive syndromes. Should we attribute this to sociocultural changes, in particular to the fact that we are according less status and gratification to hysteria than used to be the case?"[88] According to Joyce McDougall, the symptoms or the references changed, but the pathological background remained the same: "As to sexuality, all I can say as an analyst is that sexual norms change – but that castration anxiety endures. It has simply found new disguises."[89]

Another hypothesis, more sociological, was advanced, that of a shift in the clientele as psychoanalysis spread throughout French society. This was Daniel Widlöcher's position in his article devoted to classifications and their meanings for analysts; he indicated that modern nosological thinking "involved opening up what was a no man's land for classical nosology, that of the pathology of character and difficulties in life. The extension of psychoanalytic cures beyond the category of neuroses occurred primarily where patients were seeking help for problems in their lives, and where their symptoms indicated no specific mental disorder."[90] Other psychoanalysts observed an increase in the types of disorders being dealt with by psychoanalysis, notably those involving depression.[91] Psychoanalysis would more and more be faced with cases that, traditionally, were outside its purview, "where emptiness, absence, flaws in symbolization or a failure of inner temporalisation were particularly acute."[92] The increase in depression seemed proportional to the decline in an ability to express psychic conflicts. Psychiatrists noted that, during the 1970s, psychiatry was no longer content to treat mental illness but was reaching out to embrace "life support" and "the pathologies of happiness."[93]

THE POWER OF THE NEUROTIC AND THE FRAGILITY OF THE DEPRESSED

The interesting point about these nosological debates for the problem that concerns us is that neurosis was seen as the consequence of a conflict that rendered one guilty (including when depressive symptoms were dominant), while depression was experienced as a shameful flaw. Narcissism clouded the issue where the forbidden was concerned; the neurotic personality's illness was one of wrongdoing, whereas the depressive personality's sickness was one of inadequacy. It seemed to lack a well-developed Superego, and it was subject to very few conflicts. "Whereas potent individuals easily acquire anxiety neuroses," wrote Freud, "impotent ones incline to melancholia."[94] The depressed individual was immersed in a logic where inferiority was dominant, while neurotics were involved in a dynamic of transgression: they wanted, as Freud said, to be nobler than their constitution allowed. Did the disappearance of the regulatory force of the forbidden and the strait jacket of conformity open the way to depression? The depressive personality remained fixed in a permanent state of adolescence and was unable to become adult and to accept the frustrations that were the lot of every life.[95] The result was fragility, a permanent feeling of precariousness or instability. What was lacking in this posture was the guilt that would enrol it in what the "French Freud," Lacan, called the "symbolic," that relationship to the law that resulted in anxiety, certainly, but without which there was no solid structuring of one's identity, of the stable and permanent sense of one's self. All of which made suffering extremely hard to endure and provoked an unending search for a state of well-being.

These depressed individuals, whose Egos were characterized by inadequacy, underestimated the value of their experiences: "The feeling of not being as strong as one would like was often expressed in terms of 'fatigue,' as well as the sense of being less stimulated than one would prefer."[96] That is why this type of depression manifested itself less through guilt than through shame. It "is the prime emotion in the narcissistic realm … What is more, it implies that the individual feels himself to be responsible …, as if, like a god, he thought he had created himself on his own. The depressed individual feels shame because, in his fundamental megalomania, he cannot admit to his inadequacies; he does not admit to feeling limited by reality, and in particular by the constraints imposed on him by his personal history and his affiliations."[97] Guilt was related to law, while shame was related to the "social gaze."[98] The success of group therapies doubtless resided in a process of "shame removal." In fact, when the reference was no longer a fixed precept, when the impersonal law no longer counted, the other became the only means to having one's choices validated. This often pathetic quest for the other could, in the most extreme cases, turn into a dependence, an insatiable need.

The attainment of a neurotic state, enabling one's conflicts to surface, was a sign of progress in the treatment of these depressions; the individual could then heal by recognizing the limits to her being all powerful rather than permanently bewailing her powerlessness. The cure had to help the patient to transcend her submission to her feelings by making it possible for her to picture her masked conflicts.[99] The conflict served as a guide, gave her room to manoeuvre, and set her in motion once again.

Psychoanalysts had a tendency to put forward a global explanation for the increase in depressive personalities: "The exaggerated power of taboos doubtless created pathological conflicts, but the absence of any struggle or object-oriented conquest at the level of Oedipal reality risked diminishing considerably the possibility of pleasure and limited us to a *depression-antidepression* dialectic."[100] To their minds, modern society contributed to a collective devalorization of the Oedipal, that is, of the father in his symbolic function as a separation between child and mother, a separation without which the child could not become the subject of his own existence. We could be gods, but as we were human, we paid for it through pathologies in which an inner fragility was reflected in painful emotions and poor representations. "We have got to the point," wrote Bergeret, "of precipitating young people into a depressive situation ... where it is no longer possible to feel guilty of anything whatsoever."[101]

When impotence was linked to a defensive psychoneurosis such as hysteria, the conflict was visible; when it was attached to a borderline state, the conflict was masked. We were entering the modern era of depression: the individual made ill by her conflicts was giving way to the individual paralyzed by her inadequacy. Emancipation replaced constraints but, obviously, did not do away with them. It modified our culture of inner unhappiness.

COMPULSIVE HUMANITY: THE EXPLOSION OF ADDICTIONS

The craving for drugs appeared, in the eyes of psychoanalysts, like a choice equivalent to that offered by group therapies: a means of defence against depression. "The path leading from depression to different forms of drug addiction is being travelled more and more frequently," noted André Haynal in his report on depression.[102] The depressive individual, in fact, could not cope with frustration. Alcoholism or addiction to narcotics or medication was a way to compensate and could be considered as a form of self-medication for depression.[103] The addictive input was the other side of the coin to the depressive void.

Dependency: A Pathological Relationship

Addiction in the classical sense of the word was characterized medically as a physiological dependency and tolerance (the consumer had to increase his doses so that the product might maintain its effect). The substance developed a physical hold upon the individual. This hold was created mechanically by its pharmacological properties and found expression in compulsive behaviour. In the absence of these two physiological criteria, the term addiction was not used: a clear proof was required that attested to the existence of physical dependency.[104] As of the mid-1960s, the concept was extended to LSD and cannabis, at a time when these two drugs began to be widely available, and became a political problem in the United States. In other words, drugs that were not thought to induce physical dependency became themselves addictive. The concept of psychological dependency was devised for this purpose. It made it possible to stigmatize psychoactive substances that were not included in the traditional medical and social categories of dependency.

The introduction of psychological dependency as a concept also resulted in the physiological dependency on heroin being placed in a new perspective: heroin addicts were not animals but human beings. Psychological dependency reintroduced the idea of the individual in a manner analogous to that of Pinel with the insane: the individual faltered, but she was there. In fact, this dependency presupposed the idea of a *relationship* with the substance, independent of its pharmacological characteristics; one could be dependent on cannabis, and one could be an occasional consumer of heroin, including by injection.[105] But psychological dependency had another consequence as well: by minimizing the pharmacological hold of the product, it posited *a pathological relationship*, whether applied to a substance, an activity, or a person. Dependency was pathological behaviour, whatever was being consumed. One of the first books that modified the concept of addiction was *Love and Addiction* by Stanton Peele and Archie Brodsky, published in 1975. It demonstrated that love relationships could be as compulsive and destructive as a dependency on heroin, which is to say that they could result in an individual's self-destruction. A wide variety of behaviours now qualified as addictions.[106] Compulsion was the common factor in these behaviours. The loss of self-control was the key element that permitted the grouping together of everything that showed its tell-tale signs – food, heroin, or cigarettes. Addiction became a very broad concept, a class of behaviour. Twenty years after the publication of Peele and Brodsky's book, it became chapter and verse for all of psychiatry.

As of the 1970s, psychiatrists were noting more and more addictions, their having been recast as pathological relationships: food pathologies, sexual addictions, and so on. According to Stanton Peele, "The application of the notion of illness to problems linked to alcohol and drugs has increased these last decades, just as health professionals were using the illness model to describe eating disorders, destructive sexual relationships, compulsive gambling, the sexual abuse of wives and children, and even disorders as disparate as phobias, anxiety and depression."[107] However, insofar as the self-medication was successful, the overall behaviour of these dependent individuals could appear perfectly normal. This was a constant, from the bulimia of the early 1970s to internet abuse in the 1990s.[108]

Psychoanalytic writings underscore the relational problems of borderline personalities: difficulties in connecting with others and in establishing emotionally stable relationships, superficial seductive behaviour, general instability, compulsiveness. All this was the product of an inner emptiness and an absence of self-esteem, which drove the individual to constantly seek reassurance by changing his "objects." The pathology was often hidden behind a façade of good socialization and professional, even domestic accomplishment. The personality could be a "false self," an "as if." The addictive behaviour betrayed the contradictions of this type of pathological individuality, which involved "an opposition between the inflated idea they have of themselves (excessive self-obsession and a constant need to be admired), and their unusual state of dependency."[109]

Pathological Acting Out in the Place of Psychic Conflict

In the behavioural realm, dependency was a loss of control, but what was it psychopathologically? Psychiatrists frequently noted that dependency derived from a concept in Roman law that obliged the debtor unable to pay what he owed to pay with his body – a form of servitude or slavery. This non-neurotic mental pathology was part and parcel of a depressive personality: "The individual does not construct a symptom, as in neurosis, nor a delirium, as in psychosis (which already presupposes a high degree of mental processing), but *acts out* the conflict [behaviourally],"[110] through addictions, compulsions, suicides, and acting out itself. These "acts" fill the depressive void; they are a way of compensating for it.

The question of a relationship between addiction and depression was not new to psychoanalysts. Sándor Radó, who was the first director of the Psychoanalytic Institute at Columbia University (created in 1944), had, in 1933, published an article on this subject that became a classic: "The Psychoanalysis of Pharmacothymia." He described "a category of human beings who react to the frustrations of life with a special type of emotional modifications that can be called 'anxious depression.'" He showed how, for people with an acute need for stimulants, "the ego continues to sustain their self-esteem through artificial means."[111] The euphoria fended off the depressive symptoms while feeding the depressed individual's narcissism, making her feel invulnerable. Calling a halt to the medicinal intake could, depending on the case, lead to suicide or psychosis. Radó concluded his article by highlighting the existence of less serious cases, where "the patient can generally stay in tune with reality and only resort to pharmacothymics as an auxiliary or corrective. In this manner, he compensates for a lack of self-assurance in the realm of reality and covers a deficit with artifice. Through imperceptible gradations, we arrive at the normal personality who uses daily stimulants such as coffee, cigarettes, etc."[112] In 1945, Otto Fenichel analyzed at length the relationship between depression and drug addiction, and demonstrated "the significance of the narcissistic contribution to the depressed, who came to resemble individuals subject to perversions, or to drug addicts."[113] He invented the expression "drug addictions without drugs," which psychiatry later used to define new addictions. The risk was that the medication would only have an effect on the depressive feelings. They would not untangle the underlying psychic conflict but, rather, would smooth it over. The patient would then find himself in a vicious circle with no natural defences against life's difficulties.

In place of anxiety, there was the depressive void. The constant calling out to objects in the external world was a means of filling the bottomless pit that constituted the inner world of the depressed individual. As a result, antidepressive medication tended "to rapidly produce real drug addictions that artificially recreated a surface euphoria, but not happiness."[114]

There was a clear consensus on this point in psychiatry and psychoanalysis: addictive behaviour was linked one way or the other to depression. These behaviours appeared either as depressive equivalents or as a symptom of depression. One of the first empirical studies published in the United States in 1974 emphasized that depression was the most significant emotional problem in heroin dependency.[115] In 1984, a Swiss psychiatrist showed that "depression appears today to be a crucial factor in the development of drug dependency. It makes the treatment of this illness extremely difficult and explains many relapses. And so it is important to recognize the depressive states and to treat them advisedly if one wants to avoid failure in the handling of drug addicts."[116] Depression could be the cause of drug addiction, which functioned as a form of self-medication; it could be its consequence as the drug produced neurochemical malfunction; and it could be its companion as the heroine addict's lifestyle was in itself depressing (searching to score, going into debt, etc.). Drug addicts operated in a state of depressive anxiety favoured by the narcissistic structure of the personality: "They are subject, at the slightest emotional shock, to grave depressive reactions."[117] The use of antidepressants was effective in halting heroin use as it helped pave the way for the exertion of psychotherapeutic control. Ten years later, in 1993, a French addiction specialist estimated that "eating disorders, alcoholism, and drug addiction, could all be related through their connection with depression ... There is a 30% to 50% frequency of depression in eating disorders, alcoholism and drug addiction among young people."[118]

The depressive implosion and the addictive explosion were from now on inseparably linked: the impotence void and the compulsion void were Janus's two faces. In the case of depression, it was not sadness that dominated the picture but impotence – the difficulty of acting – and the inability to cope with frustrations (does not choosing imply being able to renounce?). This led to the new face of depression, which was dependency – the unbalanced action produced by the absence of self-control.

THE OTHER SIDE OF INDIVIDUAL SOVEREIGNTY

Whether it be considered the new face of hysteria or a borderline state, depression said much about the individual's current experience for it embodied the tension between the desire to be only oneself and the difficulty thereof.

Where new therapies were concerned, the dominant and happy impression was that each individual would be able to sally forth in conquest of himself without having to pay the price; therapists drew on a deficit model to increase "human potential," and their ideal was that of a complete individual, undivided – to mend was the order of the day. As for psychopathology, the proponents of the borderline state scenario estimated that the psychic economy underwent change; rather than intrapsychic conflict, there was the void that threatened the stability of the individual's identity. "Their deep demands" involved neither conflicts nor taboos but "a need to be."[119] Now it was a matter of remaking the individual, of reinserting him into the conflict, of transforming Narcissus into Oedipus – to separate was the order of the day.

If a mental disorder consisted not only of symptoms but also of ways of being in the world, depression could be considered the exact opposite of the strange obsession with being entirely oneself – of identifying no more – that took hold of our societies as of the early 1960s. "Depression" was a common – and convenient – word to describe the problems raised by this new normality. Individual sovereignty was not only a relaxation of external constraints; everyone could also take the concrete measure of the inner burden it brought into being. Depression reined in that omnipotence, which was the virtual horizon of emancipation.

In French psychoanalysis in particular, depression was regarded as a symbolic collapse: the difficulty in experiencing conflict weakened the identifying mechanisms needed to structure an identity that could live with such conflict. The style of despair changed along with the style of hope. The anxiety of being oneself morphed into the weariness of being oneself. This was the guise our inner constraints now assumed as a new age for the individual was taking shape.

These new dilemmas were not visible in society during the 1970s. They were spotted only in the psychoanalytic milieu, and at a time when psychoanalysis was widely seen as being contested by other therapies and was beginning to lose its prestige.[120] If one was concerned on the psychological front with the symbolic collapse signalled by the chronic sense of one's own inadequacy and so of a *self to be restructured*, on the medical front, as we will see, one was more and more preoccupied with a *patient to treat*.

5

The Medical Front:
New Avenues for the Depressive Mood

If the 1970s saw the dissemination of a new psychological culture, they also saw that of a new biological culture, which replaced the configuration established in the 1940s. The psychiatric approach to medication for the mind was situated along the Janet-Cerletti-Freud axis. Cerletti provided the linkage for a complementary relationship between deficit (for which Janet furnished the model) and conflict (which was part of Freud's territory). On psychiatry's medical front, the severing of this linkage would render the category of neurosis moribund.

While the techniques for self-multiplication were being developed by new therapies, the increased prominence of depression as a topic in psychopathology was an inevitable outcome of the diagnostic and therapeutic debates concerning the relations between neuroses and depressions, guilt and inadequacy, conflict and deficit. Self-esteem was at the crossroads between psychic liberation and insecure identity, which were evolving in step with one another. The medical community, for its part, was inclined to focus on a patient for whom it could care pharmacologically without any reference to conflict. And so we had two aspects of the same dynamic, both of which excluded conflict.

During the second half of the 1970s, psychiatry felt that depression was breaking new ground.[1] The disagreements concerning the biological and biochemical aspects of depression were as significant in psychiatry as they were in psychoanalysis. Here also the weakest category was neurotic depression. It was also the most widespread: it was the category found among the clientele of the general practitioner, "which [was] what ma[de] it impossible to provide a synthesis for 'the theory' of depression," declared a speaker at a 1979 conference dedicated to "a new approach to mood disorders."[2] The concept of mood disorders provided the focus for reorganizing psychiatric diagnosis. These disorders consisted primarily of anxiety and depression, which were of course the two principal emotions. Anxiety was relatively simple to recognize, even if it knew how to dissemble itself; depression, on the other hand, manifested itself through symptoms as diverse as sadness, fatigue, a variety of somatic problems, inhibition, and, of course, anxiety.

Two descriptive levels were necessary to describe the changes on the medical front. First, there was general medicine: epidemiology was better able to identify the complaints and the reasons for consultation; new antidepressants were perfected, easier to use, and had effects different from those previously on the market; and two clinical signs, anxiety and inhibition, began to redefine depression. Second, there were the diagnostic models: tripartite depression (endogenous, psychogenic, exogenous), based on an etiological diagnosis, was gradually abandoned. A description of subtypes took its place, grouped together in syndromic categories that were refined and, as far as possible, standardized.

As a result of this paradigm shift, the category of neuroses was rendered useless. The sick individual had once been subject to the following question: what underlying pathology gives rise to such and such a clinical picture? A new question confirmed the decline of the category of neuroses: what antidepressant should the doctor prescribe for such and such type of depression? Psychiatric literature advised general physicians less and less often to seek out the underlying pathology, that which affected an individual insofar as she was not simply a body. Bit by bit, psychotherapy lost its status as the treatment of choice, and psychopathology was marginalized within psychiatry.

A Tire to Reinflate and a Victim of Anxiety to Soothe

"Depression is *truly* our modern illness. That doesn't mean that we know everything about it, nor even that the term, so bandied about, means anything specific. Its vagueness provides both patient and doctor with a convenient label, justifying the former's condition and the latter's actions."[3] A convenient label indeed, for it became a generic word and a calling card. Doctors were no longer able to satisfy the demand, and therapists of all sorts entered a market whose staple was self-esteem. Gone was the argument seeking to persuade patients and those around them that this was neither an imaginary nor a mental illness.[4] Depression was comfortably installed as the disorder of modern times. As we have seen, the media urged the populace to take an interest in its inner life. The demands made of the medical community had found their language, while general practitioners now played a prominent role.

Three factors defined depression's status for general practitioners, with as background the heterogeneous nature of the pathology.[5] First, it was generally agreed that non-psychotic mental disorders would for the most part be treated through general medicine. However, the depression dealt with by the general practitioners was not the same as that treated by psychiatrists. Second, pharmacological innovations had come on stream; new antidepressants better adapted to a generalist's practice began to appear as of 1975. Third, the upshot of these two developments was that sadness and mental anguish became less prominent, losing ground to fatigue.

THE TRIAD: ASTHENIA, INSOMNIA, ANXIETY

In her 1987 essay on depression, Julia Kristeva wrote: "Sadness is the basic mood of depression."[6] However, this was a mood whose reign went into eclipse towards the end of the 1970s. The depressed individual seemed above all to be an asthenic requiring stimulus, a victim of anxiety needing to be soothed, and an insomniac seeking sleep. The triad consisting of asthenia, insomnia, and anxiety was a behavioural and affective response to the constant change working its way into daily life in democratic societies.

The first available study in France on psychological disorders in general medicine was undertaken by INSERM (the French National Institute for Health and Medical Research) during the years 1974-75.[7] Mental and psychosocial disorders (problems of family, social, and professional adaptation) were the second most frequent, after cardiovascular illness. The generalists dealt with 74 percent of these cases, and the psychiatrists 12 percent. The study confirmed that general practitioners were treating most of the population's psychopathological problems.

General practitioners (GPs) diagnosed 73 percent of the depressions, and psychiatric specialists diagnosed 16 percent. Depressions (neurotic, psychotic, or undefined) represented almost a quarter of the mental and psychosocial disorders in medicine, and nearly a third in psychiatry. Neuroses and alcoholism constituted 71 percent of mental disorders: women tended to be neurotic, whereas alcoholism was "almost exclusively" masculine.[8] The authors noted that, if the two pathologies were added together, they gave the same consultation percentage for the two sexes. Alcoholism was the principal manifestation of male depression: *women developed symptoms, men developed behaviour.*

In diagnosis, the sequence nervousness-fatigue abnormal-depression represented 18.2 percent of the cases for GPs and 0.8 percent for psychiatrists. The GPs most commonly prescribed medication, while the psychiatrists suggested another appointment. What is more, in general medicine, mental pathologies received more medical treatment than did any other.[9]

Another study, published in 1983, analyzed medical dossiers in order to compare patients' reasons for seeking help with actual diagnosis. The patients complained most often of asthenia, insomnia, and anxiety (or distress). In general medicine, depression took almost any form: exhaustion, loss of energy, fatigue, insomnia, sadness, dark thoughts, loss of appetite (or anorexia), and, more rare than the others, anguish. Diagnostically, doctors paid less attention to the pairing agitation-irritability, which was not often mentioned. They were fond of "references containing the single idea of 'a lowering.'"[10] Visits for somatic or functional problems were still in the majority, but there was a clear increase in patients complaining of personal difficulties.[11] All the studies confirmed the GPs' depression triad: insomnia, anxiety, and asthenia.[12] They were so frequently encountered in medical practice that they lacked precision: "The more traditional signs (sadness and pessimism, suicidal thoughts and attempted suicide) only made secondary appearances."[13] The depressed individual consulting a GP was rarely sad; he was limp with fatigue and seeking stimulus. Patients were clearly complaining of the problems the media found most appealing.[14] The most visible symptoms and the types of complaints being voiced derived, in the vast majority of cases, from neurotic or reactive depressions.[15]

MASKED DEPRESSION

In opening the international conference on masked depression held in Saint-Moritz, Switzerland, in January 1973, Paul Kielholz declared: "Not only has depression become more widespread over the last twenty years, but changes have been observed in the symptomatology. Especially in the psychogenetic forms of the illness, but also in its endogenous forms."[16] In fact, as many studies noted, at least since the beginning of the 1960s many patients had been complaining of a variety of symptoms that had no organic foundation: they were masks for depression. These changes involved a wide spectrum of somatic symptoms, ranging from headaches to cardiovascular and gastro-intestinal problems. Participants in this conference included the great names both of European psychiatry (Kuhn, Lopez-Ibor [one of the first psychiatrists to have addressed this problem in the 1950s], Berner, Pichot, van Praag)[17] and North-American psychiatry (Lehmann, Freedman).

During the *Entretiens de Bichat* the same year, Thérèse Lempérière, a former student of Delay and Deniker, gave a talk on this subject, pointing out that there were many depressed individuals in general medicine who were unaware of the psychogenic origin of their complaints, whether headaches, gastric/cervical, or abdominal pains. The 1960s saw many American and British studies, all of which noted the number of minor pains among the general population and their increased frequency among neurotics, whether the neuroses were hysterical or obsessive. Often they were accompanied by one or another type of asthenia.[18] At the 1972 *Assises départementales* for medicine devoted to depressive states, one of Kielholz's collaborators underlined the degree to which "the concept of depression include[d] many more things than this single psychic symptomatology." He insisted on "its immense practical impact, above all for non-psychiatrists,"[19] all the more so in that the somatic manifestations of depression were extremely diverse (constipation, palpitations, hair loss, sensitivity to cold, etc.), which made the pathology even more elusive than was thought. Psychological symptoms existed, but they were discrete and difficult to spot. Insofar as the depression was masked by a somatic complaint, it was the general practitioner who was most frequently consulted.[20] And given the difficulties in diagnosing this type of depression, it was the therapeutic proving ground that ultimately confirmed or ruled out the diagnosis.

Psychiatrists reproached generalists for treating the most obvious symptoms rather than diagnosing depressions. Still, they recognized that it wasn't exactly the same depressed individuals who consulted a family physician and a psychiatric specialist, respectively, while those treated in a hospital setting were even more different. What is more, the logic of general medicine was not the same as that of psychiatry: general practitioners tended to make sweeping diagnoses based on symptoms more than on nosology and to put more emphasis on therapy than on diagnosis. They gave "more weight to comfort and short-term satisfaction for the patient than to a long and medium-term cure,"[21] Arthur Tatossian observed in his 1985 report on the treatment of depression. And so there was no reason to be shocked by the prescriptions for medication; this practice was consistent with professional norms. Did the GP not send her patients to a specialist only when short-term treatment showed itself to be ineffective?

These procedures were all the less surprising, given how hard it was to differentiate between types of depression. The existence of "faulty" diagnoses and incorrect prescriptions could also be attributed to the fact that psychiatrists themselves did not have a clear picture of depression, which was a veritable labyrinth.[22]

NEW STIMULANT ANTIDEPRESSANTS

Masked by its somatic or behavioural equivalents (addictions), expressing itself primarily through three complaints, depression was perceived as a lowering, and it was understood as an inadequacy. This view of patients was achieving consensus just as new antidepressants were coming on the market, most of which were effective in dealing with inadequacy. At the same time, sadness and mental distress waned as growing attention was paid to anxiety and inhibition. Psychiatry's way of looking at depression was changing.

If it was hard to have a clear view of what was going on in the way of prescriptions, psychiatrists did note that, in 1978, 5 million prescriptions for antidepressants were written, consumption for this category increased more rapidly than for the average run of medications (19 percent against 6 percent), and two-thirds of the prescriptions were given out by generalists. They criticized the lack of psychopharmacological information and the way pharmaceutical companies presented their products (i.e., with an approach geared more to "marketing needs" than to "objective information").[23] Generalists were reluctant to prescribe tricyclics because of the risk of suicide, their high toxicity, their side effects, and the difficulty in monitoring treatment. For the same reason, if they did prescribe them, they prescribed small doses, which were often inadequate. Side effects presented more problems in an outpatient situation than in the hospital: patients had to continue living a normal life, and their sensitivity to the effects of the drugs was greater when the intensity of the depression was weaker.[24] And so the importance of these drugs was not to be underestimated. Antidepressants had to be easily managed by the generalist in order for her to prescribe them, and it was advisable to minimize the inconveniences and toxicity so that patients would follow the treatment. Chemists and pharmacologists sought antidepressants that could exceed the percentage effectiveness of the MAOIs and the tricyclics (60 percent to 70 percent) and that acted more rapidly.

Between 1975 and 1984, the prescribing procedures of general practitioners began to change; the quantity of antidepressants prescribed grew by 300 percent, while that of anxiolytics declined.[25] This sudden acceleration in prescriptions began in 1975, when a second generation of antidepressants, neither MAOIs nor tricyclics, saw the light of day. Some were anxiolytics and were given – a decisive innovation for the generalist – in a single dose, while others were stimulants.[26] They generally had few anticholinergic effects, and some boasted a toxicity much lower than that of the older substances.[27] If generalists continued to be criticized for prescribing too many anxiolytics, the situation did change with this new generation of antidepressants, which was more easily manageable than were the products previously available. Towards the end of the 1970s, some scientists noted signs of change in the procedures of the generalists, and in 1985 Arthur Tatossian estimated that "there has been less holding back in recent years, at least where the so-called new type of stimulant antidepressants is concerned, whose prescription by the generalists seems to account for the increasingly rapid progress antidepressant medications have made in the marketplace between 1979 and 1983, compared to the benzodiazepines."[28] This trend would accelerate with the SSRIs: with this generation of antidepressants, general medicine finally had at hand medication adequate to its diagnostic constraints.

The new products boosted the entire class of antidepressants: a single product was on the market in 1975 and thirteen in 1984, while the tricyclics went from fifteen to twenty and the MAOIs registered a steep decline.[29] The number of antidepressant prescriptions went from about 4.3 million in 1977 to about 7.4 million in 1982. The new molecules represented about 45 percent of the antidepressant market, and one of them – amineptine, a stimulant – topped the list with 20 percent, overtaking for the first time the antidepressant of choice: clomipramine. At the same time, the psychotonics (amphetamines) went from 4.3 million prescriptions to 3.7 million.[30]

ANXIETY AND INHIBITION REDEFINE DEPRESSION

The relationship between anxiety and depression presented a diagnostic problem that was particularly delicate since anxiety was also a feature of depression.[31] In such a case, the prescription of anxiolytics only masked the underlying depressive state and so blurred the depressive picture. Anxiolytic antidepressants helped resolve the therapeutic problem. But in exchange, they encouraged a diagnosis of depression in clinical instances where anxiety dominated, thus inflating the number of depressed individuals. This situation was widely recognized by psychiatry at the beginning of the 1980s: "Today's clinician," wrote, for example, Arthur Tatossian, "tends to subordinate anxiety disorders to depressive disorders, a trend that has most definitely been encouraged by the discovery of antidepressants ... because in fact, the acceptability of diagnostic guidelines, and so the choices made, are a function of the realistic options, in this case of the psychotropic drugs available."[32] The relationship between anxiety and depression became a constant point of contention, starting at least in the mid-1970s.

Anxiety was being eased into depressive territory, but a second symptom, inhibition, began to shift its position as well thanks to the stimulant effects of certain new antidepressants. As with anxiety, its status as a target, privileged or not, of antidepressants was a matter of contention. For some psychiatrists, "the products now available have improved only the tolerance and treatment of the *secondary* symptoms of depression, such as anxiety or inhibition."[33] For others, on the contrary, if the goal of treatment was "to give back to the individual his basic physiological euphoria, ... it also exerts, in varying degrees, a therapeutic influence on two *basic* symptoms of depression: anxiety and inhibition."[34] When these two symptoms were regarded as secondary, depression maintained its status as, essentially, mental distress.

During the second Conference on Psychiatry and Epidemiology held in Geneva in 1983, a psychiatrist noted a clear shift in the therapeutic approach to depression: "Up to 1977, the lifting of inhibition was a major fear of those who hoped first and foremost, by prescribing antidepressants, to relieve their patients' dark thoughts. Today, on the other hand, three of the ten most prescribed antidepressants have adopted inhibition as the most privileged target symptom in their literature."[35] The new antidepressants, the stimulants at least, favoured as their central focus a gradual move away from mental anguish and towards inhibition. All the more so in that, as we have seen, the generalists were more sensitive to complaints that spoke of a "lowering." Depression was emerging less as the opposite of joie de vivre than as *a pathology of action.*[36]

Inhibition was, along with asthenia, the primary target of antidepressant stimulants, which were replacing amphetamines (classified as a dangerous drug since the beginning of the 1970s) and posed fewer risks for the patient: "Their use is of little interest since we now have antidepressants with a strong stimulant component,"[37] such as amineptine, which "may be prescribed for depressions where inhibition is dominant."[38] Psychiatrists debated the true antidepressant status of these substances. In 1980, Julien-Daniel Guelfi, who, fifteen years later, would be the coordinator of the French translation of the DSM-IV, spoke of "substances whose actions constituted a transition between the thymoanaleptic and the psychostimulant."[39] The boundary was unclear between mood elevation and the lifting of inhibition. Did these new substances not represent an adequate response to the triad of asthenia, insomnia, and anxiety? Was this response a therapeutic taking in hand of depression or a kind of mass doping quietly introduced during the second half of the 1970s?

The model for depression that took shape between electroshock therapy and the end of the 1970s was changing. Its pathology had certainly been elusive, but it had still maintained its integrity. It was now breaking down to the point where, as we see in the following chapter, psychiatry would soon be questioning the semantic accuracy of the words "depression" and "antidepressants."

Psychiatric literature at the end of the 1970s and the beginning of the 1980s agreed on this point: the therapeutic effectiveness of antidepressants was not greater than that of iproniazide or imipramine, 30 percent to 40 percent of depressions resisted treatment, and the antidepressant effect only appeared after two, perhaps three weeks.[40] The new antidepressants, nevertheless, provided the GP with a more manageable and less dangerous tool for the patient. She therefore was less hesitant to prescribe them.

The main problem was still the lack of diagnostic consensus. Two paths were followed simultaneously, one feeding on the other, in an attempt to define with some precision, on bases that were not etiological, depression's subcategories – a task now considered "crucial."[41]

These two paths both aimed to establish *correlations*, more reliable regularities, it was thought, than those based on psychopathology. The first path was grounded in biology. Biochemistry had made enormous progress since the 1960s, both on the cellular and molecular levels. The successful search for correlations between a clinical type of depression and a biological marker would allow one to predict the effectiveness of one or another antidepressant. The clinic would then be less dependent on therapeutic proof and would have to rely less on pragmatism – that is, on the clinician's intuition. Instead of verifying the effectiveness of a molecule after the fact, one could evaluate it a priori. In terms of psychodynamics, it was also hoped, during the 1960s, that one would be able to prescribe a psychotropic drug in accordance with the individual's structure of being.

The second path was based on classification. It was grounded in psychiatric epidemiology: the objective was to create a body of trustworthy data by assembling homogeneous population groups from a variety of statistical analyses, epidemiological tools, and scales of depression that would help standardize diagnosis without having to depend on the clinical eye of the practitioner. It would guide psychiatry to what it called its "second revolution." One path involved medication for the mind, while the other involved classification. The latter resulted in the third edition of the *Diagnostic and Statistical Manual of Mental Disorders*, published in the United States in 1980.

What Antidepressant for What Depression?

During the *Journées de la psychiatrie privée* in 1977, the presentations by Roland Kuhn, Jean Oury, Pierre Fédida, and so on clearly reflected depression's decisive hold on psychiatry and psychoanalysis. The text that introduced the conference deserves to be cited as it summed up in one paragraph the state of the pathology: "A crossroads concept, but also catch-all, and not only in the mind of the layman … depression is most certainly characterized by the variety of its aetiologies, of the structures with which it interacts, of the arguments it accommodates. But we are also struck by the variableness of a semiological whole that, to appear comprehensive, tends to spread itself so thin as to entertain the dissolution of its defining mode of expression ('masked' depressions). For some, the only 'constant' data might now be the results obtained from a thymoanaleptic treatment."[42] If the heterogeneity of depression was observed on all sides, there was no consensus on a division into subgroups. The success of depression was not based on a more successful delineation of the pathology but, rather, on a nosographic opening out and a disruption in the category of mood disorders. This explained the uneasiness here and there at the idea of defining depression exclusively as a morbid entity that reacted to antidepressants. The question was: what, in a pathology so varied and deceptive, reacted to these medications?

If depressions were heterogeneous, so were antidepressants.[43] Between the clinical pictures, which were less clear than in earlier times (because the consulting patients had already consumed psychotropic drugs),[44] and the increasing number of products on the market, there was an overall increase in heterogeneity. In fact, the antidepressants, unlike the anxiolytics, had a wide-ranging impact: they acted on sadness, asthenia, anxiety, brooding, headaches, and/ or cervical pain.

Kuhn estimated, as we have seen, that imipramine was much more effective for endogenous depressions than for other depressive states. Indeed, the medication was specific for this group of depressions. For Kline, on the other hand, iproniazide was non-specific because, he thought, it was effective for all depressions. However, this antidepressant was quickly withdrawn from the marketplace because of the probability that patients would contract jaundice. More globally, the MAOIs were little used because, unlike the tricyclics, they presented significant problems not only in interacting with other medications but also with foods such as cheese. And so the tricyclics were the medications of choice. For the time being, psychiatrists agreed on their effectiveness for endogenous depression.[45]

However, Kuhn himself made clear in 1977 that "their use is absolutely legitimate in many instances of neurosis still the exclusive property of psychotherapy, preferably analytic."[46] He noted in 1973 that the antidepressant was effective in "reactive depressions, obsessive neuroses, hysteria, and certain forms of neurotic anxiety and neurasthenia."[47] The argument was that the depressive syndrome was traditionally underestimated in neuroses. In fifteen years, antidepressants had travelled the same uncertain path as did ECT between the end of the 1930s and the end of the 1940s: introduced as therapies specifically for depression, understood in the endogenous sense, they were used for neuroses with a clear depressive character or in those where depression was masked by other symptoms. The debate between neurosis and depression, which we looked at in the previous chapter, was playing itself out on the medical front as well.

Traditional psychiatric reasoning consisted in differentiating between various types of depression and seeking the underlying pathology. If Kuhn underlined the need for such a psychopathological reasoning process (antidepressants are effective in neuroses where depression is manifest), this way of proceeding did not correspond to the dominant procedures in private practice. It was also marginal vis-à-vis the kind of thinking then current in psychiatry. The question at this point was: what kind of antidepressant for what subcategory of depression? Specific antidepressants were being sought for one or another type of depression. The effect of an anxiolytic or a stimulant seemed too crude to "personalize each composite."[48] If the new products had the virtue of being more comfortable and less toxic, they also had another advantage: "These new medications offer a number of possibilities for new approaches in the understanding of depression's deep-seated biology."[49]

Two neuronal paths that could facilitate an understanding of depression's mechanisms were highlighted by biochemistry: noradrenalin and serotonin.[50] Along with dopamine, this gave us the three great systems of neurons called monoaminergics. It was soon confirmed that the tricyclics raised the rate of concentration of serotonin and noradrenalin. The researchers then hypothesized subtypes of the depressed, deficient in one or the other of these neuromediators.

Biochemical models were developed to correlate symptoms with monoaminergic modifications by borrowing from animal pharmacology and human clinical medicine. The hypothesis of subgroups of depressed individuals deficient in serotonin provoked much discussion. A growing number of articles were published on this topic during the 1970s.[51] This hypothesis inspired both strong opposition and great expectations.[52] Clinical research now tried to diversify the use of existing antidepressants. Molecules were found that improved in various ways the activity of different monoaminergic systems, in particular dopamine stimulants that,[53] therapeutically, acted more on inhibition than on sadness and mental anguish.[54] Still, the researchers noted something strange: certain molecules that

increased the transmission of noradrenalin and serotonin did not
have an antidepressant effect, while others that did not modify
transmission activity were true antidepressants. In other words,
indications of all sorts clearly confirmed the role of monoamines,
but the results seemed too contradictory.[55] Édouard Zarifian and
Henri Lôo, in a reference work published in 1982, explicitly refused
to talk about the "antidepressants' mode of action" because "such
a formulation would indicate that one is authorized to relate the
biochemical changes induced in the central nervous system by the
antidepressants to their therapeutic effects. Such is not the case."[56]
Psychiatrists were not successful in correlating the biochemical heterogeneity of depressions with that of antidepressants. An eminent
specialist in psychopharmacology declared: "Treating this problem
is humiliating for someone who had devoted twenty years to doing
so."[57] Still, the relationship between biochemical and therapeutic
action remained a fruitful hypothesis.

   The temptation was obviously strong to resort to the ever so practical therapeutic proof: the "true" depression was that on which antidepressants had an effect. This led to the tendency to reserve
depression for antidepressants. *La Revue du praticien* devoted two
special issues to depression in 1978 and 1985, respectively. The tone
changed significantly between these two dates. In 1978, Daniel
Widlöcher wrote that the biochemical and psychogenetic currents
were mutually enriching, "which ma[de] depression the psychopathological disorder for which the level of understanding and the
therapeutic possibilities [were] the most promising."[58] Seven years
later, Jean-Claude Scotto, who oversaw the dossier on depression,
wrote of psychotherapy: "This word must be taken in its widest sense,
that which privileges a 'supportive' action, one of accompaniment
…, *requiring no particular technical training*. But … the nub of the
treatment is biological: sismotherapy [i.e., ECT] and antidepressants."[59] This meant, on the one hand, that psychotherapy was no
longer to be considered as a basic treatment, and on the other hand,
that it was no longer a way of bringing to the surface unconscious
conflicts and enabling the patient to face them.

   In the mid-1980s, the deficit model produced an unprecedented
partnership between therapies of liberation and chemical medication. At a point when one still did not know how to define depression, but had in hand effective antidepressants that were manageable
and acted quite successfully on the depressive mood (whether

inhibited or anxious), what could this pathology be if not what antidepressants cured? In such cases, the notion of conflict was totally irrelevant as a guide to diagnosis. In fact, a descriptive paradigm had taken the place of an etiological paradigm.

THE BATTLE OF CLASSIFICATIONS

Psychiatry's second option for resolving the diagnostic chaos was classification. To the degree that etiological disagreements could not be resolved, one had only to ignore the etiological question and aim for the most precise clinical description possible. The major challenge was how to improve diagnostic *reliability*. This meant finding criteria that would allow clinicians independently evaluating the same patient to make the same diagnosis. The choice of treatment was left up to the clinician as the tools developed were for purposes of research.

Classification's solution to the problem of depression's heterogeneity had as its consequence the splitting off of these syndromes from the categories of neurosis or psychosis.

In 1980, the American Psychiatric Association (APA) published a classification that had required a good ten years of work: the *Diagnostic and Statistical Manual of Mental Disorders*, third edition, better known as the DSM-III. The manual was partially revised in 1987 (DSM-III-R), and a fourth edition was published in 1994 (DSM-IV).[60] The DSM was a turning point for world psychiatry.

THE CONTEXT OF A "REVOLUTION"

American psychiatry between the two wars and after the Second World War was completely different from French psychiatry.[61] The conflicts between neurologists and psychiatrists were marginal, the role of universities in the regulation of the psychiatric profession was much more significant than in France, and federal institutions made a major contribution to the development of mental health policies. Thus, the National Institute of Mental Health, created in 1946, not only had the financial means to promote ambitious policies but also quantitative research inconceivable in Europe. Also, psychoanalysts were doctors (by decision of the American Psychoanalytic Association in 1927), and psychoanalysis was integrated into medical institutions. If American psychiatrists were by and large analysts during the 1950s, the theoretical inspiration for American psychoanalysis was very different from that for French psychoanalysis. The key figure in American psychiatry during the first half of the twentieth century, Adolf Meyer,[62] organized Freud's first visit to the United States in 1909. The psychoanalysis he promoted (without being himself an analyst) was a kind of mental hygiene, a developmental technique aimed at reinforcing the patients' Ego: and it was called Ego psychology. The world explored dealt less with the patients' phantasms than with their capacity to adapt to reality.[63]

American psychiatry was not traditionally one of classification, in that its dominant conception of mental illness was "psychosocial." It had three characteristics. The first was a reactive reflex much favoured by Meyer: any person exposed to shocks that were sufficiently powerful was liable to develop a mental pathology. The second was a unitary vision of mental illness: the differences between psychoses and neuroses were quantitative and not qualitative, the pathology's degree of severity being the determining factor. The concepts of reaction and intensity implied a view of pathology that diverged from Kraepelin's picture of discrete entities. The third characteristic was a diagnostic etiology: what lay behind the symptom or syndrome?

Several factors intrinsic to American society during the 1960s led the psychiatric profession to take a radical turn where classification was concerned. The strength of the American antipsychiatric movement put the profession on the defensive: if the distinction between normal and pathological was fluid, as the psychosocial model proposed, then psychiatric diagnoses were perfectly arbitrary. The introduction of a paying third party (Medicaid and Medicare) led the administration to have diagnoses and therapies evaluated, a difficult undertaking given the lack of standardized criteria. What is more, the discovery of medications for the mind revealed a specifically American problem: an over-diagnosis of schizophrenia and an under-diagnosis of depression. Neuroleptics were prescribed for patients who were, in reality, depressive. Finally, the changes of the 1960s, which put mental disorders increasingly in the hands of doctors in private practice and community psychiatry, led to psychiatrists being regarded, to a degree, as part social workers and part psychotherapists.[64]

This reform was also related to some very clear international challenges. Indeed, it was conceived with that of the World Health

Organization in mind. In the second half of the 1960s, because national systems of description, diagnosis, and classification varied greatly, it tried to establish psychiatric categories that would make international comparisons feasible.[65] Now, with the advent of medications for the mind, psychopharmacological disciplines, as well as the markets, had gone international (the creation in 1958 of the *Collegium Internationale Neuro-Psychopharmacologicum* [CINP] served as a model). But the principal market, given its size, was the United States. And there, we find a player that could not be ignored: the Food and Drug Administration (FDA). Its standards of authorization were very strict. In particular, the medication had to be submitted for approval and had to show itself to be visibly effective. Statistical tools of evaluation were required: double blind studies comparing the medication to other products already in use (products of choice) as well as to a placebo were made compulsory.[66] For the studies to be demonstrably effective, and acceptable to all the players in the system, categories of depression and of homogeneous depressive populations were essential.

This new emphasis on classification was thus the result of psychiatry's internationalization, of the special place it occupied in the American market, and of the new difficulties encountered by American psychiatry during the 1960s.

FRENCH UNIVERSITY PSYCHIATRY AND CLASSIFICATION REFORM

French university psychiatry was not part of this vast enterprise, but it easily went along with it. There were few debates in psychiatric journals as long as the clinical tradition was strong, psychoanalysis was a reference for chemotherapy, and antipsychiatry still had little impact compared to what was happening in Great Britain and the United States.[67] INSERM's psychiatric classification, published in 1968, was a glossary, and the questionnaires and standardized scales of evaluation had little weight in France: Pierre Pichot was one of the few French figures to have developed such a scale.[68] And so the epidemiological tradition was weak.

French psychiatry was not supported by strong state institutions. There was no French equivalent to the NIMH. INSERM, founded in 1962, and whose first director general played a decisive role in the development of community mental health centres, had much less influence than did the NIMH. The most prestigious psychiatrists of the 1960s (Ey, Daumézon, etc.) were not academics, and psychiatric hospitals were not integrated with general hospitals.

The separation of neurology and psychiatry in 1968 (the 31 July law) enabled a growing number of psychiatrists to embark on a university career and to become department heads, as in any other medical discipline. They found themselves in a professional situation that favoured more academic research based on epidemiology, statistical tools, and so on, which led to departures from older clinical research. The scientific appeal of reasoning was crucial in a university setting. Industrialists found an intermediary identical to that in countries where universities had a strong psychiatric tradition and where various methods of standardized evaluation were in force. Classification reform also made it possible to provide general practitioners with a more functional model than the old three-part division.

If the psychoanalytic reference was maintained among professors of clinical psychology,[69] such was not the case in psychiatry, especially since psychoanalysis began to lose much of its prestige at the end of the 1970s. As of the 1980s, analysis was no longer a requirement for psychiatric interns. What is more, the reform of the competitions for interns in 1982 eliminated the internship specializing in psychiatry. That implied that the "choice" of psychiatry as a profession was tied less to the student's personal motivation than to her placing in the results of the competition; the culture of these psychiatrists was more medical.[70] The old style psychiatry, embodied in Henri Ey (who died in 1977) and the tradition of doctor-philosophers, insisted on the role controversy had to play because it was impossible to arrive at an etiological consensus. Epidemiological methods, the reliance on data and inter-rater reliability, together built a consensus that marginalized etiology. Not that disagreements vanished and that no trend tended to dominate but, rather, that the psychiatric milieu began to function according to "the juxtaposition of procedures and the superimposition of theories."[71]

THE AMERICAN MACHINE IS SET IN MOTION

The American Psychiatric Association's decision to develop a classification system that would serve as a true diagnostic guide was part of a strategy aimed at solidly anchoring psychiatry in scientific medicine. So said Gerald Klerman, one of the most important American psychiatrists and a world expert in depression, during a debate organized by the APA in 1982: "The decision of the APA first to develop DSM-III and then to promulgate its use represents a significant reaffirmation on the part of American psychiatry to its medical identity and to its commitment to scientific medicine."[72]

An enormous program was set in motion, with multiple ramifications. Robert Spitzer of Columbia University in New York was named to head the working group set up to prepare the revision of the DSM-II. In 1974, fourteen committees were constituted, specializing in the principal categories of mental disorder. They oversaw a number of studies in the field, organized conferences to achieve consensus, set up subcommittees to deal with litigious questions, and negotiated with various professional organizations (whether they were associations of psychoanalysts, child psychiatrists, psychologists, etc.). This procedural deployment had to produce a classification that was acceptable to all of the profession's tendencies; epidemiological data as the means and consensus as the objective were the two main axes of the DSM-III. The studies in the field, which took place between 1977 and 1979 under the patronage of the NIMH, involved nearly 13,000 patients, evaluated by 550 clinicians.

The shift in centre of gravity from the psychiatric hospital to psychiatry in the community resulted in another series of epidemiological studies bearing on the population's health problems.[73] A commission set up in 1977 to evaluate the mental health needs of the country, commissioned, under the direction of the NIMH, an epidemiological study of twenty thousand people in five locations known as epidemiological catchment areas (ECAS). Its aim was to systematically gather data concerning the prevalence of mental illnesses, as well as their syndromes and symptoms, in the general population. This research drew on new diagnostic methods developed during the 1970s to produce the DSM-III and was to contribute to a future revision of the manual. Begun in 1980, it gave rise to the publication in 1991 of a veritable "atlas" of mental disorders: *Psychiatric Disorders in America*. A clear picture emerged from this survey of American mental problems: an increase in depression, alcoholism, and drug abuse.[74]

NEVER MIND THE CAUSE
AS LONG AS ONE IS "RELIABLE"

The introduction to the DSM-III was a clear expression of its view of mental illness and enabled a good understanding of its thinking.[75] The DSM provided an approach that had implications for all mental disorders: the lack of consensus had spawned a number of different psychiatric doctrines, giving far too much weight to the psychiatrist's personal judgment in making a diagnosis. The solution was to do an end run around this judgment by applying a language shared by the entire profession, whatever the clinicians' orientations. The APA developed the equivalent of what computer experts call "an expert system" to achieve diagnostic reliability through consensus. The means it employed were embodied in the three notions underlying the DSM-III: (1) the concept of mental disorders, (2) the descriptive approach and diagnostic criteria, and (3) multiaxial assessment.

With regard to the first notion underlying the DSM, according to Spitzer, mental disorder was a "clinically significant behavioral or psychological syndrome or pattern that occurs in an individual and that is typically associated with either a painful symptom (distress) or impairment in one or more important areas of functioning (disability)." The disorder had as its source a distress that found expression as a disabling syndrome. The sick individual *had* a syndrome, as Spitzer wrote: "A common misconception is that a classification of mental disorders classifies people, when actually what are being classified are disorders that people have. For this reason, the text of DSM-III avoids the use of such expressions as 'a schizophrenic' or 'an alcoholic' and instead uses the more accurate, but admittedly more cumbersome, 'an individual with Schizophrenia' or 'an individual with alcohol dependence.'"[76] Neither the type of psychological structure nor the symptom's meaning for the individual was pertinent. Its supporters referred to this approach as neo-Kraepelinian because it saw pathologies as discrete entities.[77] However, these entities did not define illnesses but syndromes. In practical terms this changed nothing because these syndromes were treated like illnesses.

With regard to the second notion underlying the DSM, the manual was said to be atheoretical and descriptive:[78] atheoretical because it took no position vis-à-vis the various etiological theories, descriptive because its goal was to describe symptoms as precisely as possible.

The clinic alone could not provide what epidemiology called good inter-rater reliability. To carefully describe, one had to have at hand the criteria that would make possible the inclusion or exclusion of such or such type of disorder. That is why the DSM-III shifted the centre of gravity for categories from the clinic to research. Two teams of psychiatric researchers played the most important roles: John P. Feighner of Washington Hospital at the University of Saint Louis (Missouri) and Robert Spitzer (the master planner of the DSM-III) of the New York State Psychiatric Institute at Columbia University. The first team focused on the criteria of inclusion or exclusion that would determine whether an individual did or did not have mental disorder X. For that, it developed protocols enabling it to undertake epidemiological studies on a large scale, with twenty-five diagnostic categories. The second team devised statistical tools to measure the trustworthiness of the criteria and to systematize them. This method relied upon what became known as "research diagnostic criteria." It was developed by the Spitzer team in the context of a project dealing with the psychobiology of depression, the better to identify eventual subtypes. The two teams set up protocols for interviews based on this new criteria, which enabled them to reduce the variance in information.[79]

To derive clear and precise diagnostic criteria that would provide the consensus so ardently desired, it was essential to produce viable data.[80] The epidemiological studies and the structured interviews during which the clinician ticked off the symptoms made possible the assembling of homogeneous populations for each category of mental disorder.

With regard to the third notion underlying the DSM, the clinicians were subject to tight constraints but were left the possibility of making a diagnosis in terms of a number of axes: this diagnosis was referred to as being multiaxial. Axis I included all the mental disorders classified as syndromes an individual could *have*. Axis II targeted these same syndromes but from the point of view of personality: "The diagnosis of a Personality Disorder should be made only when the characteristic features are typical of the individual's long-term functioning and are not limited to discrete episodes of illness."[81] That enabled one not to forget them "when attention [was] directed to the usually more florid Axis I disorders."[82] In other words, a patient could have a disorder without the clinician needing to ask to what extent facets of his personality or his history might be playing a role. If there was a depressive episode, one treated the episode, not the individual. Axis III was reserved for physical disorders, Axis IV for the "Severity of Psychosocial Stressors" (this is where the reactive disorders were slotted), and Axis V for the adaptation and general functioning of the individual. "The multiaxial system provides a biopsychosocial approach to assessment,"[83] but only on one condition: that these three notions be taken together and not set in opposition to one another.

MOOD DISORDER TRIUMPHS OVER NEUROTIC DEPRESSION

In the DSM-I, neurotic depression "is manifested by an excessive reaction of depression due to an internal conflict or to an identifiable event," wrote Klerman. No precise diagnostic criterion was required of the clinician. Neurotic depression was put to the test of inter-rater reliability: the coefficient of reliability was very poor and, in any case, far below that which existed for schizophrenia.[84] According to Feighner, for a clinician to diagnose a depressive disorder in the DSM-III, three demands had to be met: (1) the existence of a dysphoric mood whose symptoms could be sadness, irritability, discouragement, and so on; (2) the presence of at least five criteria out of the eight in the category (lack of appetite or weight loss, difficulty sleeping, loss of energy or fatigue, agitation or listlessness, loss of interest, blaming oneself or feeling guilty, inability to concentrate, recurring thoughts of death or suicide); and (3) these symptoms had to last for at least a month.[85] The clinician only had to check off the symptoms in order to diagnose a depression. She was not to focus on an individual's history but on his symptoms.

Given that the concepts endogenous, exogenous, and neurotic imply an etiology but that it was seemingly impossible to arrive at a unanimously recognized boundary between these different types of depression, they were replaced by the notion of "major depression," which was included in the category of emotional disturbances[86] – that is, disturbances characterized by a perturbation of mood. The category of neuroses was eliminated from the DSM. The controversy following on this elimination led Spitzer to justify the action in his introduction to the third edition of the work: "Freud used the term both *descriptively* (to indicate a painful symptom in an individual with intact reality testing) and to indicate the *etiological process* (unconscious conflict arousing anxiety."[87] The DSM retained (for the time being) only the descriptive meaning under the category "neurotic disorders." This was a concession made to the psychoanalysts during the 1979 conference that gave final approval to the DSM-III project because their association was refusing to endorse it. The compromise was accepted. The great specialist in anxiety, Donald Klein, one of those responsible for the DSM-III and whose work led to the breakdown of anxiety neurosis into panic attack and generalized anxiety disorder, declared ten years later: "The neurosis controversy was a *minor capitulation* to *psychoanalytic nostalgia.*"[88]

What were formally neuroses were broken down and redistributed into the categories of "Affective, Anxiety, Somatoform, Dissociative, and Psychosexual Disorders."[89] In the DSM-II, anxiety was seen as the principal symptom of neurosis, while in the DSM-III it was just one of the anxiety disorders.[90] In the DSM-IV, the term "neurotic disorders" was eliminated.

Affect dominated the new classification landscape; it was at the core of clinical description. Most commentaries on the DSM-III, whether in the form of praise or criticism, agreed that affective, or thymic, disorders had become dominant and that depression's territory had widened.[91] Neurotic depression was the weakest link in the depressive family because, on the one hand, it was the most diagnosed,[92] and, on the other hand, it was the subject of the greatest discord among psychiatrists:[93] the neurotic depression of the DSM-II (1968) became a dysthymic disorder in the DSM III, while hysteria was broken down into somatoform and dissociative disorders: "DSM-III bade farewell not only to the psychodynamic conflict model, but also to a broader tradition in which anxiety was associated with disorders in personality structure ... Anxiety was no longer regarded as a consequence of the personality structure but primarily as a symptom in and of itself."[94] As to the concept of personality disorders, it referred to the long-term continuity of symptoms.

Given that we at last knew what we were talking about (the syndromes were clearly described), the role of the clinician now consisted only in selecting the adequate treatment, whether it be chemotherapeutic, cognitive, behavioural, or psychoanalytic, according to what he had marked off – the DSM-III-R, in any case, added a decision tree to help the clinician. These syndromes were "discrete entities." In other words, symptoms correlated systematically. The search for underlying structures was abandoned, and the term "illness" was replaced with the term "disorder." Not only was it more logical than that of "illness," but it possessed the immense advantage of being imprecise, as psychiatry explicitly recognized.[95] The DSM was characterized by stable combinations of symptoms whose formative processes, neurotic or psychotic, were of little importance. Psychiatric research based on statistical data supplanted clinical research that was no longer useful. The model for illness was a deficit model centred on affect.

A FRONTIER QUICKLY CROSSED BETWEEN RESEARCH AND TREATMENT

The DSM-III aroused much controversy because it represented a change in the conception of mental illnesses. The American psychiatrist Mitchell Wilson summed it up very well: the idea of the unconscious no longer had any importance, the temporal dimension was marginalized (the individual's history lent no meaning to the symptoms), and personality now played a secondary role: "Further, the emphasis on careful description fosters the confusion of the easily observable with the clinically relevant."[96]

One of the controversial points concerned the relationship between the ideas of reliability and validity. Reliability, as we have seen, ensured that two clinicians independently examining the same patient would make the same diagnosis. The DSM was organized, as of the third edition, in such a way as to improve inter-rater reliability. Where epidemiological research was concerned, one point was decisive: studies could now agree on the categories examined and make comparisons that led to pertinent results. This was particularly useful in spotting the risk factors so essential to epidemiology.

On the clinical side, the problem was different: validity concerned the nature of the disorder, or the value of the category that included the disorder. One had the right to talk of validity when one could establish a relationship between a syndrome and a lesion or a pathological process that was its cause (reliability being concerned only with an agreement on the identification of the syndrome). And where mental disorders were concerned, such validity could only be determined in a consensual manner.

The fact that the DSM's psychiatric thinking was based on reliability presented a clinical problem that was well expressed by a French epidemiologist in 1978: "Mood disorders, an important parameter in almost any mental illness, must not, their contents hemmed in by descriptive procedure, and rapidly halted therapeutically by antidepressants, eclipse in the mind of the researcher or practitioner the underlying mental illness or pathological structure. Otherwise, with a large proportion of pathological structures considered as depressions, noted and treated as such in the short term, one would be likely to neglect or deny the mental illnesses underlying the depressive symptoms."[97] As unimportant as this problem was for research (reliability being the condition for scientific results to be proven valid), it was crucial for the clinician, who risked, by concentrating exclusively on the syndrome, letting the pathology persist.[98] André Haynal made the same point differently: "The discussions concerning criteria make us sensitive to the fact that we do not know what we are talking about, when, for example, we speak of depressive *patients*."[99]

In fact, if we did not know what we were talking about, what was the meaning of the term "to treat"? The DSM was an instrument devised for researchers, but when clinicians used it as a diagnostic technique, it risked restricting medicine to the simple recognition of syndromes and stopping there. The psychiatrist, for her part, risked confusing her role as a researcher (reliability) with her role as a clinician (validity). Therein lay the ambiguity of the DSM: designed for research, it was also applied clinically: "The researcher's needs, are, however, very different from those of the clinician. Thus, the reductionism favouring, in aetiopathogenesis, biological *or* psychological *or* social factors, is permissible and even desirable in research, but ruinous for patient care."[100]

The Decline of Neuroses, the End of a Certain Psychiatry?

The departure from the scene of the tripartite endogenous, psychogenetic, exogenic classificatory system came about in two ways: (1) chemical treatment of mental pathology no longer required necessarily listening to the individual but, rather, simply identifying the patient's symptoms; and (2) the notion of *data* served to correlate symptoms in order to regroup them into syndromic categories. Etiology was no longer a pertinent mode of classification. Defining the type of individual who would suffer from one kind of depression rather than another had little practical importance for treating the illness. It was difficult to apply in general medicine, all the more so in that new problems appeared in psychopathology along with the debates over narcissistic pathologies, and nothing in psychiatry's internal dynamics favoured a reference to conflict as a way of dealing with pathological diversity. Conflict, perhaps satisfying on the intellectual level, had not proven itself therapeutically, and the type of neuroses it engendered was perhaps less common than were the pathologies of emptiness. Our trio's eclipse meant that the psychiatric system had become, not hostile, but indifferent to the idea of the self.

If the first psychiatric revolution, that of shock treatment and then medication, paved the way for the complementary use of a deficit model and a conflict model, then the second revolution, that of nosography, confirmed their divorce. It was the end of the Janet-Cerletti-Freud axis, which had encouraged an understanding of how the pathology of a self could be biologically cured. The period we have just examined opened the door to a new era, imbuing psychiatry with the idea that one could treat disorders of the mind or of behaviour exclusively biologically. Chemical treatment of the mind's pathology was no longer a facilitator for psychotherapy; black moods and somatic symptoms of all sorts could be treated without intrapsychic conflicts needing to be clarified.

In ten years, psychiatry had realized its *aggiornamento*: affect and mood were now the starting points for a consideration of mental disorders and their therapeutic management. The twilight of neurosis brought with it the demise of conflict. That split within the self between two terms in opposition to one other but still related ceased, in large part, to interest the medical community. This division was alien territory to the deficit model of illness when it was no longer supported by the conflict model, whether in the form of psychotherapy or biological psychiatry. The seeds were sown for future controversies regarding the boundary between the normal and the pathological. "Here there appears in outline ... the existence of a personality without conflict," wrote Lucien Israël in a sharp attack on the new classifications.[101]

The alliance between deficit and conflict enabled the psychotropic drug to be *only* a medication. Their separation raised the question: drug or medication? "Very often the depressed individual does not have to actively seek out the help of a drug; his doctors take the initiative in making him a 'passive' addict. Is that really necessary? Is that therapeutic progress, in the sense that the patient's true personality finds itself hidden from the outside world and led along a path that severs the affective connection making a psychological approach possible?"[102] The substance acted directly on the feelings but, emphasized the psychoanalysts, did not help the patient to build up her own system of defence – at least when this treatment did not also involve working with the patient in such a way that the patient was also at work. It produced a short circuit with her own self in that the individual was not presented with conditions that enabled her to distance herself, on her own, from her conflicts.

The divorce between the conflict model and the deficit model was encouraged both by the norms concerning the multiplication of the self, which sustained the illusion that one could dispense with what one could not master, and by the insecurity vis-à-vis one's identity, which served as a reminder that it was an illusion. The encounter between the dynamics of emancipation that freed the individual from discipline and conflict, and the transformations within psychiatry that furnished the practical answers to the problems created by this liberation, signalled a shift in the style of despair. The yielding of neurosis to depression marked not only the end of a certain psychiatry but also the decline of an individual's collective experience as embodied both in a deference to discipline and in conflict. It was a sea change in the subjectivity of modern humanity.

In 1973 a psychiatrist wrote, in a premonitory vein: "Under present circumstances I fear that if the concept of 'depression' were to be exploited with too much enthusiasm, it could endanger the therapeutic role that thymoanaleptic agents have played, successfully, up to the present time. In other words, raising doubts as to the diagnostic validity of 'depression' could discourage the use of antidepressants in their specific applications. We ought, I think, to be careful not to pay too much attention to the patients' mood. That could lead to forms of extremism and superficiality comparable to those we now accord to the least little indisposition resulting from minor fluctuations in blood pressure."[103] In fact, such exploitation eventually raised suspicions: did medication change the personality rather than treat pathologies? New ways of lessening or doing away with depression led to the fear that we were making of our psyche, as Pierre Legendre wrote, "an adjustable assembly."[104] If everything was possible was everything permitted? In France, the international upheavals surrounding mental disorders were viewed in the light of a venerable tradition concerning the metaphysics of the Self. One went so far as to fear its disappearance. Were we not, rather, witnessing its progressive metamorphosis?

PART THREE

The Inadequate Individual

The physiology of automatism is easier to describe than that of autonomy.
> Georges Canguilhem, *La formation du concept de réflexe
> aux XVIIe et XVIIIe siècles,* 1955 (7)

Depression is not a subjective state, it is a style of action.
> Daniel Widlöcher, "L'échelle de ralentissement dépressif:
> Fondements théoriques et premiers résultats," 1981 (56)

PATHOLOGICAL ACTION: THE SECOND SHIFT IN THE REPRESENTATION OF THE INDIVIDUAL

The first shift in direction for the system of norms defining the individual in the first half of the twentieth century involved "being oneself." This is what characterized the "general spirit" of the new normality. At the pathological level, clinical practice, especially that of psychoanalysis, altered its focus from a domain where conflict, guilt, and anxiety prevailed to a domain where inadequacy, the void, compulsion, and impulse delineated the portrait of pathological humanity. The new normative approach and the new pathology were concerned less with identification (with well-defined parental images or social roles) than with identity. Identity was the first instrument leading to the redefinition of today's individual. During the 1980s, self-affirmation worked its way into everyday life to the point where a housewife under the age of fifty did not hesitate to bare the most intimate details of her private life on television.

This decade was innovative in another way. It was not simply a matter of being oneself, of setting out blissfully in search of one's "authenticity"; one also had to act on one's own, to rely on one's own internal resources.[1] The second instrument of turn-of-the-century individuality was that of individual action.

The gospel of personal fulfilment was backed up by the commandments of individual initiative. The questions of *identity* and of *action* came together in the following way: on the normative side, individual initiative joined forces with psychic liberation; on the pathological side, a difficulty in initiating action was associated with identity insecurity. The eclipse of regulation through discipline led to the individual agent's being responsible for his own actions. At the same time, psychiatric thinking was more and more convinced that the fundamental problem in depression was psychomotor: what had been a mood disorder was now a dysfunction in mental activity. To violate the norm was less a matter of disobedience than of being unable to act. This was a new concept of individuality.

Chapter 6 puts forward the hypothesis that depression would from now on be characterized by two main attributes, one of which is entangled with the other. First, the very idea of a depressive syndrome collapsed. Second, the psychiatric gaze shifted to the pathological act: inhibition and "psychomotor slowing" took precedence over mental pain and sadness. At the same time, the pharmaceutical industry launched a new generation of molecules unprecedented in their promises of a cure. This shift in the psychiatric approach to depression was related to the context in which it occurred: a demand for action that weighed increasingly on each individual. There was a demand for medicinal assistance. Psychiatric literature spread the news, the media became concerned, public authorities set up commissions or commissioned reports that had no impact on public behaviour.

Chapter 7 shows how depression became a chronic identity pathology. This resulted from the migration of the neurotic terrain, with its long-term personality disorders, into the continent of depression. Now the distinction between a mood disorder that one had (in the course of a depressive episode) and the troubled personality that one was lost its former meaning. The chronic nature of the condition jeopardized the idea of a cure. The result was the emergence of a persona with wide implications: the valid invalid. It is not so much that it provided added evidence for the over-publicized crisis of the self as that it signalled a shift in the experience of subjectivity, a reorganization of the relationship between private and public that defined the arena in which modern intimacy would be played out. The reactions to the crisis of the cure suggested that curing something was no longer the issue; what was important was to be *accompanied* and *modified* more or less constantly – by pharmacology, by therapy, and by socio-political means.

6

The Depressive Breakdown

The traditional emphasis on mental pain has moved towards pathological action: mood disorders would be less characteristic of depression than would those involving the inability to act. The latter are
the favourite targets of molecules: by moving the individual towards
action, they improve her mood. Insecurity about identity, as we have
seen, and disturbed activity, as we will see, are the two facets of
depressive states at the end of the twentieth century. Depression
embodies not only the passion for being oneself and its difficulty
but also the need for initiative and the difficulty of carrying it
through. How can action be successfully undertaken? Each individual is exhorted to act by herself by mobilizing her affect instead of
applying external rules. This new normativity implies another interior state, another body than the one demanded by discipline.

FROM MOOD DISORDER TO ACTIVITY DISTURBANCE

Traditional psychiatry has divided depressive states into two large
entities: (1) mental pain (specifically, psychic suffering) and (2) the
general slowing of the person manifested by inhibition, asthenia,
and the slowing of the movements of both body and mind. The
second entity concerns the more bodily aspects of depression. More
to the point, it concerns what is the most animal in humans – that
is, motricity. In fact, when animal studies speak of depression, they
refer mostly to slowed or agitated behaviour. We cannot tell if a rat
is sad, but we can observe its behaviour under a series of stressors.
Movement is the issue. Depression is the absence of movement in its
mental aspect.

If, in psychiatry, there has long been a debate over which of these two entities is most characteristic of depression, slowing has been mostly considered as a consequence of mental pain. Coupled with the absence of guilt delirium, this feature made it possible to distinguish all forms of depression from melancholia. Melancholia is a disturbance of *élan vital,* while depression is a mood disorder that turns all feelings grey and, for that reason, affects movement. We have seen that the movement of sad passion towards anxiety and inhibition began in the second half of the 1970s. So, it was explained to generalists, "these rather frequent states marked by sadness more than truly depressive mood and where somatic signs are absent"[2] should not be considered as depression. Psychomotor slowing and sleep disorders form the greater part of the clinical picture. The lack of initiative is the fundamental disorder of the depressed person. Mental pain finds itself compromised by the theme of numbed affect: this sort of indifference is to mood what apathy is to action.

A new psychiatric point of view has begun to take over, especially in France and several other European countries, and it was called "transnosographic." The key concept of its analysis was no longer the syndrome, which was relegated to the dungeon because it arose from a nosography inadequate for mental disorders, but the *dimension.* Two major dimensions stand out: inhibition and impulsiveness. The latter is the flip side of the former, and they are both part of the pathology of action. In inhibition, action is absent; in impulsiveness, it is uncontrolled. The territory of apathy, whose impulse is in general the mask, now covers that of depression.

DIMENSION, OR THE EXPLOSION OF DEPRESSION

The role of fatigue in depression has long been discussed. Is it a secondary or primordial symptom in thymic disorder? Does it result from the depressed person's pessimism, disinterest, and absence of motivation? Does it precede the attack of depression properly speaking, that is, the appearance of the mood disorder? At the Salpêtrière hospital, at the end of the 1970s, Daniel Widlöcher and his team created a scale of "psychomotor slowing."[3] The statistical analyses carried out by the team on patients treated with antidepressants showed that there are close links between asthenia and slowing: "The fatigue symptom is correlated mainly to the ensemble of features that we bring together under the general term of psychomotor slow-ing."4 This fatigue shows two aspects. First, produced by ruminations and obsessions, it arises from psychoasthenia in Janet's sense and is manifested by "an incapacity for action." Second, it is the way that the person experiences slowing, his "subjective expression."5 Willy-nilly, inhibition finds itself at the centre of depression.

Mental pain is the consequence of psychomotor slowing. That is why depression is, according to Daniel Widlöcher, "a style of action."6 Like anxiety, it is an overall behavioural response. He developed this idea in a book published in 1983, in which he argues that anxi-ety and depression are "two elementary responses that function secondarily as signals regarding one's entourage and oneself. Anxiety carries out a mental behaviour of fight or struggle against internal tensions and external dangers; on the other hand, the falling back of depression constitutes a protective attitude involving retreat that allows the subject to survive when he has no more energy to fight."7 Anxiety is a mechanism for fighting, and depression is its abandon-ment. In depression there is a psychology of inferiority, a vulnerabil-ity that is much less evident in anxiety.

Widlöcher bases his analysis on the effect of classical antidepres-sants: "We know that antidepressants are particularly effective in forms where fatigue is not accompanied by mental distress, whereas they have no effect in cases involving sadness if it is not accompanied by a certain inhibition. They are neither 'euphoria agents' nor 'pain-killers' but, rather, disinhibitors."8 "Disinhibitor": that is the key word. Antidepressants treat dysfunctions of *movement* in their mental aspects. They restore powers of action and improve mood that has been adversely affected by disturbance. Besides, clinicians notice more and more that antidepressants act on morbid states other than depression and in which anxiety and mental pain are not present.

It has certainly been noted for some time now that antidepressants can be used outside of depression.9 Independently of any associated depressive pathology, today they are prescribed for panic disorders; phobias; post-traumatic stress; compulsive disorders; generalized anxiety;10 eating disorders; dependency on alcohol, tobacco or heroine; autism; Tourette's Syndrome; and so on. 11 They would also seem to act on cephalalgia, migraines, and cancer-related and neu-rological pain.12 Imipramines have some effect on enuresia, akinesia due to Parkinson's, and so on.13 Since the beginning of the 1980s, a disorder that was thought to be rare became the object of many studies: "Obsessive-compulsive disorders, that modern nomenclature placed under the heading of anxiety pathologies, have ... much to do with depression."[14] They have replaced the former obsessive neuroses,[15] and they could be sensitive to SSRIs, including in cases when they are not accompanied by depression.

Therein lies the questioning about the very word "antidepressant" that psychiatrists and pharmacologists have such trouble defining. "The use of antidepressants," notes one pharmacologist, "now goes far beyond the treatment of depression, and this poses a problem, which is knowing what an antidepressant really is."[16] The diversity of more or less definable complaints that these molecules can treat is so wide that the notion of depression overflows the banks of symptomology. Would that not be the logical outcome of depression's destiny? Is it not a pathology impossible to define, a deceptive illness, a concept that is "poorly explained but in which the individual's overall organization seems to be involved"[17] – in other words, an overall behavioural response? The disease from which all other diseases can flow is a good "field" for other psychiatric disorders.

The critique of the symptom-based concept of the DSMs is influential in France. It continues the tradition of pharmacological dissection because medication is an analyzer of behaviour. The psychotropes must be classified, not illnesses or syndromes. Medication must be prescribed for its effect on a clinical dimension, not as a function of nosography. A dimension is a feature, the way we speak of a feature of inhibited or impulsive character. It doesn't matter if we are dealing with an anxious or depressive state since the feature can be found in a multitude of syndromes, and we must act on it.

This analysis was based on psychiatry. A similar approach came into being based on biochemistry. It took its inspiration from the success of the monoaminergetic hypothesis and the practical results that work on serotonin led to with regard to SSRIs. A work on serotonin, published in 1991 in the United States, described its role in numerous psychiatric symptoms and offered an analysis.[18] Insufficient or excess serotonin does not signify that it is the cause of these multiple disorders, nor does it indicate that other neurotransmitters are not involved. Serotonin is considered as the neurochemical vector of a person's equilibrium. Equilibrium dysfunctions form a couple consisting of opposing dimensions: inhibition and impulsiveness. The dimension-based hypothesis takes us back to the notion of reaction, as both van Praag and Widlöcher pointed out,[19] a notion that dominated American psychiatric reasoning before the discipline converted to biological psychiatry.

This approach certainly owes its success to its adaptability to the work of general practitioners, whose tendency is to produce diagnoses based on dimensionality.[20] As well, unlike specialists, general practitioners grant more importance to the short term than to the long term as well as to the patient's comfort.

INHIBITION AND IMPULSIVENESS: THE TWO FACES OF PATHOLOGICAL ACTIVITY

If we are dealing with a "hyposerotonin" patient, the impulsive dimension is dominant, with its sudden violence, suicidal ideas, explosive acting out, bulimia, and addictive behaviours (alcoholism and pathological gambling). If we are dealing with a "hyperserotonin" person, inhibition is massive. Impulsiveness is the difficulty of controlling an action, whereas inhibition is action hindered. It is "the cardinal concept of depression."[21]

The first French colloquium on this theme took place in 1978. The speakers pointed out with near unanimity that inhibition is as frequent as it is non-specific: "The concept of inhibition cannot be applied to something that is in the order of personal initiative ... Inhibition holds back the act, the expression, the behaviour."[22] Holding back, freezing, braking, suspension of activity, and so on are all part of the language of apathy. Impulsiveness is also part of it as it is not the opposite of inhibition but, rather, the mask behind which apathy is hidden,[23] a secondary reaction. Polymorphous, it possesses a function: to protect from anxiety[24] – hence the traditional fear of suicide with antidepressants that reduce inhibition before improving mood. This fear lessens, so we have seen, with antidepressants marketed after 1975. This has no doubt contributed to increasing the role of inhibition and to restricting that of mental pain.

The three interdependent areas of (1) clinical reflection, (2) biological work on monoamines, and (3) pharmacological research practised by pharmaceutical companies all combine to put forward these two concepts. Indecision, hesitation, avoidance, along with physical, emotional, or cognitive blockage, on the one hand; inability to wait or accept constraints, risk-taking, instability, and irritability on the other. Excess and lack of self-control are disorders of the will:

the very ability of the self is constrained to varying degrees. Their transnosography would reveal "the stability of certain behaviour profiles all through the person's life."[25] In other words, it reveals what, classically, we would call a *character trait*. There seem to be strong links between dimensions and *temperament*. We can then envisage a hereditary vulnerability. Do we not find in psychiatry these narcissistic pathologies and character neuroses, suddenly discovered by French psychopathological analytic practices?

The notion of inhibition has a double advantage that makes it very useful. Observed in a multitude of syndromes, it is very general, and antidepressants have the common ability to work well on it. We can see why it became an inflationary concept.[26] Inhibition seems to have become the major complaint among more than a third of people consulting general practitioners during the 1990s: fatigue and insomnia, a feeling of being blocked, difficulties with memory and concentration describe the mental landscape of the inhibited person.[27] Epidemiology has taught us that general practitioners are more attentive to phenomena of lowering (inhibition, fatigue, moral suffering) than to those of heightening (hypomanias, etc.). Anxiety, insomnia, and fatigue are the complaints most frequently expressed and are each, in different ways, associated with inhibition. It seems coherent to make a common dimension out of them. This construction also has the big advantage of overcoming a common problem among general practitioners: determining the difference between asthenic neurosis and the depressive state.[28] It is now no longer necessary to distinguish between neurosis and depression. Finally, the problem has been solved.

Antidepressants are regulators of action. They modify mental states by dividing in an optimal way the energy flows between high and low. But the distinction between antineurotic and disinhibitor is difficult to establish because inhibition is also a characteristic of neurosis: the self protects itself from anxiety resulting from an intrapsychic conflict through inhibition. It drives neurotic individuals into disinhibition through drugs and, especially, alcohol.[29] Dependency is one of the risks of this self-medicating.

In neurotic action, "inhibition," writes Guyotat, "appears as a defence mechanism against drive."[30] But if we concentrate on inhibition alone, in Janet's perspective, the pathology is in the difficulty of taking action: the deficit is its cause. Inhibition is very clearly one of the reasons for the tipping of neurosis into depression.

ASTHENIA: NERVES, MIND, AND HYSTERIA

The fashion of inhibition in psychiatry simultaneously marks the return of both neurasthenia and psychoasthenia. But instead of the old language of nerves (Beard) or of obsessive ideas (Janet), we have the language of neurochemical transmission.

"Neurasthenia," wrote Pierre Pichot in 1994, "will be found behind the mask of depression." Isn't the feeling of fatigue and weariness found everywhere in general medicine?[31] It appears under a different name in the DSMs,[32] but it is included in the mental illness section of the WHO classifications, which state that this diagnosis is no longer used and has been replaced by the use of depressive or anxiety disorders. Classifications featuring physical and mental exhaustion are more common.[33] And so we get to chronic fatigue syndrome.[34]

But those who conjure up hysteria are there to respond to those who invoke asthenias. As always, the unclassifiable illness appears in multiple forms (in depression, food pathologies, eating disorders, or multiple personality).[35] However, hysterical persons are above all fatigued and inhibited; they demand medication that brings them into addictive patterns. Their depression is dominated by asthenia and various physical suffering. Among certain hysterics, we can observe addictive personalities as "pain is an excuse for demanding barbiturates, anxiolytics and amphetamine stimulants."[36] They need tonics to fight fatigue, analgesics against headaches, anxiolytics for their anxieties, and so on. We find these people more often with the general practitioner than with the psychoanalyst.[37] Hysteria no longer shows itself through the spectacular cases of paralysis among women raised in a culture of sin and duty. Instead of bodily delirium, we have piercing fatigue; instead of physical paralysis, we have spectacular weariness, recognizable in the language of depression. Fatigue, anxiety, and insomnia are expressed in the consultation rooms of general practitioners, and the magazines in the waiting area feature articles on just these problems.[38] "The desire for rivalry and struggle and the fear of confronting it appear to us as one of the essential conflicts of the fatigued self," wrote two psychiatrist-psychoanalysts.[39] The psychic conflict has not disappeared; it has hidden in the loss of energy on which antidepressants act so well.

AN EXCELLENT TIME TO SUFFER?

"Act so well." The words are no exaggeration if we believe the good news trumpeted forth by the prophets of biological psychiatry: the nay-sayers are mostly to be found in the psychoanalytic groups. "You couldn't have picked a better time in human history to feel miserable,"[40] wrote the American psychiatrist Mark Gold in the very first line of his book *The Good News about Depression*. The first good news came from pharmacology. A new generation of antidepressants entered the market during the 1980s: the selective serotonin reuptake inhibitors. According to Gold, they changed "the way we diagnose depression — and may even change the way we define it."[41] The second bit of good news was institutional: the recognition of biological psychiatry (which should be called, he pointed out, "medical psychiatry") as a professional norm and its integration into medicine. In fact, and here's more good news, "many, many psychiatrists have returned to being doctors and to thinking like doctors" because "depression can be a biological illness for which you need a doctor."[42]

In the third version of the DSM, Robert Spitzer pointed out that there existed "no satisfactory definition that specifies precise boundaries for the concept 'mental disorder' (also true for such concepts as physical disorder and mental and physical health)."[43] In the fourth version, Allen Frances regretted not having abandoned the term "mental disorder" because it "implies a distinction between 'mental' disorder and 'physical' disorder" that is "reductionistic": "We have persisted in using the term because we cannot find an adequate substitute."[44] I do not mind risking the hypothesis that we will never find this substitute. No doctor would ever speak of an illness by labelling it as "a physical disorder." To get rid of the dualism, we would need a language that does not force us to use the words "body" and "mind." The mind cannot be observed the same way as can a physical phenomenon. There is a purely rhetorical effect that identifies mental medicine with the rest of medicine because its specificity disappears: the disorder of the mind no longer concerns a person's difficulties but, rather, an illness that affects a patient deprived of his capacity as an agent. This effect is the result of the rebiologization of psychic processes.[45] Rejecting dualism in any form is the axis of the medicalization of psychiatry: the pathology of the mind is that of a sick organ – and all the more so, let us remember, because affect is the most "corporal" part of the mind. That gets us out of a problem in which the pathology is also an experience in which we can learn something in order to be "cured." Nowadays, diseased nerves have become neurochemical disorders. "What science has found …," writes an American journalist, is that "[w]hat people experience when they plummet to the depths or fear airplanes is not 'neurotic.' Scientific data indicate that these illnesses are no less 'physical' than diabetes, no more 'mental' than migraine."[46]

The tendency towards the rebiologization of mental disorder is heard loud and clear in French university-based psychiatry. It works through a kind of magic thinking that identifies illness and syndrome, as is shown by the titles of several books published since 1980 about the depressive *illness*. No one is writing treatises on psychiatry any more; rather, they are penning specialized works on schizophrenias, anxieties, depressions, and addictions. Psychiatry is fragmenting into specialized clinical fields.[47] Depression naturally falls into this tendency, with the triple decline of the notions of neurosis, conflict, and guilt. The victory of the deficit model is made obvious by the statement that individuals are the objects of their illness rather than participants; they are the victims of a process. Depression becomes an illness like any other.

If it is a great time to suffer, the interpretation of those words is full of ambiguities. Do the new antidepressants act more effectively on depressive states or do their advantages make it possible to extend the treatment to categories of illnesses that were not at issue before? In order to answer this question we need to evaluate the progress of psychiatric therapies brought forth by the biochemistry of depressions. The key point is the analysis of mechanisms that block the transmission of information in the neuronal systems.

SEROTONIN, OR A NERVOUS FASHION

In his introduction to a special issue of *La Revue du practicien* on depression in 1985, Daniel Widlöcher notes that "antidepressants are not a medication designed to bring comfort; their effect as a psychostimulant is very specific. Administered to persons who present no signs of depression, their side effects add to a specific effect that is not pleasant at all."[48] This situation was modified by the launching of selective serotonin reuptake inhibitors.

Serotonin has been the page-one subject in psychiatry for some time now. The volume of articles dedicated to its involvement in any number of pathologies is unimaginable. Entire works have been written about it. Serotonin and anxiety, serotonin and obsessive-compulsive disorders, serotonin and obesity, serotonin and phobias, and so on: this neuromediator, which includes numerous families of receptors that have been listed since the 1980s, appears to be the crossroads of a multitude of symptoms. "Serotonin is an enigma. It is at once implicated in virtually everything but responsible for nothing," said two neurobiologists in 1995 in a highly technical volume that brought together the cream of psychopharmacology.[49] At the nineteenth Congress of the Collegium Internationale Neuropsycho-pharmalogicum (CINP) in Washington in June 1994, sixty-nine papers were given on serotonin and only two on noradrenaline. This neuromediator mobilized not only specialists but also, in the United States at least, the public at large. With serotonin, the highly technical entity known as a neuromediator came out of the scientific closet via Prozac and became the subject of numerous articles in daily papers and magazines, including works for the general public such as Peter Kramer's famous book, which kicked off the series. Published in 1996, *Serotonin Solutions* told the public about several simple ways to fight "unbalanced chemicals" that were "the cause" of all mood disorders.[50]

THE KEYSTONE OF PSYCHOPHARMACOLOGY

To escape therapeutic empiricism and reduce the failure rates of antidepressants, psychiatry was forced to hypothesize about subtypes of depressed people and their depressions. Two methods used by psychiatry to resolve these issues were examined. The first was the clinical and psychopathological analysis dominant in the 1950s and 1960s. It sought out the underlying pathology behind syndromes, basing itself on a three-part division of depression: endogenous, neurotic, and reactive. The second method was the syndrome-based reasoning of the DSM-III, which used standardized diagnostic tools and epidemiological studies. The third method – the biochemical – emerged at the end of the 1950s after the discovery of the antidepressant functions of imipramine and iproniazide. It questioned whether the diversity of reactions to antidepressants was not linked to the diversity of neuronal pathways on which these medications work. If we could discover a biological criterion linking the deficit of one type of neuronal pathway to a type of depression, we could predict the response to the antidepressant. It would then be possible to find the molecules that would correct "as specifically as possible the groups of symptoms that make up different depressive situations."[51] In the 1970s, this hypothesis, uncertain yet full of promise, was discussed once more. Yet no acceptable answer was supplied by neuroscience.

Biochemical research shows that psychotropic drugs stimulate to varying degrees the transmission of information in the neurons. Our moods and behaviours flow from their workings. Among the fifty categories of neurons discovered, the three top ones are monoaminergic: noradrenaline, serotonin, and dopamine. At the end of the 1950s, clinical and experimental observation suggested that a neuroleptic (reserpine) had as a side effect deep depression among psychotic patients – not only that, but it emptied the brain of monoamines. The mechanism at work inhibits their capacity to transmit chemical information.[52] This discovery was "the keystone of psychopharmacology."[53] Researchers put forth the hypothesis that antidepressants acted on transmissions of serotonin (discovered in the 1920s) and noradrenaline (discovered in the 1930s).[54] Depression was correlated with the inadequacy in the concentration in one and/or the other of these neuronal channels.[55] This correlation has mobilized psychopharmacological research for more than forty years.

A synthesis published in 1970 recognized that, though these neurons do play a decisive role, nothing proves that syndromes actually result from similar physiological mechanisms.[56] For such a possibility to exist, the syndromes would have to be illnesses. That is why a depressed individual may react well to a certain antidepressant without us being able to say exactly why. Despite the progress in the knowledge of how information is transmitted through the central nervous system, no biological anomaly constitutes a marker for depression.[57] Psychiatric literature has been completely consistent on this theme, as much in the 1980s as now:[58] "A considerable amount of work has tried to explain the biochemical mechanisms of antidepressant drugs, but all attempts to correlate neurochemical data with a clinical effect observed in a depressed individual have remained a guessing-game."[59] This statement, published in *L'Encéphale* in 1994, couldn't be clearer.

French university-based researchers were happy echoing the international consensus. Most major biochemists, neurobiologists, and psychopharmacologists all agreed on their uncertainties: they did not know if serotonin variations were responsible for antidepressant action, or whether it was just a simple concomitant effect, or whether it was a marker of more complex mechanisms.[60] Biology's contribution to psychiatry, to the diagnosis of mental pathologies and the effectiveness of antidepressants, is rather thin. The neurosciences progress, while psychiatry goes in circles.

All the same, work on serotonin has helped us to understand side effects and to develop molecules that are better tolerated and that psychiatrists refer to as "clean" molecules. The serotonin system "is the only working model of antidepressant action that has generated a novel treatment modality that has proved effective."[61] This is reason enough to explain the serotonin fashion.

THE IDEAL ANTIDEPRESSANT: CURING WITH PLEASURE

At the end of the 1960s and the beginning of the 1970s, a number of pharmaceutical companies attempted to develop molecules by starting with biochemical hypotheses and not with the usual procedures: modification of the "chemical chain" of existing molecules,[62] experiments on animals, and clinical trials on people. A therapeutic test to prove the hypothesis of serotonin deficiency was lacking because tricyclics and monoamine oxidase inhibitors act on several monoaminergic systems. We did not have, as one of the inventors of the first serotonin-system molecules wrote in 1982, "the proof of an improvement in the depressive state due to a substance acting as selectively as possible on the central serotonic system."[63] At the end of the 1970s, chemists and pharmacologists found some fifteen molecules, chemically heterogeneous by the way, that acted specifically on serotonin receptors. Two French researchers developed indalpine, one of the first SSRIS to be marketed and created by a French laboratory. In 1977, the first clinical tests comparing imipramine and indalpine showed that the antidepressants' effects were similar but that the comfort factor of the latter was clearly superior to that of the former. They proved that the low side effects, cardiovascular tolerance, and rapid effect result from the selective action on serotonin.

One thing surprised the doctors working on the experiments: change of mood and lessening of inhibition occurred at the same time:[64] "The patients were cured with pleasure."[65] The doctors were immediately enthusiastic: "This therapeutic drug created less problems for them and less anxiety than classic antidepressants" and led to "more fruitful psychotherapeutic contact."[66] The molecule was presented at the Entretiens de Bichat in 1983. It does not preferentially act on one type of depression (endogenous, reactive, or neurotic). It is effective in cases of mood disorders, whether they "be a reaction to a traumatic event, or accompanying a 'difficult' period of existence, such as menopause or retirement, or associated with organic illness or in the typical framework of depression."[67] By acting *specifically* on serotonin, this new molecule was effective on *all* depressions. Psychiatrists were enthusiastic: in 1991, one evoked "the happy days of indalpine."[68] It offered, or so it was written in *Elle* in 1983, "great hope to the therapeutic treatment of depression."[69] Yet indalpine was withdrawn from the market in 1985 because of a grave problem of toxicity that had not appeared in clinical trials.

Zimelidine,[70] a molecule developed by the Swedish firm Astra, created the same hopes at that time. Its inventor, Arvid Carlsson, hypothesized that variations in serotonin concentration explained the effects of antidepressants. The first publications about this molecule date back to 1972. Launched in several European countries, but not in France, at the beginning of the 1980s,[71] it was withdrawn because it caused cases of the flu and, in rare cases, a fatal neurological syndrome.

The research that led to Prozac began at the Eli Lilly drug company in 1970. Because researchers were starting out with theoretical hypotheses and not clinical tests, within Lilly the molecule was called a compound in search of a disease.[72] "If we could find," declared one member of the team that invented the molecule, "a compound that has the same therapeutic effectiveness as tricyclic antidepressants without the fatal anticholinergic and cardiovascular effects, such a compound would constitute major progress."[73] The research protocol was developed based on the problem of side effects, not in order to reach greater effectiveness. One of the researchers was impressed by Carlsson's work. At the beginning of the 1970s, the team began to search for substances that would inhibit the reuptake of serotonin alone. At the end of the decade, research was almost halted because of zimelidine (since the information about indalpine hardly got out of France). The first clinical tests were disappointing but were continued all the same. Preliminary therapeutic trials showed not only that the molecule had antidepressant effects but also that it led to weight loss among patients and was effective in the treatment of bulimia, alcoholism, and tobacco addiction. Large-scale tests carried out at the beginning of the 1980s revealed another unsuspected factor: the prescription of this antidepressant did not have to be followed up in order to reach maximum therapeutic effectiveness, unlike tricyclics, which had to be ajusted. A single dose was generally sufficient. The product was promoted to general practitioners and received FDA approval in December 1987.[74]

THE FANTASY TRADE: YOU HAVE THE POWER

Even if there remained a number of questions that still did not have answers, Mark Gold believed that, all the same, soon "we [would] be able to prevent depression from taking its deadly toll. By identifying certain chemicals in the blood, we may even soon be able to predict who is at risk of suicide."[75] In 1987, with unshakable optimism, the most famous "receptologist" in the world, Solomon Snyder, predicted in a collaborative work about the progress of psychopharmacology that "new psychotropic agents with extraordinary strength and selectivity [would] emerge … These medications [would] allow us to selectively modulate emotional nuances that [were] so subtle that they currently reside[d] in the language of poets rather than psychiatrists."[76] Ten years later, though no progress had been made, researchers from pharmaceutical labs went so far as to predict a different molecule for each different depression. The director of neuroscience research at Eli Lilly in Indianapolis stated that the next generation of psychiatric drugs would "be ten times better than those that we currently have," whereas the director of Pfizer (the manufacturer of Prozac's most serious competitor) happily declared that they would be "far superior to those we now have at our disposal." Molecules were announced for every type of serotonin (some fifteen had been discovered) and noradrenaline receptor.[77] "For different depressions, different antidepressants," wrote one French medical journal in 1996. We would soon be able to choose the right antidepressant according to the type of depression and the profile of the depressed person.[78] The more neurobiology (especially the molecular branch) progressed in its knowledge of neuronal channels and in its discovery of the multiplicity of receptors, the more chemists and pharmacologists could invent powerful and precise molecules. We could then finally answer the question that had emerged in the 1970s: which antidepressant should be prescribed for which depression?

In the end, what we have today are products, apparently harmless and effective for the different symptoms of depression. "Being rid of depression is as simple as birth control: take your pill and be happy," one author wrote in the *Lancet* in 1990.[79] The antidepressant market continued its strong growth, which began in 1975, but consumers' habits changed: sales of Prozac grew by 37.15 percent per year.[80] In 1995, this molecule held down second place among the most popular medications in France.[81]

A serotonin economy has developed over the last ten years. Given the high direct and indirect costs of depression for social service budgets and business productivity, health economists have shown that it is cheaper to use SSRIs than tricyclics, even though each pill is eight to ten times more expensive, because the treatment is followed up better and, thus, its effectiveness is increased.[82] SSRIs would be the closest thing to the ideal antidepressant.[83] New molecules that received the go-ahead in 1997 gave comfort to this therapeutic optimism. They acted specifically on serotonin *and* noradrenaline, had even fewer side effects than SSRIs, acted more rapidly, and proved more effective in cases of severe depression, including among hospitalized melancholic patients.[84] These products had the traditional strength of antidepressants because they acted on several monoamines, and they were well tolerated, just as were serotonin drugs. As an advertisement for one of them pointed out: "Now you have the power." Is the pharmacological dream to reach the impossible? Has science begun to "believe in the potion that will change fate?"[85]

ACT AT ANY COST: THE INDIVIDUAL AS ARC

When it comes to the depressed mind, science promises results that are only comprehensible in the language of magic. Before evaluating these miraculous promises, let's remember that they respond to social aspirations and are in synch with new problems that individuals are encountering. First, new attention to suffering in the social domain sets off the pathologies of the economic crisis whose traumas and distresses are translated in psychiatric terms into depression. Next, the individualization of action creates new pressures on the individual, who must now provide constant effort where once she could simply obey.

THE FASHION OF SUFFERING

According to the CREDES (Centre d'études et de documentation sur la santé), between the beginning of the 1980s and the beginning of the 1990s, the rate of depression increased 50 percent in France. If part of this increase is due to the fact that people admit more readily to being depressed today than they did in the past, "the increase in the prevalence of depression appears to be an established fact ... The prevalence grows with unfavourable situations – solitude, low salaries, unemployment – situations that in themselves are clearly increasing."[86] Overall, the percentage of depressed people at any given moment has gone from 3 percent to a little under 5 percent (in some research, it is estimated at from 6 percent to 7 percent).[87] The few comparative studies that exist in Europe show notable statistical differences that have not been explained.[88]

As well, suicide, drug and alcohol abuse, and non-psychiatric illness accompany depression. Depressed people report much more illness than do non-depressed at the same age (seven to three). Depressed people between twenty and twenty-nine years old have as many health problems as do non-depressed individuals between forty-five and fifty-nine years old; depressed women aged forty-five to fifty-nine have the health profile of a person over eighty. "Depressed people," the authors write, "are old before their time."[89] They have three times more digestive, urinary and genital, and cardio-vascular disorders; twice as many cancers, endocrine system diseases, osteo-articulatory problems; and so on. Their medication consumption, including non-psychotropes, and visits to the doctor are clearly higher than are those of the rest of the population.[90] The direct costs (doctors' visits, treatment, etc.) and indirect costs (absenteeism, low productivity, etc.) appear enormous. Depression seems to be at the centre of a completely heterogeneous pathological dynamic.

Depression has been analyzed as a common state in many psychopathological problems: alcoholism, violence, drug addiction, and suicide. Drug addiction and violent behaviour are often interpreted by psychopathology as defence mechanisms against borderline states of depression. In 1997, the report of France's second National Health Conference pointed out that health education for children and teenagers should integrate "the understanding of psychological and social behaviours, such as violence and depression,"[91] as well as aggression towards oneself and others: "The detection of behavioural problems is a priority."[92] In situations of poverty and exclusion, study groups and official reports point out the criss-crossing of multiple disorders in which violence, depression, psychosomatic illness, and repeated trauma interfere constantly. All reports on public psychiatry now say that it is essential "to consider that certain life problems that are not mental illness, and do not necessarily lead to it, can involve recourse to health care."[93] The job of the public psychiatrist today is centred less on psychoses and more on the delicate inter-relation between social and psychopathological problems that must be both brought together and set apart – unless we agree that the psychiatrist becomes part of social welfare programs. Depression reveals or is associated with a multitude of social and medical problems that are obviously costly for our societies, more particularly for the social service network.

The Commissariat au Plan (a French government think tank for modernizing society, today known as the Conseil d'Analyse Stratégique) sees "a radically new phenomenon ... in the increased vulnerability of the working population."[94] The economic crisis appears to have caused a doubling in the number of suicides in the aged thirty-five-to-forty-four population since the 1980s. Isolation worsens this sense of fragility.[95] An office offering help in the area of the psychopathology of work receives "people who still have a job but are so afraid of losing it that they need help."[96] According to the High Committee for Public Health, "psychological suffering is now, in the health field, the main symptom of financial insecurity."[97]

Public psychiatry is increasingly called upon by people who are suffering, but not from cases of mental illness. Trauma cases caused by financial insecurity have become the main work of psychiatrists in institutions – depression, chronic anxiety, drug addiction, alcoholism, and long-term self-medication – since psychoses have remained stable in absolute numbers but have lowered in relative importance:[98] "The loss of hope becomes a major risk."[99] Depression, and not anxiety, is at the crossroads of well known multiple traumatic and addictive pathologies. It is the description that brings everything together. Not only the attention to suffering but also suffering's cognitive use for understanding and defining social problems are both wholly recent.[100]

THE INDIVIDUALIZATION OF ACTION

Action these days has become an individual enterprise. It has no other source than the agent who accomplishes it and who takes sole responsibility for it. Individual initiative has moved to the top position among criteria that measure a person's value.

At the beginning of the 1980s, two symbolic events occurred in France: (1) the left took power and (2) its collective project (what made it "left") failed, with the result that the entrepreneur became everyone's role model. These two events are related since both the reformist and the revolutionary utopias at the heart of the idea of progress declined – both the society that assured the well-being of its population and the alternative to capitalism. The image of the entrepreneur was no longer that of the big fish swallowing the small or the man enjoying his trust fund. It turned into a style of action that each individual was exhorted to use. The business mentality was also the response to the weakening of the state, which, in France, had always looked after the society's future. The notion of the entrepreneur became a reference point for socio-political action. This was a definite change for a country like France: private action took over the state's collective mission, while the public sector began using private models. Citizen-oriented concerns had to ally themselves with administrations functioning like businesses.

Winners, athletes, adventurers, and other fighters took over France's imagination. They found their embodiment in a character who today is disgraced but who nevertheless symbolized France's entry into the culture of competition: Bernard Tapie. Does anyone still remember that he was the number-one host on the TF1 network in 1986 and that, in prime time, he presided over a variety show, with the evocative title of *Ambitions*, about businesspeople? This was more than just a show. The first wave of emancipation invited viewers to set out and conquer their personal identity, while the second wave preached social success through personal initiative.

In business, disciplinary models (whether Taylor's or Ford's) of human resource management lost ground to norms that incited personnel to take on autonomous behaviour patterns, even if these people were low on the hierarchical ladder. Participative management, group expression, quality circles, and so on became new ways of exercising authority and were designed to inculcate the entreprenurial spirit into each employee. The means of regulating and dominating the workforce were based less on blind obedience and more on initiative: responsibility, ability to evolve and create projects, motivation, flexibility, and so on. This was the new managerial liturgy. Gone was the pattern of the mechanical, repetitive person; at hand was the dawn of the independent mind doing flexible jobs. At the beginning of the twentieth century, engineer Frederick Winslow Taylor attempted to make the worker docile, like a patient ox, as he himself said. But nowadays the engineers of human relations are working to produce autonomy. They are not trying to make the body submissive; they are hoping to mobilize the affect and mental capacities of each employee. The constraints and ways of defining problems have changed. From the middle of the 1980s, industrial medicine and sociological research about the workplace noted a major increase in anxiety, psychosomatic disorders, and depression. The business environment is the antechamber of the nervous breakdown.[101]

With the increased amount of involvement demanded by workplaces from the 1980s onward came, from the end of that decade, a clear decrease in the degree of stability. First unskilled workers were affected, then those higher up on the ladder were threatened, with the top executives being reached in the 1990s. Careers became volatile things.[102] The style of inequalities changed, and this had an impact on collective psychology: there were inequalities between social groups, of course, and to those were added internal conflicts within the groups.[103] The increase in unequal success, in cases when education and social origins were equivalent, could only add to frustration and hurt pride because my next-door neighbour, and not some distant competitor, was the one who was superior to me. The value that people give themselves turns fragile when this kind of inequality is in play.

Schools underwent transformations that had similar effects on student psychology. In the 1960s, social selection generally operated outside of school.[104] But today, as the sociology of education has proved massively, the swelling of the high school population means that selection has to operate all through the person's educational career. In a parallel fashion, "exacerbated imperatives of individual and educational success fall heavily on the shoulders of children and teenagers."[105] The demands that weigh upon the student increase as the young assume responsibility for their failures, which creates forms of personal stigma.[106] Once more, we find changes in the ways of being unequal.

Beginning in the 1960s, the institutional functions of socialization exercised by the family were, to a great extent, carried over to the school. The development of children, greatly encouraged by psychology (Dr Spock, Laurence Pernoud, etc.), became a parental mission of the highest importance. Today, clinicians are noticing pathologies involving identity problems among patients born during that period. They may result from "a sentimentalization, no doubt excessive, of the parental functions."[107] The couple and the family became more autonomous, creating the process known as "demarriage," and this led to new insecurities that blurred the symbolic values of everyone's role. Sex roles became more equal, as did the generations, and this led to a balancing act between generalized contractualism and daily power struggles. When hierarchical borders fade, the symbolic differences with which they are synonymous also break down.[108]

In all areas – be they working life, family, or school – the world was changing its rules. Gone were mechanical obedience, discipline, and moral conformity; they had shifted to flexibility, change, quickness of reaction, and so on. Self-control, flexibility of mind and feeling, and the capacity for action meant that each individual had to be up to the task of constantly adapting to a changing world that was losing its stable shape, becoming temporary, consisting of ebb and flow, something like a snakes-and-ladders game. The social and political game was not so easy to read any more. These institutional transformations made it seem as if each person, even the humblest and lowest of the lot, had to take on the job of *choosing* and *deciding* everything.

Change had long been a desirable thing because it was linked to the idea of progress, which was meant to continue unabated, and to social protection, which could but increase. Today, change is perceived in an ambivalent way because the fear of falling, of not emerging unscathed, has taken over from hopes for upward social mobility. Change has given way to notions of vulnerability, insecurity, and a precarious existence. We are changing, of course, but that does not necessarily mean we are progressing. Combined with all the forces that today exhort us to look into our own private lives, the "civilization of change" has stimulated a massive interest in psychic disorders.[109] It can be heard from all quarters, and it takes form in the many marketplaces that offer inner balance and tranquility. Today, many of our social tensions have been expressed in terms of implosion and depressive collapse or, in a similar way, its flip side: explosions of violence, rage, the search for new sensations. Contemporary psychiatry has taught us that personal impotence can lapse into inhibition, or explode into impulsiveness, or fall into the endless behavioural repetition of compulsion. Depression stands at the crossroads of norms that define action as well as in the heightened use of the notions of suffering and disorder with regard to how we approach social problems and the new solutions proposed by pharmaceutical research.

THE IMAGINATION OF DISINHIBITION

We can understand that the energy promised by antidepressants that have such small negative effects on the quality of daily life gave unexpected hope – hope that had not existed fifteen years earlier. Their marketing responded to the constraints and aspirations of acting by oneself, while the doctor's office became the intersection between these problems and medical supply.

At the end of the 1970s, certain types of advertising, especially for stimulant antidepressants, had as their theme an action to stimulate rather than a pathology to cure. That period also saw the launching of new molecules whose status vacillated between psychostimulants and mood adjusters. One of these ads evoked both psychic suffering and action ("The patient whom you can now quickly return to a normal family and professional life"), while another was exclusively centred on performance ("Get back that taste for action and the freedom to move forward"). Twenty years later, "Claire got back her taste for business" thanks to an MAOI, while an ad campaign for an SSRI that "reawakens inner strength" featured a slogan that proclaimed "This is the real Me," combining high-tech with the natural life.

The year 1988 saw the publication in France of 300 *Drugs to Push Your Intellectual and Physical Limits*. It caused a scandal. The authors – who preferred to remain anonymous – lobbied for "the right to performance enhancement" in a society of heightened competition. They differentiated between drug-taking, which involves withdrawing into one's private universe, and performance enhancement, which involves one's confronting the growing pressures that everyone feels. The upsurge in the use of stimulants like psychotropes was striking, including the use of anxiolytics, since diminished anxiety can disinhibit the self.[110] A calm person is able to act.

In France, in the journal *L'Encéphale*, two psychiatrists pointed out that "the necessity for performance for the subdepressive subject" who does not fulfill the criteria that would allow a diagnosis of episodic depression "would lead to a prescription of a stimulant antidepressant. In a less constraining context, we would not have prescribed an antidepressant, but several elements of psychotherapy should help the person get through a rather difficult period. It is easy of course to denounce excesses and promote the idea of individual effort and natural evolution without medical help. But who can boast of the ability to evaluate the exact level of another person's suffering?"[111] The question is very well put.

In 1991, the introduction to a special issue of a psychoanalytic journal devoted to medication pointed to the importance of the reference to breakdown in psychiatric practice: "The increasing demand for psychiatric comfort and normality, as well as the need for rapid and efficient results, creates among doctors a therapeutic response based on somatic medicine ... In the end, the ideal of chemical mastery over cognitive aptitudes, emotional life and behaviour is what is sought."[112] Feelings of comfort are indeed indispensable for taking action. Do we not need to mobilize our affect in order to act? Can people afford to wait for a solution to their conflicts when the demands for action and adaptation are ever increasing?

This was the context in which Prozac was launched via a marketing campaign aimed at general practitioners. After a series of articles in professional psychiatric journals on the theme of "mood improvers," an article in *Newsweek* in March 1990 entitled "The Promise of Prozac" set the stage for public discussion about depression. The article described people going to see their doctor to ask for a prescription for this pill that would apparently let them face the vicissitudes of daily existence without having to pay the psychic price. Peter Kramer also wondered about this ideal of chemical mastery. His book is not dedicated to finding the means to get happiness via prescription, despite the impression the French press tried to give. His is a practical reflection on the type of self demanded by "today's high-tech capitalism": "Confidence, flexibility, quickness and energy ... are at a premium."[113] Let's just say that these attributes let us stay in the race longer. Because it was effective with people who were not "really" depressed, the product called Prozac got the reputation of being able not only to improve mood and to facilitate action but also to transform personality in a favourable manner. The patients described by Kramer were able to "be productive" with Prozac. But so what? What is wrong with careful manipulation of our moods as long as the molecules are not toxic? What kind of problem would this cause?

Prozac is not the happiness pill but, rather, the initiative drug. From there to saying that it could be a stimulant is a long step. Don't MAOIS, as psychiatrists already noticed back in the 1960s, sometimes make patients feel "better than good?" That's the way Daninos described the antidepressant that got him out of the dark tunnel. From the 1960s on, pharmacologists, chemists, and psychiatrists were all hoping for molecules of this kind, molecules that were easier to prescribe and more efficient. The step turned out to be an easy one to make, and people wondered if the end of the "subject" had finally arrived. Easy to use, this molecule reduced the individual to her body.

"The issue cannot be contained within the medical world alone," an author wrote in *L'Encéphale* in 1994, and this we have forgotten: "Patients need results depending on the time they have and their other obligations. Not to take this into account might expose them to socio-professional difficulties that would turn into depressive complications."[114] These remarks open onto practical issues: psychiatry and general practitioners are seeing patients who demand pharmacological and psychological supplements, the better to master their multiple difficulties.

MIRACLE POWERS OR A BAND-AID SOLUTION?

Psychomotor slowing, inhibition and impulsiveness, asthenia: these notions could refer to any nosographical model, but all are concerned with pathological action. Frozen action sculpts the depressive universe. It is a kind of "stoppage of time,"[115] whereas impulsiveness is time accelerated. Apathy takes the place of mental pain since, clinically, it is the true target of antidepressants, and socially it joins the new problems that people face when it comes to taking action. The depressive breakdown accompanies the individual arc like a shadow. Psychiatric categories, therapeutic means, and social norms reconfigure individuality.

The miracles foretold might well respond to the aspirations for better "functioning," but they are truly the fruit of advertising campaigns. Though some prestigious researchers (such as Snyder) held these beliefs, most did not, at least not publicly. Arvid Carlsson said it some years ago: "In light of the formidable progress in basic knowledge, it is remarkable to see how modest the developments in pharmacotherapy really are since the 1950s."[116] Jonathan Cole and Donald Klein, for example, thought that a number of people taking Prozac were waiting in vain for the miraculous effects of the product – either that or its supposed effectiveness depended more on wishful thinking.[117] A sociological study conducted via interviews with people taking antidepressants showed that Prozac's effect was quite variable and that disappointment was not rare at all.[118] SSRIs are exactly like all other antidepressants: their effectiveness varies.

The mastery of the human mind through pharmacological means will not happen tomorrow – or even the day after. In 1964, François Dagognet wrote some excellent pages about the ancient mythologies of curing. The ideal antidepressant is the modern version of such myths. It carries us into the magic of miracle powers, the power of "the shaman who could cure us with a simple breath, a potion, a mixture, an incisive destructive force." "Now we must," he wrote, "reject that senseless belief that could … take root: that a pill could straighten the soul, give back the taste for living, create sudden and utter joy."[119] No medication, psychotrope or not, is an all-powerful potion that can be applied to an illness (or any other sick entity) and so cause it to end.

Please forgive me, but I have bad news: the supposed all-curing properties of antidepressants are simply band-aid solutions to an incurable illness, as we are now beginning to see. Everything becomes depression because antidepressants act on everything. Everything can be treated, but we no longer know what can be cured. The conflict is hidden as life becomes a chronic identity illness. That is not necessarily a bad thing, for our individualities are perfectly built to stand such "diseases," but we're better off knowing what they are hiding.

7

The Uncertain Subject of Depression, or End-of-the-Century Individuality

The ability to act by oneself is at the heart of socialization, and the breakdown of action is the fundamental disorder of depression. There are two ways of understanding the situation: one is concerned only with the subject of conflict, the other has nothing to do with conflict. The controversy between Janet and Freud was played out a century later in a completely different normative and psychiatric context. If depression really is the double pathological manifestation of psychic liberation and individual initiative, then, necessarily, internal splits other than those of conflict will be played out. At the psychiatric level, today the main controversy over depression centres on the role of antidepressants in these indefinable "states," classifiable according to a variety of bases but, above all, chronic and recurring.

The delicate relation between inadequacy and conflict becomes apparent with particular sharpness when it comes to the new molecules, launched with suitable marketing acumen. On the one hand, they create fantastic hopes because, as a number of articles have pointed out, they seem to effectively separate the quantities of energy in the "psychic apparatus" by acting on anxious and depressive affects – that is, on practically all possible pain and dysfunction. These molecules make the individual more lively and less anxious, more a master of himself or herself, whether he or she is sick or not. On the other hand, from the point of view of psychopathology, the tone is much more worrisome. In 1996, the *Revue internationale de psychopathologie* wondered, "Is it necessary to have in hand a diagnosis of psychopathology when the product is no longer designed as a *response* to these states (depression, anxiety, dissociation, etc.), but rather as a way of creating new mental states without dependency or threat to the physical integrity of the subject?"[1] The substances that produce such states were supposed to present no danger of addiction or toxicity, so there was no need for a diagnosis that would uncover the pathology underlying the symptom. We needed only to reapportion the decreased or poorly regulated energies with the help of a psychotrope. We swam in the mythic waters of the perfect drug, which meant it was impossible to determine whether it was a drug or a medication.

SSRIs created the fear of a chemical abrasion of the dilemmas that make our subjectivity. Insofar as we possess medicines that can be applied as much to serious pathologies as to small cuts and scrapes, the loss of the need for a diagnosis would mean that the nightmare of a society of "pharmacohumans" would finally come to pass. I hope I may be allowed to use that expression to speak of a category of persons who would no longer be subject to the usual condition known as limits.

This belief in the infinite possibilities of the neurosciences and pharmacology is perfectly unrealistic. It invests these disciplines with power over pathologies and, more broadly, over people without them. This power is a long way off as biologists and psychiatrists recognize that the attempt to link a "biological marker" to a clinical entity is a failure. Nor does it seem that the new paths and new hypotheses being explored are very promising. Besides, this belief arises from a confusion between the progress of biological research and that of psychiatry. The latter is a branch of medicine, and its function is to treat patients. It is not situated on the same plane as biological research. Whether we hope for the subject's complete mastery of herself (by awakening her inner strength through a molecule), or whether we fear it (because it would reduce the human being to her physical well-being instead of freeing her), we're fooling ourselves in both cases.

First, it is obvious that, in pharmacotherapy, antidepressants are far from being ideal medications. Three obstacles stand in their way, if we are to believe the main article in a 1996 issue of *Drugs*: (1) they need to obtain an effectiveness superior to that of tricyclics; (2) they need to provide more rapid action at the beginning of treatment; and (3) they need to produce regular effectiveness in the case of resistant depression.[2] Antidepressants have become a comfortable medication, which is a whole other issue.

From the 1980s onward, psychiatric epidemiology began to realize certain things about the difficulties of treatment – for example, resistant depression and chronicity were the rule. Cure entered a crisis. This has been a recurrent theme in the literature, but I have seen hardly any public polemic about depression, at least not in the press. Thus, people's opinions have not been well informed: what should have been discussed in practical terms was framed as a moral issue. This kind of discussion confused advertising messages with what psychiatric research, including the kind sponsored by industry, has described and whose results can be consulted. So there is no reason to fear the eclipse of the old self, the one that was the subject of her conflicts. Quite the contrary: we can now measure the transformations of subjectivity. The association of long-term states and the ambiguous status of antidepressants between drug and medication will be the centre of discussions.

The crisis of cure and the decline of the reference to conflict suggest that contemporary individuality is simply no longer part of cure; it is accompanied and transformed in all sorts of ways as it moves through time. Simultaneously, from the political point of view, our societies have left behind the idea of the right solution (this accounts for the breakdown in the traditional French left-right divide). Conflict no longer seems to structure the unity of the person with his or her social world, and its messages no longer seem to provide adequate guideposts for action. The two levels of the crisis of cure in psychiatry and the "deconflictualizing" of the psychic realm (as well as the social zone) lay down the main lines for our new collective psychology. The subject does not emerge from this process moribund, just changed.

MENTAL DIABETES

Doubts began to emerge in psychiatric literature.[3] Psychiatrists – and this was a change in the field compared to the 1960s and 1970s – started asking questions about cure. Depression became a disease of neurochemical transmission, but, at the same time, it built up resistance.[4] Today it has been redefined by psychiatry as a recurring disease with chronic tendencies. Has the duration of depression increased? Were we too optimistic after the discovery of antidepressants? Let's look at the facts before the explanations.

THE CRISIS OF CURE

Three-quarters of patients who have experienced an episode of depression will not recover the psychological equilibrium they possessed before. Twenty percent of depression cases become chronic and another 20 percent resist treatment.[5] According to the Epidemiological Cathcment Area studies in the United States, 50 percent to 85 percent of patients will experience new episodes or will reach a lower state than the one they previously occupied. The frequency of relapses and setbacks was noted by all practitioners. A conference organized by the American Psychiatric Association evaluated at between fifty and eighty the percentage of persons who will have at least one relapse in their lives after an episode of depression. Fifty percent will do so in the two years following it.[6] All epidemiological studies confirm this unfavourable situation.[7] A synthesis of these studies shows that depression, despite heterogeneous results due to different populations, nosography, and methods, has a recurring feature in three-quarters of cases. Fifty percent of patients suffer relapses within two years after an episode of depression, 20 percent become chronic, and 15 percent to 20 percent achieve only partial remission.[8]

The consensus on these proportions leaves no doubt: most patients do not recover their past equilibrium, a good minority will experience only partial remission, and a large majority will fall into relapse and depression as a chronic condition. Hence, prescriptions grow longer, which is made possible by the comfort provided by antidepressants marketed over the second half of the 1970s, and especially ssris at the end of the 1980s. "Depressive disorders, frequent though they are, are curable through treatments whose comfort and tolerance continue to grow," wrote two psychiatrists.[9] But they went on to add, "Can we still speak of a cure, or would it be wiser to use the term remission?"[10] The hope for long-term improvements began to appear modest. The comfort of ssris and their low toxicity reduced the problems of the chronic condition. This is certainly not a negligible factor, but we can, on the other hand, ask ourselves whether there are not numerous cases in which they maintain and do not facilitate the confrontation with possible conflicts whose outcome is depression.

Not only did the duration of treatment increase, but so did the percentage of patients gobbling low-dose antidepressants for years after the first episode of depression. The result: symptoms returned after treatment was halted. Disorders, it seem, grew chronic. The lessening of symptoms under the effect of antidepressants is not the same as a cure.[11] The growing number of inadequate prescriptions, the poor observation of treatment in general medicine,[12] associated pathologies (especially chronic alcoholism), pathological features of personality, and so on – the reasons for this situation are numerous. But most of all, the very notion of a cure is uncertain as it "can be confirmed or denied depending on the criteria used."[13]

Many authors have turned their attention towards maintenance treatments[14] – prophylactic treatments for recurring depression. Most of the patients concerned should benefit from such treatments, and only the duration remains to be determined. For some, the treatment can be continued all through a lifetime; for others, the cut-off date is five years.[15] However, these criteria arise more from clinical intuition than from standardized results. In any case, we can imagine a life-long treatment for a single episode of depression if the patient is over fifty years old, for two episodes if she is over forty, and for more than two if she is under forty.[16]

When it comes to evaluating the long-term effectiveness of antidepressants, Pringuey et al. sum up their position with an obvious rhetorical contortion: "Survival analyses carried out over five years of follow-up among patients responding to imipramine show an increased risk of depressive relapse upon halting of the treatment, but do not show a true prophylactic antidepressant effect, while not proving that the treatment is not effective, which should lead us to revise the clinical notion of response."[17] We should also note the questioning of the nature of antidepressant action and clinical response. In 1993, a working committee of the Collegium Internationale Neuro-Psychopharmacologicum expressed its interest in the chemical therapy of maintenance but left full latitude to the prescribing physician. Studies carried out during the 1980s "showed only relative success of psychotropic maintenance, most notably when compared to the placebo effect."[18] One is sometimes satisfied to designate as "antidepressant any molecule that improves those symptoms characteristic of depression more effectively than a placebo."[19] But what is the percentage? And for which patients? And what do we do when the placebo is more effective than the medication?

Though the emphasis on the necessity of associating psychotherapeutic help with the antidepressant cure remains a constant, it "does not appear to lessen the risk of relapse. It may simply lead to the patient sticking to the cure in a better fashion."[20] Psychotherapy becomes an enabler for chemical therapy. Besides, the psychotherapies most recommended today are behavioural or cognitive. And they are based on an exclusively deficiency-based model.

The excessive use of prescriptions is a well known risk. Antidepressants "have their side effects and long-term possibilities that we as yet know nothing of."[21] Prolonged treatment can have negative effects on memory and cognitive function, and the suicide rate seems higher among patient groups treated with antidepressants than among those treated with placebos. And we do not know much about the long-term effects on monoamines in the brain and the receptor sites of the neurons that synthesize them. There are no set criteria for an overall therapeutic strategy: it is up to the clinician to evaluate the benefits and drawbacks in discussion with the patient.[22] Yet too few depressed patients see doctors. Some of them receive a faulty diagnosis, and those who receive a correct one are too rarely given adequate treatment.[23]

The problems caused by withdrawal after prolonged treatment with antidepressants are now well known. They "have been pointed out by numerous authors and can be observed among more than 20% of patients." Therein lies "the issue of a possible physical or psychic dependency on antidepressant treatment."[24] Syndromes of addiction can be observed with MAOIs because of their psychostimulant effects, and they can lead doctors into giving long-term prescriptions.[25] These prescriptions can themselves lead to dependency: "All these data seem to describe a high-dose physical dependency."[26] Obviously, to effectively treat depression means reducing the intensity of the symptoms and the length of the episode, but this is not the same as progression towards a cure. As two psychiatrists have written, "It's not easy to clarify the notion of cure in psychiatry."[27] There is, then, a very clear contrast between the promises of pharmacology and the psychiatric consensus regarding the crisis of cure. Between the end of the 1970s and the beginning of the 1980s, a complete turn-around took place concerning antidepressant molecules.[28] Prescribed for most mental disorders, at best they made up for personal inadequacy without curing anything.

DYSTHYMIAS AND ANXIODEPRESSIVES, OR THE BURIAL OF NEUROSIS

The growing length of depressive episodes was not suddenly revealed by an awakening in epidemiology; rather, it resulted from an attraction to that part of the depressive constellation that was concerned with neurosis. "Many resistant depressions occur in neurotic psychic structures," declared Deniker in 1986.[29] This was a constant,[30] based on the realization that antidepressants act on numerous anxiety disorders in a much more effective way than do benzodiazepines (BZDs) and on the new popularity of terms such as "anxiodepressive" and "dysthymia." The extension of the targets of antidepressants and the recoding of neurosis turned depression into a chronic identity pathology.

Antidepressants "seem more and more to be 'antineurotic' medications."[31] Antineurotic medications – here is an essential vector with regard not only to the increase of diagnoses of depression but also to the change in depression's meaning. Herman van Praag said it very clearly: "The SSRIs might be the first generation of drugs that, indeed, affect personality."[32] Indeed, as Thomas Ban put it: "SSRIs are forcing us to face the issue of whether the use of psychotropics should be restricted to the treatment of disease or extended to the modification of behaviour, or even to render life more pleasurable."[33] For psychiatrists, acting on a neurosis was the equivalent of acting on the personality.

The DSM-III divided the neurosis of anxiety into panic attacks and generalized anxiety disorder as it had been proven that antidepressants acted effectively on the former. Today, they would be equally effective on the second category and, indeed, on most anxiety disorders. To finish the portrait, they would also act on cases of defence psychoneuroses (hysteria and obsessional neuroses). Two psychiatric categories provide the key to depression's redefinition of neuroses: (1) *anxiodepressive* disorders and (2) *dysthymic* disorders.

Ever since antidepressants were discovered, it was generally considered that patients responded better to these molecules if the depression could be classified as endogenous (something like melancholia but less serious) rather than as a neurotic depression (i.e., as psychogenic). Neurotic depression tended to be chronic – and not a depressive *episode* – since it sprang from the person's personality. It could be seen in terms of unresolved unconscious psychic conflicts (Freud) or deficiencies (Janet). These chronic depressions, considered as personality disorders, were subject to psychotherapeutic treatment.

The distinction between anxiety and depression, which creates, we will recall, diagnostic difficulties in general practice, disappears with the invention of anxiodepression.[34] It takes over from the notions of neurotic depression and reactive depression.[35] Very common in general medicine, these states are chronic and render daily life extremely difficult. These "states once labelled as neurotic" are "a bottomless grab-bag."[36] All psychiatric epidemiology recognizes the important comorbidity of anxiety and depressive disorders.[37]

The notion of dysthymia belongs to the psychiatrist Hagop Akiskal and appears in the DSM-III.[38] In the 1970s, Akiskal demonstrated that a major number of chronic depressions of psychogenic origin were part of mood disorders. Patients "appeared to be depressed for life … and were sentenced to the couch because there was no other treatment."[39] The 1987 DSM-III-R did away with neurotic depression and replaced it with dysthymic disorders. These patients responded better to SSRIs than to other antidepressants.[40] Dimensional reasoning as well as syndrome-based thought made reference to neurosis invalid. The dysthymia-SSRI pairing opened the door to chemical therapy for personality disorders. What is specific about this type of personality? Not conflict, whose lack of resolution explains its chronic nature – but temperament, character. In other words, a destiny. The difficulty of differentiating between endogenous and exogenous can be overcome because it no longer plays a part in the choice of treatment.

The distinction between the DSM's Axis I, which lists pathologies, and its Axis II, which lists pathological personalities, was challenged insofar as the long duration of the disorder seems to indicate that the patient's personality is at the heart of the matter.[41] These type of depressions create consensus on one point: their prognosis is very bad. Therapy is a long-term affair, and its objective is "to maintain remission through disallowing the symptomatic expression of a process that is presumed to still be active."[42] Yet there has not been any evaluation of prescriptions over such long durations, and the long-term effects are not known, as is pointed out from time to time. Since we cannot cure, as in the case of madness, we can at least support.

Comfortable molecules represent ideal products for these pathologies not because they are more effective but, rather, because they are more adaptable to chronic disease than are the old antidepressants. Dysthymias and SSRIs reinforce each other: the former is a light depression of long duration, while the latter is a comfortable molecule and has fewer addictive effects than do the older molecules. Psychiatry believed that antidepressants could either help a neurotic individual get past a particularly rough patch or help him confront his unconscious conflicts. Depression became an aspect of neurosis, and today neurosis has dissolved into the field of depression. On the other hand, both neurosis and depression have become chronic: everything can be treated, nothing can be cured.

At the start of this sixty-year-old trajectory we find a sick yet curable self with painful moods. At the finish line, we find action that is regularly disrupted and individuals who are chronically affected by their pathology.

AN EXPANDING SPECIES: THE WALKING WOUNDED

On the deficiency front, the tendency towards chronic disorder pushed psychiatrists into using the theme of patient quality of life instead of the idea of cure through the therapeutic encounter.

The Deficiency Front: Quality of Life or Dependency?

In medicine, quality of life is a classic theme in cases of chronic illness. The diabetic patient dependent on insulin is the typical example. In the 1960s, in psychiatry, this theme appeared in the United States and was applied to psychoses. It was used to criticize the mass deinstitutionalization from psychiatric hospitals and to highlight the inadequate network of halfway houses.[43] Great Britain, Scandinavia, and then the rest of Europe got interested in the question since it seemed to involve helping psychotic individuals to live their daily lives outside of a psychiatric hospital. The quality of life issue was later extended to two types of disorders that, from the 1980s onward, were considered chronic: anxiety and depression.

Neither health nor welfare tools were developed to measure standard ways to determine "what the subject lives inside"[44] and to reorient attention towards "the overall state of the patient."[45] Questionnaires evaluate the distance between the aspirations of patients and what they feel they are experiencing, the tolerance regarding this distance, value judgments regarding their ways of acting, and so on. "The notion of satisfaction ... matters,"[46] and so does that of happiness.[47]

Ensuring an adequate quality of life is a way of making patients more autonomous within the constraint of chronic illness.[48] The ideal patient is "an active interactor."[49] She can recognize the signs of a relapse on her own and quickly make an appointment with her psychiatrist, who need only readjust the dose of the antidepressant being used: "Orderly self-medication is a good indicator of the patient's psychological maturity, much more than the talent of his doctor. It expresses ... the patient's integration of his therapeutic program and his understanding of it, including his transgressions and the necessary justified adjustments."[50] The ideal therapeutic alliance involves transferring the doctor's medical knowledge to the patient. Depression is one of those chronic illnesses that finds its solution in the patient's own initiative.[51]

The problem is that some of these patients fear becoming dependent on medication, just as they tend to fight the guilt that their desire for dependency creates. This association with 'drugs' is reinforced by relapses when treatment is stopped. This type of resistance often appears in long-term treatments. In *L'Encéphale*, we read this restrained conclusion: "True progress has been achieved in the treatment of depressed patients, but it is paradoxical to see that imipramine remains the molecule of reference. We have gotten interested in prolonged antidepressant treatment in the prevention of relapses, but we really don't understand the duration or the long-term effects. We can recognize the value of antidepressant molecules in certain anxiety disorders, but at the same time we've increased the risks of self-prescribing and turning the medication into an ordinary procedure."[52] On the one hand, there is better quality of life for improved patients; on the other hand, there is fear of dependency. These two phenomena are intimately related. Doesn't cure assume the stoppage of treatment sooner or later?

Psychiatry tends to use the model of insulin-dependent diabetes to neutralize the difficulties raised by the idea of a cure, but depressed people now find themselves in the same situation as do psychotic patients. The acute phases of the pathology are well treated, but chronic illness is the rule. Psychiatrists who work in the psychodynamic and psychopharmacological currents have realized this.[53] In the end, two psychiatrists from the Sainte-Anne hospital in Paris write: "Benzodiazepins have lost their status as medications ... and become simple domestic helpers. We are afraid that antidepressants will come to the same point and that, as with benzodiazepins, some of them will create dependency with withdrawal problems and abusive use, including addictive symptoms."[54] The problem is well put, and not in some marginal psychiatric journal but in *L'Encéphale*, where almost all French university psychiatrists publish, with each special issue being sponsored by a pharmaceutical company. Anti-depressants leave the category of medication the way depression leaves the category of illness.

Antidepressants more or less diminish the identity insecurities of individuals who feel chronically inadequate,[55] and they regulate action for as long as they are ingested – at least when the depression does not resist them. Long-term treatment takes over from cure because, indeed, antidepressants are antineurotic medications: they place conflicts at a distance. Extending their use makes it hard to distinguish between a mood disorder a person might have during a depressive episode, a neurotic symptom expressing a person's unconscious conflicts, a temperament resulting from the chance effects of family genetics, or, very simply, various social traumas linked to contemporary lifestyles. This analysis can be found in the most prestigious psychiatric journals as well as in psychiatry text-books and literature for general practitioners.

This paradoxical situation, in which the medication is invested with magical powers while the pathology becomes chronic, should move us to ask questions about the limits of illness. The distinction between the normal and the pathological has become a moral issue. In 1985, Daniel Widlöcher, introducing a special issue of the *Revue du practicien* on depression, sounded the alarm: "When it comes to therapy, we need to ask the question: what degree of intensity and what duration should provoke medical treatment when it comes to depressive states?"[56] This question was asked before the SSRI fashion by one of the leaders of French psychiatry. The launch of new mol-ecules only served to accelerate this movement, casting the issue into public view. This ambiguity accompanied the issue, which combined inadequacy with conflict. Its flip side involved the questioning of people's identity: were they comfortably drugged? The decline of the concept of conflict contributes to a rapprochement – both rightly *and* wrongly – between drugs and psychotropic medication.

Antidepressant abuse, difficulties in stopping, and risks of depen-dency are all linked to the weak therapeutic results in the progress of the neurosciences. Pierre Pichot pointed out this fact: "The work produced by the neurosciences is extremely impressive. I'm not contesting that, but for the time being, very little of anything useful has emerged in terms of concrete clinical applications for psychia-try." He added: "This brings us back to the definition of the concept

of illness and its limits. There is no truly satisfactory definition."57
Such comments – and they are not rare – point to the weakness of
theory in contemporary psychiatry. On the one hand, insofar as it
has no autonomy in relation to them, psychiatry is a satellite of the
neurosciences; on the other hand, insofar as it is obliged to respond
to social demands, psychiatry is faced with the need to rethink its
references. How can it define and conceptualize the notion of
mental pathology in today's world?

THE FRONT LINES: CURE IS COMPROMISE

The conflictual approach to mental pathology is, of course, represented by psychoanalysis: "The psychoanalytic cure has shown that
we must live with the shadow of despair. Our demons can neither
be expelled nor pushed under; they are precious to us as an attribute of human existence. If we can learn to live with them, they
will come to our aid."58 Here we encounter the issue of reorganizing the relation with the self, not primarily the search for well-being.
Instead of aiming for a cure, we move towards relativizing the need
for well-being (animal) with the benefits of freedom (human). The
ill individual is a self who is suffering and who can recognize her
own cure only through integrating illness into her experience and
self-history.

  The idea of cure would then be characterized not through a
return to some former time (i.e., before the illness) but, rather, by
the fact that the doctor, psychotherapist, or molecule would no
longer be necessary. That moment is of course difficult to isolate,
and it presupposes a kind of practical wisdom, a compromise in
which the self participates along with his or her therapist. According
to Georges Canguilhem, who explicitly refers to psychoanalysis as
work, the role of the doctor is to practise a pedagogy of cure: "This
pedagogy should work to help the subject understand that no technique, no institution, present or future, can provide him with the
guaranteed integrity of his relational powers with other people and
things."59 Canguilhem adds that this limit is inherent to every living
being and is its natural law: "Health after recovery is not a past state
of health. The lucid awareness of the fact that cure does not mean
returning to the past will help the patient in his or her search for
the least amount of renunciation possible, by freeing him from a

fixation with a former state."[60] There is no cure without work, without development, without a story – a fiction in which the person is involved through the use of the I.

One thing seems certain in the conflictual model: well-being is not a cure. This is because being cured involves the ability to suffer and to tolerate suffering. From this point of view, being cured is not at all the same thing as being happy. It means being free, recovering a power over the self that will let us "decide if we want this or that." If we accept the idea that health is the ability to go beyond our own norms, we need to distinguish between happiness and freedom, between well-being and cure. If an individual in good health is up to the various bumps and bruises of existence, and able to go beyond his norms, I would also add that, in terms of psychic disorder, he can do so *only because* he is conflictual. Conflict is both engine and brake.

Hence, the virulent opposition to the DSM that places before the clinician "an ethical option: the choice between an animal and a human ideal."[61] The choice is between an approach that would have no concern for the self as a subject of conflict and an approach that would be concerned only with this self. But today, we cannot settle for such a radical choice because it excludes animality – possessing a body – without which we would not be alive. Medication relieves suffering that reveals a conflict, or so it is said among psychoanalysts. It keeps the conflict alive without our knowing and is nothing more than a prosthesis. Yet it makes it possible for a person to put off confronting his or her conflicts to some more favourable time. If we are to believe one of the finest critics of psychoanalysis, François Roustang, human animality simultaneously fell through the hatch and was cured. Isn't neglecting animality a form of "spiritualist" reductionism? Must everything go through consciousness in order for cure to be possible? Roustang evokes "certain truths that have been neglected by psychoanalysis, which considers the psyche in isolation and must give it a reality it could not have except through the soma."[62] In some psychoanalytic circles, isn't there an avoidance of the body and the social realm similar to the avoidance of the psyche in biological psychiatry?

What can we say about these endless cures that accompany a "patient" over many long years, if not through a lifetime, because "the knowledge it brings does not lead to modification,"[63] does not lead to change, without which there is no cure? Cure seems reduced to an "initiation into the mysteries of the unconscious."[64] The patient remains dependent on the therapist, a dependency similar to that experienced by those who ingest a certain molecule on a long-term basis. The chronic mode is certainly not the monopoly of biological psychiatry. As François Roustang remarks, in his ferocious way: "If analysis has no limit in time and space …, analysis will not only last as long as life does, it will absorb all of life."[65] The figure of the walking wounded appears in all the markets of inner equilibrium.

To resolve conflicts, we need to question the self. "Is it normal … to put oneself in question?" Joyce McDougall wondered, and she was right to so wonder.[66] Right, because she raised the problem of today's client groups in psychiatry and the types of requests that are formulated. Is standard therapy relevant to those who live in economic insecurity and exclusion – and to the many wage-earners who use and abuse tranquilizers and antidepressants (not to mention alcohol, the great French taboo) in order to face the increasing constraints that act upon them as they wait for the storm to pass? Is it necessary – and, if so, in the name of what principle – for all of us to face our conflicts? Are there not countless cases in which the cure is worse than the disease?

If conflict is the honey that feeds psychoanalysis, it is obvious that new demands are always being made of it. These demands don't have the open face of conflict but, rather, the more slippery visage of the void. They emerged during the 1970s and polarized the debate around neurosis and depression. These days, they are phrased in vague terms of a sense of malaise arising from new economic and social constraints and the insecure nature of private life. Psychoanalysis and addiction specialists have been thinking hard about the pathologies of emptiness, the void, and absence. But such reflection has also been developing among the hard core, if you like: among societies of analysts.[67]

A practitioner working at a centre for psychoanalytic consultation and treatment, who receives a thousand demands a year, has noticed the increase in requests for analysis motivated by lay-offs, unemployment, and financial insecurity: "We have seen the emergence of a *new traumatology*, in which the repetitive and painful reference to factual reality has conferred a character of *current-affairs neurosis* to the symptomology."[68] To be more precise, this would be "a form of 'economic war neurosis.'"[69] This patient group is often unstable when it comes to following a cure, including when the patients' projects have been "worked on and planned for some time."[70] They have a pronounced difficulty with long-term involvement. But the most significant aspect of this group, according to the author, is that "the problematic centred on desire and the forbidden ... has given way, in terms of frequency, to the problematic centred on the loss of object and subjective identity ... Above all, groups of symptoms appear to blur, become polymorphous, with somatizations and marked acts," and the patients are at times "captives of an eternal present."[71] Hence, the need to adapt the classic framework of cure by diversifying the means of treating such patients. There is one more point that should be brought up concerning the tonality of malaise: after the preliminary interviews, analysts do not know how to define the references to these patients' suffering: "We don't really know *where* it hurts, *how* and when."[72]

Just as public psychiatry is seeing the number of psychoses diminish relative to the multiple traumas created by insecurity, psychoanalysis is no doubt noticing the relativization of defence psychoneuroses (hysterias, phobias, obsessive disorders) among its clientele.

Pathological Humanity: Traumatized, not Neurotic

In psychoanalysis, it is suspected that acquiring greater lucidity does not necessarily lead to cure, whereas in psychiatry, it is believed that abandoning conflict in favour of well-being would make cure impossible.

The elements that pried psychiatry away from the reference to an ill subject contribute to a declension of treatments, ranging from the micro-management of moods to maintaining the very idea of cure. The first brings us to the horizon of well-being, a quality-of-life issue we may wish to see as dependency; whereas the second offers a perspective in which the freedom to choose one way or another dominates the desire for well-being. We certainly can't act *as if we could deliver people from their conflicts*, as depression's tendency to become chronic clearly shows on the deficit front, but nor can we act *as if there was nothing but conflict*. This is because to narcissistic pathologies that can be more easily discovered because of the domination of norms of initiative and interdiction are added the many forms of psychic suffering arising from the insecurities of life, expressed through types of despair that are often not the fruit of conflict. Often they are not pathologies at all. On two fronts, pathological humanity has changed.

The relative decline in psychoses in public psychiatry and of psychoneurotic defences in psychoanalysis arise from the same dynamic. The varying degrees of intensity of the pathologies notwithstanding, they do resemble each other on one point: the importance of trauma. Today, the pathological person is more likely a trauma case than a neurotic (or psychotic) one; she is jostled, empty, and agitated. And, in conditions of financial insecurity, she has trouble fulfilling the material, social, and psychological conditions that would enable her to reach the register of conflict. The new threats from within and their treatment sketch out the portrait of an individual whose inner identity is chronically fragile but who can be treated perfectly well over the long term.

The debate over the specificity or non-specificity of therapy, which divided Jean Delay and Henri Ey over electroconvulsive therapy, then Nathan Kline and Roland Kuhn over antidepressants, has now been settled. Non-specificity has won the battle. The new molecules are closer to Kline's psychic energizers than to Kuhn's thymoanaleptics. In that they act on most non-psychotic mental disorders, they are truly the aspirin of the mind. But this victory took place in the context of the over-extension of chemical therapies. Improvements to these molecules have made them today's "ideal" medication – as long as we understand that they're ideal for chronic illness. This redefinition "helps the medicine go down" insofar as the inadequate curative power of molecules is concerned, in the sense that they rid the person of his or her mental problem. Today's individual is neither ill nor cured; rather, he has just signed up for one of the many maintenance programs on offer.

We can now better understand how the history of depression reveals the type of person we have become as a result of the demands of psychic emancipation and individual initiative. Depression is to inadequacy what madness is to reason, and neurosis to conflict. Depression is the historical mediator that forces conflictual humanity to retreat, threatened by neurosis, to the benefit of fusional humanity, searching for sensations to overcome an endless lack of tranquility. Deficit filled, apathy stimulated, impulses regulated, compulsion tamed – all of this has made dependency the flip side of depression. With the gospel of personal development on the one hand and the cult of performance on the other, conflict does not disappear; however, it loses its obvious quality and can no longer be counted on to guide us.

LEAVING BEHIND THE REFERENCE TO NATURE AND ILLNESS IN PSYCHIATRY

Moving from the crossroads to the grab-bag, only to fragment into dimensions (dysthymia and anxiodepression), today depression brings together a group of personal difficulties concerning all pain-producing aspects of life. It traces the line of our existence by giving a generic name to most mood disorders and action dysfunctionalities. The difficulty of defining this deceitful malady has allowed extreme flexibility in the uses of its name. Its core, still unknown, is tenacious to the point that it creates relapses at best, chronic illness at worst. Maintenance treatments, even if they still create controversy, are generally approved. Antidepressants are effective for a wide array of symptoms and make a diagnosis founded on etiology no longer necessary. But in exchange for abandoning etiology, the illness is now situated at the borders of the person who is pathological and the person who has a pathology.

When Nature Is No Longer the Base, Illness Is No Longer a Criteria

Depression shows that psychiatry's evolution is crisscrossed by the same tendencies as we find in the other life sciences. We can act on nature, albeit the psychic kind, and not only on sickness and hereditary dysfunctions, which we used to suffer through the best we could. References have changed for living beings, but psychiatry's problem is that these illnesses are "special." They concern the potential uses of the notion of personality via two questions that underpin the biological, medical, and psychopathological history of depression: *what* are we treating? *Whom* are we curing?

The syndrome-based and dimension-based approaches to depression have provided tools that have an indispensable descriptive value in epidemiological and pharmacological research, but they have not moved us any closer to a cure. The same goes for progress in neurobiology and pharmacology. Worse still, university-based psychiatry has found itself boxed in by the insulin-dependent model, which justifies chronicity. It could have chosen the model of psychosis, but that would have created, as you can imagine, a negative effect on the clientele. It's hard not to conclude that the program was a failure, but a *failure in this precise way*: it did not succeed in advancing a cure. There is one good reason for recognizing this: it enables us to draw conclusions as to the significance of what occurred and to better understand why, and in the name of which common reference, we chose one way over another.

The SSRIs were the first antidepressants that acted on the personality and modified it to the point that, in a certain number of cases, people believed they were finally free to be themselves. They awoke "their inner strength," and advertising for *all* antidepressants changed: we now had ads that promised "the reopening of human relations," that clamoured for the title of "the well-being tricyclic," or that claimed to deliver "that feeling of being yourself again." Omnipotence, relations with others, well-being, emotional authenticity – we heard it all. The American press often gave its articles on Prozac such titles as "A New Self" and "A New You." Yet, we already knew that the old antidepressants could have the same effect. However, generally speaking, on the one hand they weren't effective for healthy people, and, on the other, they were meant to prepare the patient to confront her conflict. Psychiatry situated itself with reference to nature and sickness. As a result, the SSRIs were the first antidepressants that acted on the personality – as long, at least, as we understood this: we had to be in a context where the illness model was not a reference and where nature itself was no longer a base value. Our normative beliefs about what a person should be in order to be considered a true person were shaken to the core.

We know we can act upon ourselves, whatever the pathology and its reason, thanks to molecules that lessen the intensity of conflicts and the consequences of trauma. We know that our psychic nature is no longer a substructure without qualities. We leave behind both nature and illness. Must we fear that "the appearance of transnosographic medications will lead to effects of desubjectification,"[73] as the Lacanian psychoanalyst and professor of law Pierre Legendre put it? These medications could well put an end to the self (as it would no longer be the theatre of conflict and renunciation) and of the laws of desire. "In the name of what do we want?" Legendre asks.[74] The question is political, and with good reason, since it brings us back to the common world. Unfortunately, Legendre does not propose any solution other than to return to the era of canon law.

I don't think that the decline of the self – that is, the self of conflicts – is equivalent to desubjectification. Instead, it demonstrates
that today's human being is not the same as the one we knew at the
end of the nineteenth century or even in the middle of the twentieth
century. This is because the conditions and forms of finitude have
changed. When thinking about the "self," we need to integrate a
few new arguments that might have been set aside too hastily, at
least in France.

AMERICAN ARGUMENTS
FOR A FRENCH CONTROVERSY

In 1997, Peter Kramer added an afterword to the new American
edition of his work. Insofar as it is impossible to base oneself on a
strict definition of pathology, he asked outright "whether to broaden
the definition of illness or to concede that biological treatments are
being used to influence normal mental states."[75] Unlike most psychiatrists, especially French ones, who settle for recognizing the
inadequacy of the concept of illness in psychiatry without proposing
a solution, Kramer advances arguments to help us reflect on the
prescription of psychotropes outside of any reference to a diagnosis.
Kramer should interest the French because he is, if I may put it this
way, a real American: his arguments are pragmatic, he offers a choice
and evaluates the consequences, and his vision of the subject is
utilitarian (i.e., one builds a society through the wise use of humanity's penchants). His arguments are delightfully free of moral or
metaphysical heights. They are down to earth, and that is what is so
good about them: he says out loud what people on the ground are
actually doing.

The very worthwhile final chapter of his book, "The Message in
the Capsule," attempts to see behind the hopes and fears inspired
by the new molecules. Kramer tries to develop criteria to justify
treating a person who is not sick by differentiating antidepressant
molecules from drugs. Prozac is far from being a drug because "it
induces pleasure in part by freeing people to enjoy activities that
are social and productive. And, unlike marijuana or LSD or even
alcohol, it does so without being experienced as pleasurable in itself
and without inducing distortions of perception. Prozac simply gives
anhedonic people access to pleasures identical to those enjoyed by
other normal people."[76] He believes that this generalized use does

not represent a major break in our societies because such uses are well established in medicine – products for baldness or teenage acne, plastic surgery, estrogen to limit the effects of menopause, and so on. He could have chosen other examples, too – aspirin, which is essentially a symptom-based medication or, more spectacularly, medically assisted procreation that helps people overcome physiological inadequacy. These examples are widespread and are anything but rare. Medicine is no longer the domain of sick people alone.

Kramer offers a choice: use molecules to treat depression, which would be paid for by health authorities, or for the improvement of the psychological comfort of "normal subjects," which would not be reimbursed. What is important is that these molecules increase individual abilities without the toxicity and drop-out risks associated with drugs and alcohol. Kramer is perfectly right when he situates psychiatry among the current tendencies of medicine. In fact, today's psychiatric reasoning legitimizes the prescribing of antidepressants to any person suffering from any sort of incapacity. Dysthymics; anxiodepressives; inhibited, panicked, or subsyndrome individuals of all kinds who show up in the offices of general practitioners (but who also consult cardiologists, rheumatologists, etc.) should be treated with antidepressants *as a first step*. The prescribing of molecules with a wide spectrum of effects responds to an increase in today's normative demands; the difficulty of confronting them can be costly to an individual caught up in a world where professional, family, and emotional failure can add up quickly. Such failures can lead to social rejection much faster now than in the past.

The critical reaction in France to his book shows that Kramer's questions were not understood. His utilitarian perspective ran into a wall of French metaphysics. The very dubious belief, questioned by many psychiatrists, is that a miracle pill could exist that would make the person who ingests it feel "better than good" most of the time.[77] That belief is a trap because, like any antidepressant, Prozac has varying therapeutic effects and is far from being ideal. The French press saw in Kramer's book a promotion of happiness on prescription, and I doubt that the work was truly discussed in psychiatry. Neither journalists nor psychiatrists picked up on the questions that concerned Kramer. His interesting pragmatic reasoning had no appeal in a country that has turned the Self into a sacred being, so much so that the slightest puff of cannabis is an attack on human dignity. Yet Kramer was advancing arguments that could have launched a worthwhile discussion about antidepressants and could have enlightened opinion about the complexity of treating mental states.

Psychiatrist and historian David Healy, in a very well-informed work about the history of antidepressants, asked the same sorts of questions at the end of his inquiry. He was quick to point out that "the role of drug treatments would be to facilitate the resolution of a disorder rather than to specifically cure it."[78] He also proposed practical criteria that would help replace the now untenable reference to illness. He commented: "As a prescriber I enjoy considerable advantages that are denied to others. I can take a minor tranquilizer before a public address or interview if I wish, without having to display my 'weakness' to another. I can treat my tendency to dry skin with a steroid ointment of my choice."[79] This could be said of all of us, as long as we are well informed by our doctors as to the risks and advantages of each choice. Instead of calling molecules "antidepressants," we could simply opt for the word "tonic" – since tonics don't treat a disease.

As for Kramer, he hit the nail on the head: "There is no privileged sphere of the mind, no set of problems that is the exclusive domain of self-understanding. We are not formed of experience alone."[80] In effect, neurochemical imbalances and the difficulties in transmitting information between neurons is also part of who we are. He reminded us of the importance of our animal nature in any definition of the self and of how its treatment can improve the "higher functions," to use the old way of speaking. Kramer is defending a medicine of behaviours. The dissolution of psychiatry that Henri Ey feared is no doubt one of the consequences of this, but psychiatry no longer treats illness, and maybe not even syndromes. Édouard Zarifian has criticized psychiatry's tendency to regulate behaviour. He also noted the decline of psychopathology within the teaching of psychiatry. We are still following the conflict between specific and non-specific, the conflict that, from ECT to Prozac, has haunted psychiatry. Today, are there any new elements that can help us understand the controversy?

French psychiatry, especially in the university world, would do well to remember an old political lesson given by Henri Ey. "Of course," he declared in 1947, "we can't debate until we're all in agreement, nor find answers to all the problems at hand! Of course not! The debate will have to stop when a certain number of coherent *doctrinal* positions have been defined and will be available for all to choose among them."[81] To enlighten positions and to clearly present arguments is the only thing that counts as the heterogeneity of mental pathologies will not allow agreement between schools and currents of thought.

The new antidepressants are certainly excellent medications, as long as we understand the limits of their therapeutic use. To hold up the prospect of miracles that the profession does not even believe in can only produce disappointment. In France, for example, has anyone catalogued the disappointments caused by medical therapy? In a society where constraints on individual initiative are strong and where responsibility for failure weighs more heavily on groups that are socially weak, the medicine of behaviour has a legitimate place, and I see no moral argument for giving it a bad name. The only thing that matters is to understand the stakes and indicate the limits, instead of blundering on into dangerous confusion. Let's not forget that the sociologist and the historian are not here to tell people how they should think and live their lives.

LET'S NOT FORGET WHAT JANET SAID

When it comes to pharmacological treatment, we find the same charge of moral abjection that was levelled against hypnosis. Janet believed that this criticism was based on a faulty idea: "In suggestive therapy we use powers that are dishonourable or without moral values ... Suggestion is contemptible because it acts only on the surface of the mind and not on the basis of the soul, it modifies only symptoms and does not transform the very heart of the patient's spirit." "Even if that were true," Janet retorts, "is it then forbidden to make use of symptomatic medication, and isn't the treatment of other illnesses full of such use?"[82] His remark is well taken. The opposition of superficial and deep, higher and lower, voluntary and automatic underpins moral criticism. There is a constant conflict between the higher and lower parts of human beings: the superiority of the mind over the body must be maintained. That is the meaning of the question, "Is the patient comfortably medicated?" The new molecules are more effective than the old, the percentage of resistant depressions has not diminished, the effects on patients are hard to predict, and we are a long way from a molecule that could control affect and let us transform ourselves according to our desires. What remains of pharmacology's miracles now that depression has become a chronic illness? "Even when the medication succeeds," wrote François Dagognet back in 1964, "we shouldn't conclude that it delivers us."[83] A good medication does not need to be associated with a magic potion.

Antidepressants cannot make the dream of "mental disinfection" come true. They suggest instead that the naturalization of the psyche will run up against a new obstacle – at least outside of psychoses – which is chronic illness. Unless it wants to take refuge in magical thinking, which is still hoping for the invention (always put off until some future time) of a "specific redeemer" that would guarantee a perfect cure, psychiatry will not advance by completely rebiologizing mental disorder, by renaturalizing the mind and forgetting that the type of pathology it is treating has a specific uniqueness (in that it stands at the crossroads between the medical and the moral). Biologists have pointed this out: human beings are characterized by having the possibility of escaping their genetic destiny.[84] This possibility imposes technical limits on the therapeutic effects of the progress of pharmacology: programming the mind is just not possible from the practical point of view. If there is no white magic, why fear black magic?

The conflict is suspended thanks to a molecule, and, in the best cases, from time to time a change of personality may occur. Practitioners such as Guyotat and Lambert already noted this at the beginning of the 1960s. Considered as a type of mental disinfection along Janet's lines, the treatment can improve a person's possibilities by acting on his or her psychic nature. Taking an antidepressant is not an issue as it was never in contradiction with a desire for self-knowledge or conflict resolution. The individual has the material means to put off conflicts, perhaps for the term of his or her lifetime. This distancing is more or less effective depending on who is doing it, and when, but it does locate the core of the person's problem. The molecule does help us overcome what we suffer from in depression, which is, according to psychoanalysts, the feeling of not being up to our ideal of the Ego, an ideal that, unlike the Superego, puts us into a position to act. The conflict has not disappeared; it is simply less visible because less obtrusive.

Here, the base has split, a new psychiatric situation has opened up before us with, on the one hand, chronic states, and, on the other, the comfortable effectiveness of molecules. Pharmacology lets us act on an inadequate mind, be it ill or not. By reducing the psychological inequalities handed down to us by nature or filiation in order to improve upon ourselves, the new molecules prove that it is possible to act on a person's nature – his or her temperament or character (i.e., that which does not change with time). Leaving behind our dependency on nature places us firmly and forever on the borders. It reminds psychiatry that it is a special branch of medicine, at the crossroads of the medical and the moral. If psychiatry does not recognize its special nature without increasing its therapeutic effectiveness, it will be suspected of hiding "a deficit with an artifice," as Sándor Radó put it.

"Our greatest fear," wrote Kramer, "was that medication would rob us of what is uniquely human: anxiety, guilt, shame, grief, self-consciousness ... In the end, I suspect that the moral implications of Prozac are difficult to specify not only because the drug is new but because we are new as well. Like so many of the 'good responders' to Prozac, we are two persons, with two senses of self. What is threatening for the old self is already comforting, perhaps eagerly sought after by the new. Here, I think, is Prozac's most profound moral consequence, in changing the sort of evidence we attend to, in changing our sense of constraints on human behaviour, in changing the observing self."[85] The key phrase is "two persons, with two senses of self." Instead of a conflict that creates the unity of the subject, a double identity is offered to the person in the form of a choice. Insofar as the person is healthy with the molecule but unhealthy without it, which person is the real person? The neurotic subject was built by leaving behind the double (Janet) in favour of conflict (Freud). The latter's decline allows the return of the question of double identities. But this questioning is expressed in terms that could not have existed at the beginning of the twentieth century: being more than oneself (until what limit?) or other than oneself (who?). We know that kind of language very well: it belongs to the world of drugs.

Dependency, like depression, is both an illness and a state of mind. It covers territory that goes far beyond psychotropic medication and illicit drugs. The innocent techniques of self-improvement that were popularized in the 1970s have, today, turned into a mistrust of cults whose marketing is centred on personal transformation: at the horizon of personal liberation is the dependency on a master. The fear of cults is to psychotherapy what the fear of drugs is to psychotropic medication. And it does not matter, as far as that point is concerned, whether we are talking about chemistry or organization.

CONFLICT IN DECLINE, FROM THE PSYCHIC TO THE POLITICAL

The quarrel between Janet and Freud rages on more than a century later but in a pharmacological context that uses substances to let us act on our temperaments as much as on our pathologies and in a normative context that beckons us to become ourselves and to surpass ourselves through action. Leaving behind the reference to illness and nature while invoking the crisis of the forbidden displays an astonishingly parallel path. Psychiatry abandons its references just as we seem less divided by conflict – and more empty and agitated. If nothing is written as destiny, nothing is permanent either. The contemporary self is caught in a process of "deconflictuation" in the psychiatric and socio-political realms.

The "Deconflictuation" of the Psychic Realm, or Janet's Posthumous Revenge on Freud

Conflict was structured on two levels, the first political and the second individual. On the political level, the invention of the welfare state (insurance for workers and assistance for those who could not work), its formation by political representation (parliaments and parties) and mass organizations (unions, youth movements), allowed societies to overcome a risk associated with class struggle: that of slipping into civil war. This gave conflict a political stage that accorded it meaning by setting down the lines of confrontation and accord between various actors. Sharing wealth more fairly and fighting inequalities between social classes were the two great political compromises that dominated the second half of the nineteenth century. Conflict conditioned social unity, and it allowed the existence of human groups without them having to justify their meaning by referring to an outside term (or a sovereign who would decide for everyone). Therein lies the very core of political action in a democracy.[86]

On the individual level, conflict fulfilled the same symbolic function as it did at the political level: it structured a division of the self in which elements were both in relationship and in conflict. In fact, they were *in relationship because of their conflict.* The division of the self is a constitutive part of the unity of the person. This division is born on the borders of the subject of madness and becomes the centre of the subject of neurosis. It is the dimension that is not private (we don't choose it) or even intersubjective (we don't negotiate it), but, rather, it founds the self. "The satisfaction of desire," wrote Legendre, "is not on the program for the reproduction of humanity, but without desire reproduction would not take place. It is impossible to eliminate this contradiction."[87] This law can be transgressed but not abolished.

Depression is one of the markers of the difficulty conflict has in producing relations. Conflict no longer seems to be the great province of the unity between social and individual realms. What, then, are the ingredients that create, destroy, and renew intimate and social relations? The two realms have to be understood together.

The recent inundation of our societies by depression includes the process of the decline of the notion of the self, which held centre stage since the end of the nineteenth century. Freud, and not Janet, gave the modern subject its ideal form. Ideal for two reasons, the first of which has a universal character for modernity: Freud integrated human animality (the Id) with civilization (the Superego). We are all made up of drives and instincts, like all mammals, but our particularity is that moral law divides and engenders, to speak as Freud did, this topical variation of guilt that is known as anxiety. The experience of conflict structures the subject's identity whose unity it maintains, but the intensity of the conflict can be such that the person fragments into psychosis and the Ego scatters into identity dissociation (the heart of schizophrenia, according to Bleuler).

The second reason that the form of the modern subject is ideal stems from Freud's considering the human being from the person's indetermination, as Jacques Lacan pointed out in his 1959 and 1960 seminars on *Civilization and Its Discontents.* In the French use of psychoanalysis, guilt is central; it is a way of giving form to this indetermination. Psychiatrist Angélo Hesnard introduced Freud's ideas into France (one day we'll have to reevaluate the former's role), and he emphasized the issues of fault and guilt from his very first work, which was published in 1913. And he continually went back to the theme thereafter: it is the centre of his work.[88] Psychoanalysis provides, he wrote in 1946, a moral code for "humanity that tends to remain absolutely ignorant of its own basic animality."[89] Analysis will help it cure itself of infantile fantasies centring on imaginary faults and will help it recognize adult moral values. The notions of fault and morbid conflict formed the introduction of Freud's thought into France, whereas they were secondary in the American history of psychoanalysis.

According to Lacan, Freud thinks that the human being is searching for happiness but that, with regard to attaining it, "nothing is prepared for it, either in the macrocosm or the microcosm."[90] The Id-Superego pairing is inscribed in a tradition of the metaphysics of the subject, which, in order for society to exist, puts necessary limitations on humanity's natural penchants. In France, starting from the 1950s, when Lacan took on such institutional weight that all French psychoanalysis was organized around him, the relation to the forbidden dominated thinking in the field. Lacan made reference to Hesnard's morbid conflict and showed that the subject must risk castration anxiety in order to attain, simultaneously, desire and law. The Lacanian subject does not know the body; rather, it is bound to the law. The child becomes an adult subject by sensing the difference between the castrating (and thus imaginary) father and the father at the origin of the Superego (and thus symbolic). "Psychoanalysis," he wrote in 1960, "teaches that in the end it is easier to accept interdiction than to run the risk of castration."[91] To become a subject, we have to face the anxiety of becoming ourselves. The neurotic individual adopts a convenient strategy: she attains neither desire nor law. Psychic conflict, which Lacan radicalizes to the point of negating human animality, is essential to French thought. It is used differently by American psychoanalysis, which is looking to help people perfect themselves by themselves. The way of conceiving individuality, be it pathological or not, is completely different in the United States then it is in France. Castration anxiety is to France what Ego mobility is to the United States. It occupies an essential space in France's psychoanalytical mechanism.

French psychoanalysis shares in this metaphysics of the Subject, even beyond Lacanian circles. It defines a national psychiatric style – a Republican style, I would say. The normative Republican system involves tearing away the individual from his private dependencies in order to make a citizen out of him, whereas the American political norm means allowing the expression of private interests in public space. The identification of the subject of desire and the subject of law, which seems to be a French invention, is analogous to the relation of the citizen to the law. The American Declaration of

Independence speaks of "the pursuit of happiness," while French citizenship is organized by an impersonal law. Obeying the whole through this law, the French citizen depends on no person and hence obeys only her/himself. Therein lies a way of viewing the psychological and social self that we find in numerous areas, particularly in the contemporary investment in penal law. Today, is it not invested with the mission of structuring the self,[92] something which other institutions seem unable to do? In France, the relations between desire and law are a problem that goes far beyond psychoanalytic circles.

Freud made neurosis a reference in order to speak of the dilemmas of the normal individual – a role that madness, by its excess, could not fulfill. The decline of neurosis is the decline of an experience of the world that placed conflict at the centre of the human condition and gave it meaning. Conflictual humanity was still cared for by an external force superior to it. The individual submitted to strong laws and hierarchy, her body made docile by discipline. The notion of law refers to both freedom *and* social control. It brings order to the self and society.

Inhibition is a norm integrated into a culture of the forbidden and obedience; it moderates the personal ambitions of the working class. The neurotic individual suffers, then, from too large a load of the forbidden. His Superego is too harsh, and what is usually a condition of civilization turns into a personal defect. In a culture of performance and individual action, in which energy breakdowns can cost dearly, and in which we always have to be running at top speed and efficiency, inhibition is pure dysfunction, an inadequacy. The individual has an institutional need to act at any cost by being able to count on his inner strengths. He inhabits initiative more than obedience; he is caught in the question of what it is possible to do and not what it is permissible to do. That is why inadequacy is to the contemporary person what conflict was to the person of the first half of the twentieth century. From neurosis to depression – that is Janet's posthumous revenge on Freud.

THE MELANCHOLIA OF THE EXCEPTIONAL MAN AND THE PASSION FOR EQUALITY

By attracting neurosis into the orbit of depression and attempting to get rid of it for a multitude of practical reasons, including the embarrassing issue of etiology, psychiatry finds itself with the uncomfortable problem of chronic illness and dependency. Of course, it has been facing psychoses for some time now. But here is another mental pathology, and another type of society, another experience with the uncontrollable, the unknown. Depression is less of an "other," certainly less radical than madness, and at the same time different from the familiarity of neurosis. It has none of the fearful abilities of madness or the ambivalences of the old melancholia. Yet there is a relation between melancholia and depression: both are the unhappiness of self-consciousness heightened to the extreme, the awareness of being *only* oneself. If melancholia was the domain of the exceptional human being, then depression is the manifestation of the *democratization of the exceptional.*[93]

We live with this belief and this truth: each person should have the possibility of creating his or her own history instead of submitting to life as if it were a matter of destiny. Humanity "put [it]self in motion" by opening possibilities and playing out individual initiative, while carrying this process to the individual's most intimate places. This dynamic increases indetermination, accelerates the break-up of permanence, and multiplies the supply of reference points even as it blurs them. The man without qualities – the novelist Robert Musil drew his portrait – is the man open to the undetermined – progressively, he is emptied of all identity imposed from the outside that might have helped structure him. "People," Musil wrote, "used to be like the stalks of corn in the field. They were probably more violently flung to and fro by God, hail, fire, pestilence and war than they are today, but it was collectively, in terms of towns, of country-sides, the field as a whole."[94] The feeling of being shaken is now personalized; it comes from within.

When, in 1887, Nietzsche announced the arrival of the sovereign individual, "with the help of the morality of customs,"[95] he saw in him a strong being: "The proud knowledge of the extraordinary privilege of responsibility, the consciousness of this rare freedom, of this power over himself and over fate, has sunk right down to his innermost depths, and has become an instinct, a dominating instinct." "But there is no doubt about it," he added, "the sovereign man calls it his conscience."[96] The individual, free from morality, creating herself by herself and aspiring to the superhuman (acting upon her own nature, surpassing herself, being more than herself), is now our reality. But, instead of possessing the strength of the masters, she turns out to be fragile, lacking in being, weary of her sovereignty and full of complaints. She does not inhabit Nietzsche's gay science and laughter. Depression, then, is melancholia plus equality, the perfect disorder of the democratic human being. It is *the inexorable counterpart of the human being who is her/his own sovereign.* We are not speaking of the human being who has acted badly but, rather, of the human being who cannot act. Depression is not conceived in terms of law, what is allowed and what is forbidden, but in terms of *capacity.*

The individual is now neither with nature nor ruled by a superior, impersonal law. He reaches for the future, whose labours he must face, made heavy by internal responsibility. He is less governed by constraint (that which is permitted or forbidden) and more by limits (the possible against the impossible). When is it *possible* to act on nature, on emotional syndromes we know little about, whether we have them or whether they are intimately part of us, or even whether it is *normal* to act on them? Are we allowed to do it and, if so, in the name of what? In psychiatry, the reference issue arises once we no longer have nature or illness to lean on, or the authority of tradition, of which society has freed itself. If everything is possible, is everything then normal and, therefore, allowed? These issues are political insofar as they refer to a society's founding principles – that is, the horizon of a common world. The trouble we have answering these questions results in our concern about dependency. The sovereign individual is both depressed and dependent.

DEPENDENCY, OR NOSTALGIA FOR THE LOST SELF

The critique of moral abasement once levelled against hypnosis has been reformulated for antidepressants, but in a whole other context. Identity worries caused by a chemical substance acting on states of consciousness is, in fact, not a new problem in our societies. For some thirty years now, we have had on hand an antimodel: illegal drugs. They are the perfect cognitive tools for designating a kind of misconduct that consists in manipulating our own states of consciousness, whatever the danger the product poses. The drugged person is the ideal antimodel for defining a way of being oneself that, thanks to the ingestion of a substance, avoids the pathways that lead to conflict. Changing the personality of truly ill people means giving them back their health, but changing the personality of those who may not be ill is equal to drugging them, even if the drug is not dangerous. The patient who has been given a good quality of life can be said to have been comfortably drugged. And this is what constitutes the damage done to the *ideal* of who or what a person is.

Dependency, which is a pathological relation to a product, activity, or person, is, with depression, psychiatry's other big obsession.[97] For biological and behaviourist psychiatry, it is risky conduct. For our societies, since the stakes are less medical than symbolic, dependency has become something more essential. The drugged individual is the person who has crossed the border between "everything is possible" and "everything is allowed." She has pushed the limits of the sovereign individual. Dependency is the price of limitless freedom that the self has granted itself; it is a form of slavery. If madness is the first, then dependency is the second way of saying what can occur when freedom vacillates within the self. But madness and dependency say this in completely opposing languages. The first reveals the dark side of the birth of the modern self; the second sheds harsh light on its decline.

In the most extreme cases, madness takes on the form of a dissolution of identity – the distance between the self and the self is at its maximum. On the other hand, dependency tends towards an identity fusion, with distance being minimal. Madness has two centuries of history behind it, while dependency is only some forty years old. The notion of dependency was first developed around illegal drugs, which are a concern of rich societies. They spread across the United States and Europe during the 1960s in the name of the right to choice, which was alienated by bourgeois morality, capitalism, and the overall conditioning of the masses by consumerism.[98] Later, the notion of dependency was extended to designate any pathological relation, no matter its object.

In order to move from madness to dependency in fewer than two hundred years, neurosis had to be invented at the end of the nineteenth century and then be converted into depression in the last third of the twentieth century. Dependency is to psychic liberation and individual initiative what madness was to law and reason: a self that we can never find sufficient (identity insecurity), a demand for action to which we can never sufficiently respond (the indecision of inhibition, the uncontrolled action of impulsiveness). If the aspiration to be oneself leads to depression, depression leads to dependency, to the nostalgia for the lost self.

The Declaration of Human Rights states that human beings are the owners of themselves. The French Revolution politically instituted the modern self. Madness was transformed into an illness with a specifically human freedom, inherent to the indetermination that characterizes its reason and its law. Two centuries later, the ownership of the self has become our lifestyle; it has been sociologically integrated into our mores and is at the very heart of our intimate sovereignty. At the beginning of democratic modernity, humanity was divided and split apart; during the last third of the twentieth century, humanity entered a relationship of fusion and became dependent.

Madness was the underside of reason, Freudian neurosis was the underside of the conflictual self, and depression was the underside of an individual who is only himself and, as a result, is never enough himself (as though he were always running behind his own shadow, on which he is dependent). If depression is a pathology of a consciousness *that is only itself,* then dependency is the pathology of a consciousness *that is never enough of itself,* that is never adequately filled with its identity, that is never adequately active – too undecided, too explosive. Depression and dependency are the two sides of the same pathology of inadequacy.

The overwhelming advertising images created for certain antidepressants are the reply of the norms inherent to our lives. But these norms are strangely reminiscent of what accounts for the popularity of drugs: the multiplication of the self through the manipulation of one's own states of consciousness. If there is one caricature in private life in France, it is the "addict." The imagery developed around drugs has penetrated our societies much more deeply than have the actual problems caused by them or their users. The new molecules open up a new horizon: the unlimited possibility of manufacturing your own mental landscape without the risk of toxicity or side effects associated with the old classes of antidepressants. This possibility can create a sense of moral revulsion because, since there is no longer any illness to refer to, we find ourselves in the imaginary world of drugs. Imaginary indeed, because danger is not the only issue when it comes to drugs. They are "grace without merit," as the poet Octavio Paz put it – that is, without work, without development, without personal effort. With drugs, the self is simply not answering the call.

Depression is the mediator that allows us to clearly see the processes by which the person ill with conflict, who once risked madness, today suffers from an inadequacy that sets off dependency. Madness is an event that befalls us; drugs are an action that makes things happen. I go mad, but I take drugs. Drugs are a behaviour, implying an intention and an action. Unlike madness, they challenge the will whose pathology they are. Are not drugs ways we have of increasing our personal capacities, whether we're hoping to improve our endurance, our concentration, our imagination, or our pleasure? For us inhabitants of the modern age, as Jean-Pierre Vernant reminds us, the will "is the person conceived of in his role of agent, the Ego envisaged as a source of action for which he is responsible not only in the eyes of others, but in which he is personally involved." Will, Vernant goes on to say, presupposes "a recognized superiority, when it comes to action, of the human subject as its origin, the productive cause of all actions that flow from him."99

The many factors that separate the action and the agent in religious societies have been wiped away. Action has no other source than the agent who carries it out and who is responsible for it. The figure of the self emerges wholly changed from this. The question behind action is not: "Do I have the right?" but, rather, "Am I able to?" We are now caught up in a profound and shared process in which reference to what is permitted is subordinated to a reference to what is possible.

A double movement ensues. First, technological excitement over the definitive restructuring of the self, a cyberhuman wave, as pointed out in the catalogue of the "Post-Human" exhibition in Lausanne, Switzerland, in 1992: "More and more people are understanding that there is no longer any use in trying to 'cure' a personality disorder. On the contrary: it would be better, it would seem, to try to modify rather than treat the personality."100 In parallel fashion, a sense of moral excitement has arisen. We can see this in the over-investment in penal law concerning the "limits" that the subject must not transgress in order to remain a subject. What, then, is the "limit" between a little bit of plastic surgery and the android creation that Michael Jackson has become; between the wise management of one's moods through psychotropes and the excesses of the "chemical robot"; between seduction strategies that are just "too much" and sexual abuse. The borders of the person and those that divide people, one from the next, have preoccupied us to the point where we no longer know *who is who*. Is not incest, like dependency, "a short circuit with oneself?"101 A society of individual initiative and psychic liberation, insofar as it forces each person to make constant decisions, encourages the practice of self-modification and, in so doing, creates problems with the structuring of the self – problems that attracted no attention at all in a discipline-based society. The continent of the permitted has been absorbed by the greater domain of the possible, and the result is, if I may say so, that no one can plead ignorance of the law.

This concern with "limits" confirms, it would seem, that contemporary individualism is simply the triumph of the private person, right down to her deepest suffering.[102] We seem to be facing a complete reformulation of things. Public action is also involved in refashioning intimate space in the great transformation of the ways we see ourselves.

The Decline of Conflict in the Social Sphere:
The Personal as the New Political Constraint

The new attention being paid to anxiety arising from social issues has led to the development of mechanisms of psychological help for traumas of all sorts, from victims of terrorism to people who have been laid off. This support is a way of regulating those vulnerabilities that have become the subject of endless works and studies. Let us not sink into the realm of anxiety and suffering without first asking ourselves why this attention is being paid. Too often it leads to the critique of the elites who have abandoned the poor, whereas political action is facing new difficulties. What does politics have to do with mental suffering?[103] Suffering is individual and normally the business of personal resourcefulness or of professionals in the particular field at issue.

This concern for suffering is part of the decline of the conflictual dimension in the social sphere, and the rise of intragroup inequalities reveals this. Instead of struggles between social groups, individual competition affects people in different ways – less "municipally," as Musil would have put it. We are witnessing a double phenomenon: increasing universality (globalization), which is abstract, and acute personalization, which is felt much more concretely. We can fight a boss or an opposing class, but how do you fight "globalization"? It is much more difficult to demand justice in this context or to pin the responsibility for a situation that has victimized us on an adversary we can name. Besides, it is ever more difficult to separate suffering from injustice, compassion from inequality, legitimate conflicts that strive to share the wealth from the illegitimate kind that arise from a corporatism that is well placed within power relations. Resentment turns towards oneself (depression is an attack on the self) or towards a scapegoat (the anti-immigrant Front National in France has conjured up the Enemy, a figure who disappeared at the end of the Second World War),[104] or, within identity politics, it is played out in the search for the self.

Instead of a crisis in the political realm and the self resulting from the rise of individualism, we are witnessing a two-pronged change in the figures of the personal *and* the political. Common action is no longer built with mass movements, marshalled by an organization against an identifiable adversary. Political representation is no longer distributed according to which class one belongs, as electoral sociology has unanimously shown. Citizenship no longer means bracketing off one's private interests. Certainly, there is no political action outside the common world, but today this world moves through the individualization of action. Political action is now less an issue of resolving conflicts between adversaries and more an issue of collectively facilitating individual action. This is a new political constraint.

Today, particularly in the social realm that has become a veritable place of experimentation and reflection on the issue, we are seeing new forms of political action whose basis is not conflict but partnership and mediation. Conflict is not posited; it must be built, or *situated*. In conditions of insecurity, when it comes to long-term unemployment, the service centre where the welfare recipient went to pick up his check while waiting to be offered work is no longer relevant. This social safety net has been replaced by integrating people into a network of partners. The goal is to help people solve their problems themselves, while assisting them along their way. By producing individuality, we hope at the same time to produce society.[105] Recipients take an active role in their integration and, as a counterpoint, the role of institutions is now to provide the conditions that enable this to happen: remove shame and help restore dignity, create respect where contempt once dwelled, rebuild individuals when they have been reduced by despair and unlawfulness.

The transformations in the struggle against drug use reveal much about how social action is being restated. Certain products (methadone, antidepressants) that help reduce risks find an echo in certain "community-based healing" structures. Supporting people in the long term, with their difficulties in finding autonomy (living with drugs), and integrating them into a system of guilt are both ways of regulating behaviour. And, in France, they are developing at the same time, often in the greatest confusion.

A new youth-court strategy is to consider delinquent minors as adult subjects who have rights. The goal is not only to break the sense of impunity by imposing sentences but also to "explain what the law is, [to] explain [the] legal consequences and social consequences of law-breaking."[106] Commissions that give out welfare payments redefine the individual living in insecure conditions by turning to this idea: "Exclusion is defined by the loss or the impossibility of attaining the usual factors of social identity."[107] In both cases, the target is the ability to project oneself into the future. And in both cases, social action rebuilds from the inside by integrating into strategies of resocialization what personally matters to the failing individual. This is done by displaying the internal elements upon which he or she might be able to rely.

These methods are certainly no panacea. The demands they make on more fragile individuals, when it comes to the social integration contract, can have disastrous results. A recent report on mental health among financially insecure groups pointed this out: "The effort demanded of people who need to integrate is in general much greater than that demanded of those who are already part of society."[108] The commodification of this partnership project is no rare occurrence, and real solutions can be in cruelly short supply, but what is important here is to grasp the new direction. A new public space may be opening up. It would stress the *common* subjectivity of people rather than the objectivity of contradictory influences, and it would create autonomy rather than resolve conflicts.

What is interesting about new social policies is this: they make us think that there are procedures put forward by organized groups whose goal is to help individuals take responsibility for their own lives, including those who are at the bottom of the ladder. These state-supported methods help produce individuality, including through long-term support. They maintain a common reference that might guide the actions of each individual, each one as herself, all sharing common rights, yet singular when it comes to the problems she has to solve. Individual difference is no longer wholly subsumed by collective inequality. The relations between inequality and difference become political issues. Contemporary individualism is less the triumph of egotism over civic spirit and more a change in the way we experience the world.

The Individual: Institutions, Not Subjectivity

New figures of individuality spring from everything from self-medication to individual-based political action. Their way of being is no longer a matter of class conflict or of individuality caught in a society of discipline. The aspirations, problems, and solutions that shape them are quite different. We have changed our "world of meanings," our ways of understanding truth and error. The institution of the self enters at this point. This notion, it seems to me, will help us understand that individualism cannot be reduced to the privatization of existence and that it presupposes "a world that is shared and public."[109]

From obedience to action, from discipline to autonomy, from identification to identity: these movements have swept away the border between the public citizen and the private individual. We may well regret that, but it is useless, and even politically dangerous, to keep our heads in the sand. This situation is the result of conflict's productivity. Its decline does not necessarily mean that we are inexorably drawn to stop sharing the world with our counterparts. The individual is not left to himself, as if he were alone to face his choices. Nor, on the other hand, is he simply a patch job between subjectivities that choose their lifestyles as if they were in some great supermarket.

If moral constraints have grown lighter, psychic constraints have taken their place. Emancipation and action have stretched individual responsibility beyond all borders and have made us painfully aware that we are only ourselves. The private sphere has entered the dimension of history and shares in its tumult. Hence that feeling of massive deinstitutionalization that sociologists often interpret a little lazily as a psychologization of social relations. Today's social relations are psychologized (because they are based on something "personal," whereas before they were "governed"), they involve links between an Ego (a subjectivity) and another Ego (the relation between the two creating intersubjectivity) in a kind of generalized contractual relation whose final goal is the (mutual) realization of the self. Traditionally, the individual was handed the characteristic of selfishness (and had to be governed by the community), but now the individual receives empathy (which can create a society on its own). Scientific methods, though often irreproachable, cannot mask the confusion of concepts. A society is composed of actors and is maintained by institutions. As Marcel Mauss wrote in *Œuvres*, it is "a set of actions and ideas, already in place, that individuals encounter, and that more or less imposes itself on them."[110] What individuals find themselves surrounded by is an ensemble whose references all converge on modification and relations of support.

The convergence of the State, the professional sectors, the educational system, and private enterprise on personal initiative, combined with unprecedented moral leeway and a growing numbers of openings, gives the psychic realm a social, and therefore personal, signature that is completely new. The types of responses to the new problems of the self take on the form of helping relationships offered to individuals, sometimes all through their lives. These relationships become a sort of maintenance system that can be administered in a myriad of ways – pharmacological, psychotherapeutic, and socio-political. Products, persons, and organizations can be their avenues. These various actors, who come from public health or private services, all refer back to the same logic: produce individuality that can act by itself and transform itself based on its inner resources. This logic can serve as an instrument of domination as much as a pathway to reintegration and therapeutic care-giving. The confrontations, strategies, and judgments of these actors take place in this imaginary field and not in the classic "class struggle" model or the one provided by life insurance. Part of our lives and our ways of acting, having created a vocabulary we all use on a daily basis ("motivate," "facilitate," and "company"), this logic is part of our very being. It has instituted itself. These new shared forms of the production of individuality are our new institutions.

In less than half a century a major redirection has taken place in the style of the institutions of the self. We were prepared by the first wave of emancipation, which involved the revolt of the private individual against the obligation to work towards common goals. This was the work of the gurus of personal liberation. Way back in 1966, Philip Rieff was already announcing their coming victory. Today we are involved in the second wave, that of personal initiative and submission to the norms of performance. Individual initiative is necessary if people are to remain in the social group. Inhibition and impulsiveness, apathetic emptiness and the stimulation that fills it, follow them like a shadow. Both ideals and constraints have changed.

At the end of the 1960s, "liberation" was the word that brought young people together. Everything was possible. These movements fought institutions. The family stifled you, school was another form of barracks, work (and its product, consumerism) was alienation, and the law (the bourgeois variety, of course) was an instrument of domination that had to be thrown off. Unprecedented moral freedom united with improved economic conditions, and the opening of lifestyle choices, always upwardly mobile, became a tangible reality during that decade. Madness did appear in the landscape of public debate at the beginning of the 1970s, as a symbol of modern oppression rather than mental illness, but only because everything was possible. The madman wasn't sick, he was simply different, and he suffered from the non-acceptance of this difference. Nearly fifty years later, quite another message is often heard: nothing is possible. People feel as though they have collapsed into the present. The shutting down of the economy and the dropping out of a segment of the population reinforces this feeling. The demands on our cognition are many. The theme of respect-the-limits runs up against the collective aspirations of those who want no limits placed on their freedom of choice.

The history of depression has helped us, I believe, understand this social and mental turnaround. Its irresistible rise permeates the two pairs of changes that have affected the individual in the first half of the twentieth century: (1) psychic liberation and identity insecurity and (2) individual initiative and the inability to act. These two pairings display the anthropological stakes at play in the movement from neurotic conflict to depressive inadequacy in the field of psychiatry. The individual emerges from the battle to face messages from this unknown person she cannot control, this irreducible part that Westerners call the unconscious. Instead of a personal *breach*, where the elements are in relation because of their conflict, they are facing an inner *chasm*, where there is neither conflict nor relation. We are not less loaded down with laws than was the kind of individual that has disappeared, but these laws have changed. They create fewer neurotic pathological conflicts than they do dependent pathological relations. It is no use yearning for a return to the forbidden, or endlessly repeating that limits have to be placed on subjects that have never known any. We can't go back in time.

We need to understand that the unknown being within us is changing, and the costs, just like the gains, are moving house.

In the end, the story is very simple. Liberation might have gotten us out of the drama of guilt and obedience, but it has taken us straight into the demands of responsibility and action. And so the weariness of depression took over from the anxiety of neuroses.

The Weight of the Possible

Everything has become so intricate that mastering it would require an exceptional intellect. Because skill at playing the game is no longer enough; the question that keeps coming up is: can this game be played at all now and what would be the right game to play?

Ludwig Wittgenstein, Culture and Value, 1937 (27e)

Without family, without a name, the Cronenberg hero tries to build himself … an essence through technological incantation alone.

Serge Grünberg, *David Cronenberg*, 1992 (118)

Depression threatens the person who resembles only herself the way sin haunted the soul turned towards God or guilt gnawed at the person torn by conflict. More than a source of mental pain, it is a way of life. The major fact of individuality during the second half of the twentieth century was the confrontation between the notion of limitless possibility and the notion of the uncontrolled. The rise of depression set off the tensions produced by this confrontation, as the realm of the permitted crumbled before the onslaught of the possible.

This book took inspiration from an intention found in science fiction,[1] particularly in the work of David Cronenberg. This film-maker has explored interiors but not those of sensitive, nervous beings, and he has ignored the walking wounded of the marriage bed who made up Freud's patient base (mostly female) in the past century. Cronenberg's surgical camera reaches into the mutant flesh of the vertiginous mental landscape that belongs to the person of all possibilities. It grapples with "his animal part."[2] The gemellary state, teleportation, drugs, video and car crashes are Cronenberg's ways of describing the mutations of inner states, the sudden changes in the body. Identity swings between man and fly in *The Fly* (1968), and drugs are part of the trip the hero takes between humanity and monstrosity. At the start of his transmutation, his capacities grow tenfold, he is the powerful sovereign of himself, for him everything is possible: this is his Nietzschean moment. The "biological homosexuality" of the gynecologist twins in *Dead Ringers* (1988) short-circuits the minimal distance that would have let each live without the other and so become true individuals. In this "journey to the end of the flip side,"[3] there are no conflicts, only a fused couple that no woman can separate and that ends up lapsing into drug use. If the man who resembles himself is the ripest fruit on that tree, it comes as no surprise that he is the first to fall. That is his democratic moment.

Identity hesitation between human and insect (*The Fly*) echoes the abrasion of personal identity expressed by the double (*Dead Ringers*). These films explore two facets of our perplexity: the doubling of the same (instead of conflict) and the absolute strangeness that brings conflict back (is he a monstrous insect or is there still some human part, a self, in the fly?). The furthest and closest mingle their blood. This work of science fiction dissects the border between human and non-human for the viewer's cerebral pleasure. Cronenberg has a theory: things mutate in us, but we never leave the human sphere.

That is exactly what depression and addiction teach us. They make us travel across the regions of the realm of the possible, which have progressively taken over after the decline of the old moral systems. In this new space, "transgression without the forbidden"[4] is added to choice without exclusion and to abnormalities without pathology. Therein lie several burning and intimate issues that anthropologists of democratic societies have started to explore. I was less interested in offering solid conclusions than in simply wishing to put forth some of the transformations of "this nodal point of the mind," as James G. Ballard put it, "where *the inner world of the mind and the outer world of reality meet* and fuse."[5] Therein resides psychiatry's and psychopathology's endless need to understand human affairs. Their language is designed to speak of these impalpable vibrations that create personhood. Rather than repeating the incantatory rituals over the self-in-crisis, I preferred to use these disciplines to put into perspective the transformations of subjectivity that they have shown us.

From the unfindable subject of depression to the nostalgia of the self lost in addiction, from the passion of being oneself to the enslavement to oneself, we have carried out this "journey to the end of the flip side." In 1800, the issue of the pathological individual appeared with the madness-delirium pairing. In 1900, it was transformed by the dilemmas of guilt that shook the person made nervous by her desires to free herself. In 2000, the pathologies of the individual involve the responsibilities of a person who has freed herself from the law of her fathers and the old systems of obedience and conformity. Depression and addiction are the two sides of the sovereign individual, the person who believes herself to be the author of her own life, whereas she remains "the subject in both senses of the word: the agent and the patient."[6]

Depression reminds us in no uncertain terms that to be the owner of oneself does not mean that everything is possible – all that rises and falls within us, that contracts and expands. Because it *stops us*, depression holds our attention: it reminds us that we have not left the human realm and that the latter remains chained to a system of meanings that simultaneously go beyond it and constitute it. The symbolic dimension, which was once the property of religious authority and gave meaning to each person's inexorable destiny, permeates the human species, which has control not only over its history (in traditional democratic logic) but also over its own nervous corporality (in contemporary technological logic). Depression portrays for all of us the style of the uncontrollable in the age of limitless possibilities. We can manipulate our bodily and mental nature, we can push back our limits by all sorts of means, but this manipulation won't save us from anything. Constraints and freedoms change, but "that irreducible part" is not diminished.[7] It can change – no more and no less – and it is that change that I have tried to map. If, as Freud thought, "a person becomes neurotic because he cannot tolerate the amount of frustration which society imposes on him,"[8] he becomes depressed because he must tolerate the illusion that everything is possible for him.

As addictive explosion reflects depressive implosion, so the drug-taker's search for sensation reflects the depressed person's lack of feelings. Depression, that crossroads pathology, serves as a canvas upon which to sketch out the changes in modern subjectivity, the displacement of the hard task of being healthy. In a context in which choice is the norm and inner insecurity the price, these pathologies make up the dark side of contemporary private life. Such is the equation of the sovereign individual: psychic freedom and individual initiative = identity insecurities and the incapacity to act.

In this movement we find what is at stake in our own collective psychology. No doubt we are still too psychologically caught up in a rigid perspective of the conflictual self. For we certainly don't lack ways of reflecting on the new issues of the self and illuminating our pathway, inventing our future instead of regretting the good old days when borders were clear and progress could be counted on. Isn't that a bit of retrospective illusion, "the crisis of modernity" being a recurrent theme? Borders are also sites, and you can live in the labyrinth if you find Ariadne's thread. A society of individuals is not designed only to create monads that meet one another in the marketplace to negotiate contracts among lawyers, imploding in depressive emptiness or exploding through impulsive acting out. This society has witnessed its political landscape change, and its forms of public involvement take on other shapes, its ways of acting redesigned.

Depression and addiction are names given to the uncontrollable, which we encounter when we stop talking about winning our freedom and start working on becoming ourselves and taking the initiative for action. They remind us that the unknown is part of every person – and that it always has been. It can change but never disappear: that is why we never leave the human realm. That is depression's lesson. The impossibility of completely reducing the distance between us and ourselves is inherent to any human experience in which the person owns herself and the individual origin of her action.

Depression is the guardrail of the person with no road map. And it is not just a source of pain; it is the counterpoint to the individual's expenditure of energy. The ideas of project, motivation, and communication dominate our culture's norms. They are the passwords of our time. Depression is a pathology of time (the depressed person has no future) and a pathology of motivation (the depressed person has no energy, his movement is slowed, his words slurred). The depressed person has trouble forming projects; he or she lacks energy and the minimum motivation to carry them out. Inhibited, impulsive, or compulsive, she has trouble communicating with herself and others. With no project, motivation, or communication, the depressed person stands in exact opposition to our social norms. We should not be surprised at how the terms relating to depression have exploded into everyday language, and not only in psychiatry: responsibility can be assumed, but its pathologies must be treated. The deficient and the compulsive human being are the two faces of this new Janus.

Notes

PREFACE

1 Nietzsche, *Twilight of the Idols*, 59.
2 Office of the Surgeon General, *Mental Health*, 4.
3 M. Barke, R. Fribush, and P.N. Stearns note this absence in note 30 to "Nervous Breakdown in Twentieth-Century America," 576. There, they refer readers to E. Shorter, *History of Psychiatry*, commenting: "But a fuller historical perspective on the rise of depression and its public resonance in the United States remains vital." For a very general history, see Jackson, *Melancholia and Depression*, 1986. On antidepressants, the most complete work is by the Englishman David Healy, *The Antidepressant Era*, 1997.
4 On 27 February 2009, *The Guardian* published "The Creation of the Prozac Myth," by Darian Leader, a dossier on about twenty years of Prozac. The day before, the online journal PLOS (Public Library of Science) had published a study by Kirsch et al., showing that, outside of severe depressions, Prozac was hardly more effective than a placebo.
5 Fluoxetine was marketed by Eli Lilly but was revealed to the general public by Peter Kramer's *Listening to Prozac* and, in 1994, by novelist Elizabeth Wurtzel's *Prozac Nation*. In the *Guardian* feature (see note 4), Wurtzel addresses the degree to which her memoir has become synonymous with Prozac, attributing this, in part, to her book's original title, "I Hate Myself and I Want to Die" (this became the title of the book's prologue), which was replaced at the behest of her publisher.
6 Kramer, *Listening to Prozac*.
7 Pachet, *Le premier venu*.
8 Coblence, *Le dandysme, obligation d'incertitude*.

9 Bercovitch, *The Puritan Origins of the American Self*; and Pétillon, *L'Europe aux anciens parapets.*

10 Baudelaire, *Artificial Paradise,* 17.

11 *Ibid.,* 80.

12 Some works do escape this tendency, for instance Allan Young's *The Harmony of Illusions.* Young is content, and he is correct, in my opinion, with simple description, which, according to Marcel Mauss, is the main work of sociology and anthropology: "Sociological explanation is completed when one has seen *what* it is that people believe and think, and *who* the people are who believe and think that." (Mauss, quoted in Dumont, *Essays on Individualism,* 192).

13 This long-standing problem with mental-health insurance coverage and the resulting stigmatization of mental il lness was a major motivation for the Mental Health Parity Act. It was central to the advocacy and debate surrounding this legislation (S.558), which was first passed in the Senate in September 2007.

14 Horwitz and Wakefield, *The Loss of Sadness,* 22–3; Ehrenberg, "Les guerres du sujet."

15 Ehrenberg, "Le sujet cérébral."

16 See Lovell, "Mania and the Making of Contemporary US Culture." On several other books about the bipolar issue, see Sacks, "A Summer of Madness."

17 Martin, *Bipolar Expeditions,* 28.

18 *Ibid.,* 10.

19 *Ibid.,* 29.

20 Self-help groups can be understood as part of those associations that, in *Bowling Alone,* Robert Putnam describes as "binding."

21 Sociologist Lydwin Verhaegen points to three psychiatric careers in 1985, one of which involved the functional use of the psychiatric hospital. She supports her claim with the example of a bipolar patient who declared himself to be ill but who thought his illness was the price of his talent. He was a well recognized artist. See chapter five in Verhaegen, *Les psychiatres: Médecine de pointe ou assistance?.*

22 Martin, *Bipolar Expeditions,* 279.

23 Karp, *Speaking of Sadness,* 178.

24 *Ibid.,* 15.

25 *Ibid.,* 168.

26 *Ibid.,* 167.

27 Except Phillip Rieff, the most pessimistic of them all.

28 Karp, *Speaking of Sadness,* 187 (emphasis in original).

29 "In greater or lesser degree I have grappled with *depression* for almost twenty years" (Karp, *Speaking of Sadness,* 3 [emphasis in original]). For Emily Martin, depression is also a business card that allows her into the life of the groups she has studied. I thank Anne M. Lovell for this remark. Martin points out that she was forbidden to take notes during her ethnographic observation of bipolar and hyperactive groups.

30 On this theme, see the story of musician and music critic Allan Shawn, *Wish I Could Be There.*

31 Anonymous, "Why Having a Mental Illness Is Not like Having Diabetes," 846–7.

32 Thompson, *The Beast,* 14.

33 See Bercovitch, *The Puritan Origins of the American Self.* Most of Karp's chapter 1 is a story of this type while also being an explanation of the interview method used. See also the work of Andrew Solomon, *Noonday Demon,* which the author refers to as "an extremely personal book" (12).

34 I refer to Hannah Arendt, *On Revolution,* which compares the American pursuit of private and public happiness with the French pursuit of social issues.

35 F. Zimmerman, "The Love-Lorn Consumptive."

36 The work even received the approval of the head of DSM-III, Robert Spitzer, who wrote the preface. A young French historian and philosopher, Steeves Demazeux, wrote an illuminating review of the work entitled "Cachez cette tristesse que l'on ne saurait voir."

37 Horwitz and Wakefield, *The Loss of Sadness,* 205.

38 Ibid., 205.

39 Ibid., 201.

40 Ibid., 202.

41 Ibid., 219 (emphasis in original).

42 Wakefield, "The Concept of Mental Disorder," 374.

43 Ibid., 384.

44 Cavell, *The Claim of Reason,* 111. French philosopher Pierre-Henri Castel discusses transsexualism in great detail from this perspective in *La métamorphose impensable.*

45 See Vincent Descombes, *The Mind's Provisions.* For more on this book, see R. Brandom's "From a Critique of Cognitive Internalism to a Conception of Objective Spirit."

46 Putnam, *The Collapse of the Fact/Value Dichotomy and Other Essays.*

47 Ibid., 61–2 (emphasis in original).

48 See E. Martin, *Bipolar Expeditions,* 40–2. In my book, these factors occupy a more central position simply because of my historical perspective.

49 Wittgenstein, *Philosophical Investigations*, 42ᵉ.
50 In an interview with Jerome Wakefield, Steeves Demazeux, referring to
   this book, asked him if he wasn't focusing too much on reducing depression to sadness. He pointed out that I had argued that its manifestation
   today is inhibition, the difficulty of taking action. Wakefield, who did not
   know my book, replied that that brought to mind French existentialism,
   something like a *mal du siècle*. My concern is exactly how not to fall into
   this generalizing trap. I hope to have avoided it. See Demazeux, "Pour
   une critique constructive de la psychiatrie américaine."
51 Klibansky et al., *Saturn and Melancholy*, XXX.
52 The comparison of the history of depression in the United States and in
   France is relevant because autonomy as a value doesn't have the same
   importance in the latter as it does in the former. I return to this issue
   when it comes to narcissism, narcissistic pathologies, and borderline states
   in a comparative anthropological and sociological perspective regarding
   the two countries. See Ehrenberg, *La grande névrose*.

INTRODUCTION

1 De Fleury, *Medicine and the Mind*, 265.
2 Because it has become a symbol, Prozac is the only brand to which I will
   refer in this work. For other psychotropic medications, only the name of
   the molecule will be given. Prozac is the brand name for the molecule
   named "fluoxetine."
3 Ehrenberg, *Le culte de la performance* and *L'individu incertain*.
4 Montesquieu, *Montesquieu*, 315.
5 Lefort, "Reversibility," 165.
6 How each person puts it into practice is another matter.
7 "Institution" emphasizes the social nature of the notion of self or of
   being oneself. Here we refer to Vincent Descombes' notion of institution, which is based on the writings of Wittgenstein and Mauss. On the
   one hand, the notion implies that there are "meanings that people must
   recognize" without a prior consensus; on the other hand, the meanings
   are externalized, which is to say, that "each person recognizes the idea
   as a firmly established rule that is independent of the individual." See
   Descombes, *Les institutions du sens*, 288. The notion of person is neutral,
   meaning that each culture has its own interpretation. On the other
   hand, the notions of personality, subject, and individual are "modern."
8 I refer to Gladys Swain's thesis on madness, *Le sujet de la folie* (1977 and
   1997). See also Marcel Gauchet's essay, *De pinel à Freud* in the 1997 edition. For the importance of this thesis, see chapter 1.

9 Conversely, for psychiatrists to be debating it strikes me as decisive. But this is rarely the case nowadays (in university psychiatry, at least). For an exception, see Zarifian, *Le prix du bien-être.*

10 Except in cases where the pathology results from a toxin (e.g., alcohol, drugs) or from an infection.

11 A symptom is an isolated sign, whereas a syndrome is a group of symptoms systematically correlated with one another.

12 As Daniel Widlöcher reminds us: "Above all, the notion of illness relates to practical means. It is a matter of recognizing and treating an identified condition. The problem does not consist of differentiating a normal condition from a pathological one" (*Les logiques de la dépression,* 31).

13 For more on heterogeneity as an ontological constraint of psychiatry, see Lantéri-Laura, *Psychiatrie et connaissance.*

14 From France, *L'Encéphale* and *L'Évolution psychiatrique* especially, as well as surveys from other psychiatric magazines. The Anglo-American works used are textbooks, commonly cited articles, and authors who are either regarded as authorities in their profession or who have been the subject of discussions. The first chapter is a synthesis of works from the history of psychiatry and mental illnesses in the nineteenth century.

15 *Elle* and *Marie-Claire,* from 1955 to the early 1980s; *L'Express* from the 1960s to the early 1980s.

CHAPTER ONE

1 See chapter 6.

2 As for the United Sates, see Speaker, "From 'Happiness Pills' to 'National Nightmare.'"

3 There are only a few such observations in this investigation. The matter is a monumental work in progress, as much for the history of psychiatry as for the history of psychoanalysis.

4 Rouart, "Dépression et problèmes de psychiatrie générale," 461, from "Symposium sur les états dépressifs" (21 November 1954), organized by *L'Évolution psychiatrique, La Société psychanalytique de Paris,* with the participation of the *Société française de psychanalyse.*

5 See chapter 4.

6 "Possessing bodies is precisely what persons ... are" (Ricoeur, *Oneself as Another,* 33). The notion of the unconscious is at the heart of this tension. It has been a means of integrating animality into a global conception of the human. And this to such an extent that François Roustang considers that "the role of the notion of the unconscious could be better played by that of human animality." See Roustang, *Influence,* 8. See also a

certain number of premonitory remarks on the relations between reflex psychology and guilt in Canguilhem, *La formation du concept de réflexe.*

7 The Greek person suffers from something (i.e., an object is required for the suffering to exist), whereas the modern person simply suffers. She herself can be the object of her suffering. See Vernant, "L'individu dans la cité."

8 Assimilating the words "unknown" and "unconscious" is fairly common in psychiatry. In 1960, Henri Ey opened a famous symposium on the subject with these words: "The unconscious is defined by the fact that it is *unknown* to the consciousness" (*L'inconscient,* 13 [emphasis in original]).

9 "The psychological fact is neither spiritual nor corporeal, but rather, it occurs throughout a man's being; it is his behaviour viewed in its entirety" (Janet, *De l'angoisse à l'extase,* 36)

10 For the history of culture, see Glaser, *Sigmund Freud et l'âme du XXᵉ siècle;* Schorske, *Fin-de-siècle Vienna;* Le Rider, *Modernity and Crises of Identity;* and Seigel, *Bohemian Paris.* For a social history, see Corbin, "Backstage"; and Vincent, "A History of Secrets?"

11 Corbin, *"Backstage,"* 525. The silent interlocutor was the doll.

12 German scientists recently found a virus known as Borna in the blood of the depressed. See "Un virus responsable de la dépression?" *La Recherche* (October 1996):. See also *Le Quotidien du médecin,* 30 July 1996.

13 Ey, "Commentaires critiques sur *L'histoire de la folie* de Michel Foucault," 243.

14 Foucault, *The Birth of the Clinic,* xii. The clinic is equated with the patient's bedside. For the contextualization of psychiatry in the realm of medicine in the late eighteenth century as well as debates on physical and mental issues, see Goldstein, *Console and Classify.*

15 "In our eyes, the demons are bad and reprehensible wishes, derivatives of instinctual impulses that have been repudiated and repressed. We merely eliminate the projection of these mental entities into the external world which the middle ages carried out; instead, we regard them as having arisen in the patient's internal life, where they have their abode." See Freud, "A Seventeenth-Century Demonological Neurosis," in *The Complete Psychological Works,* 19:72.

16 Gladys Swain showed that Pinel's importance does not derive from having freed the insane from their shackles but, rather, from having invented modern psychiatry; that is, from treating the ailing subject as a patient (Swain, *Le sujet de la folie*). This theme was prevalent in Toulouse in December 1969, in the *Journée annuelle de l'évolution psychiatrique,* which was devoted to the "ideological conception of 'L'Histoire de la folie.'"

Georges Daumézon insisted on the fact that "Pinel's merit is other (than the freedom from the shackles); Gusdorf calls him the Lavoisier of medicine" and not only a philanthropist. ("Lecture historique de *L'Histoire de la folie*," 235). He adds that Pinel's psychiatric *oeuvre*, far beyond the supposed liberating of the insane, lies in the application of his method (236).

17 It is, in Hegel's words, "a simple contradiction within the realm of reason, which is still present" (quoted in Swain, *Dialoque avec l'insensé*, 143). Paul Bercherie contests this argument. According to him, Pinel rejected the dominant notion of his time: that alienation resulted from an affliction of the brain. "His taking this stance had a first consequence, namely that of supplying a theoretical basis for the idea of curing mental illness: it is not the brain that is afflicted, but the spirits alone, leaving us with the possible act of treating the mental issues and the potential for curing madness" (Bercherie, *Les fondements de la clinique*, 36–37).

18 Swain, *Le sujet de la folie*, 143.

19 De Quincey, *Confessions of an English Opium Eater*, 46. This matter was studied in Ehrenberg, *L'individu incertain*.

20 Ey, "Commentaires critiques," 258. Ey applies this formula only to the psychotic.

21 Mauzi, *L'idée du Bonheur*. This work contains several references to melancholia.

22 Roustang, *Influence*, 65.

23 Mauzi, *L'idée du Bonheur*, 590.

24 Bonnefoy, Preface to *La mélancholie au miroir*, 7.

25 Klibansky, Panofsky, and Saxl, *Saturn and Melancholy*, 228–40.

26 In the preface to the 1989 French edition, *Saturne et la mélancholie*, 19.

27 Klibansky, Panofsky, and Saxl, *Saturn and Melancholy*, 232. "With the exception of France, who waged 'war on sadness' and who opted resolutely for health," Marc Fumaroli writes, "it is celebrated throughout Europe as the sublime misfortune of a soul feasting on its own suffering." ("Nous serons guéri si nous le voulons,").

28 quoted in Klibansky, Panofsky, and Saxl, *Saturn and Melancholy*, 232.

29 "The nerves and the brain govern the intellectual and physical conduct of an individual" (Starobinski, *Histoire du traitement*, 49).

30 Starobinski, *Histoire du traitement*, 83.

31 "With monomania and melancholia, the disorder stems from mental affections influencing the individual's ability to reason. The mania is characterized by a general delirium, stemming from a rational disorder, which leads to the disorder of the mental affections" (Jean-Étienne Dominique Esquirol quoted in Gourévitch, "Esquirol et lypémanie," 14).

32 Esquirol, quoted in Lantéri-Laura, "Introduction historique et critique," 12.

33 Gourévitch, "La dépression, fille de l'art romantique," 705.

34 Gourévitch, "Esquirol et lypémanie," 17.

35 Ibid., 18; and Swain, *Dialogue avec l'insensé*, 168.

36 Swain, *Dialogue avec l'insensé*, 179.

37 Lantéri-Laura, "Introduction historique et critique," 13–16. This point has been emphasized by the few historians who take psychiatric thought seriously. Gladys Swain refers to it (in the article cited above) as does Paul Bercherie. Pierre Janet notes that Guislain "put the life of the emotion at the root of all mental illness." See Janet, *De l'angoisse à l'extase*, 10

38 Séglas, "De la melancholie sans délire," 34. Séglas pays tribute to Guislain and Griesinger.

39 Ibid., 33 (emphasis mine).

40 Ibid., 36. Here, Séglàs is citing one of his patients.

41 Zeldin, *Intellect, Taste and Anxiety*, 783. In 1973 (when it was first printed), Zeldin was undoubtedly one of the first historians to have touched upon "personal anxiety," which, he pointed out, was "uncharted territory" (823).

42 Canguilhem, *La formation du concept de réflexe*, 7.

43 Zeldin, *Intellect, Taste and Anxiety*, 784.

44 "Deemed the inevitable accompaniment of illness, pain was usually acknowledged and then relegated to a place of secondary importance, rather than studied for its own intrinsic qualities" (Rey, *The History of Pain*, 6).

45 Canguilhem, *La formation du concept de réflexe*, 149.

46 Clarke and Jacyna, *Nineteenth-Century Origins of Neuroscientific Concepts*. The authors point out that reflex activity has received more attention than any other subject. They attribute the fact that reflex action also appears in the consciousness to Wilhelm Griesinger, the dominant figure in German psychiatry in the nineteenth century. According to Griesinger, mental behaviour consists of "psychical movement" (see Clarke and Jacyna, *Nineteenth-Century Origins*, 137). Physiologist William Carpenter promoted a notion that defined the reflex as a basal biological function and extended it to the "psychological realm" (see Clarke and Jacyna, *Nineteenth-Century Origins*, 139). See also Chapter 4, "Les voies du reflexe," in Marc Jeannerod's, *De la physiologie mentale.*

47 Gauchet, *L'inconscient cérébral*, 82. As the author states, the cerebral unconscious refers to the "unconscious cerebration" first mentioned by William Carpenter.

48 Freud wrote that Brücke was "the greatest authority that worked upon [him]," quoted in Gay, *Freud*, 33.

49 Canguilhem, *La formation du concept de réflexe,* 153n5; and Gauchet, *L'inconscient cérébral,* 122. The quote is from Jules Soury's *Le système nerveux central.* This work, which is both historical and critical (and touches upon the problem of the reflex), is widely used by historians of the sciences of the brain.

50 About Carpenter, Crabtree writes, "The word 'cerebration' referred not to thinking but to the reflex action of the brain. Unconscious cerebration was intended as an explanation for automatic actions that seem to be intelligent but do not come into the agent's awareness"(*From Mesmer to Freud,* 256).

51 "Whenever we deal with sensation, we are in the realm of psychology. It makes sense that we would try to situate the psyche somewhere, even if it's in the spinal cord" (Canguilhem, *Études,* 301).

52 The discovery of the nerve cell, near the end of the nineteenth century, made it possible to trace the progression of the reflex. See Clarke and Jacyna, *Neuroscientific Concepts,* chap. 4.

53 Rare, because they required considerable investment. See Goldstein, *Console and Classify.*

54 Zeldin, *Intellect, Taste and Anxiety,* 82.

55 During the nineteenth century, a first model linking the syndrome with the lesion became necessary. Then, at the end of the century, came a model based on a cause, in line with pasteurism and the progress of psychology as predicated upon the work of Claude Bernard. See Lantéri-Laura, "La connaissance clinique."

56 *Frankfurter Zeitung,* 8 February 1893, quoted by Glaser, *Sigmund Freud,* 98.

57 See Pachet, *Les baromètres de l'âme.*

58 Essentially, I used Zeldin, *Intellect, Taste and Anxiety;* Rabinbach, *The Human Motor,* chap. 6; Ellenberger, *The Discovery of the Unconscious;* and Huguet, *L'ennui et ses discours,* particularly chap. 5. Aside from Gosling, *Before Freud,* I failed to find a book that systematically recounts the history of neurasthenia.

59 This book is cited by every historian of that time.

60 Quoted in Zeldin, *Intellect, Taste and Anxiety,* 840.

61 Rabinbach, *The Human Motor,* 160.

62 Nevertheless, in France, because of the importance given to the hereditarian tradition, social and heredtitarian causes were often mistaken for one another. See Rabinbach, ibid., 156–7.

63 Durkheim, *On Suicide,* 46.

64 W. Erb, *Sur l'accroissement de la maladie nerveuse à notre époque* (1895), quoted in Freud, "'Civilized' Sexual Morality and Modern Nervousness," 13.

65 Freud, "'Civilized' Sexual Morality and Modern Nervousness," 12.

66 See Schorske, *Fin-de-siècle Vienna*; Glaser, *Sigmund Freud*; Le Rider, *Modernity and Crises of Identity*; Seigel, *Bohemian Paris*; and Huguet, *L'ennui et ses discours*. The latter evokes Zola when speaking of "the boredom of the new heroes of doubt" (163). Let us add to this list the stimulating chapter by Pétillon devoted to Musil in *L'Europe aux anciens parapets*. This is the empire of the Ego.

67 Quoted in Glaser, *Sigmund Freud*, 59

68 Ibid., 61.

69 Otto Binswanger, quoted in Freud, "'Civilized' Sexual Morality and Modern Nervousness," 13.

70 Richard von Krafft-Ebing quoted in Freud, "'Civilized' Sexual Morality and Modern Nervousness," 13–14.

71 Wilhelm Erb quoted in Freud, "'Civilized' Sexual Morality and Modern Nervousness," 12.

72 Dubois, The *Psychic Treatment of Nervous Disorders* (1909), quoted in Lambotte, *Le discours mélancholique*, 29.

73 Janet, *La force et la faiblesse psychologiques*, 12.

74 Carroy, *Les personnalités doubles et multiples*, xiii.

75 Starobinski, "Le mot réaction," 5. See also Starobinski, "La notion de réaction psychopathologique," *Confrontations psychiatriques* 12 (1974). This is the issue in which Starobinski published a first version of this source article.

76 Bernheim, quoted in Starobinski, "Le mot réaction," 12.

77 In "Rewriting the Soul," Hacking cites the "the definitive historical study" (183) of Esther Fischer-Homberg, *Die traumatische Neurose*.

78 Hacking, "Rewriting the Soul," 185.

79 Swain, "De la marque de l'événement à la rencontre intérieure: Images populaires et conceptions savantes en psychopathologies" (1983), reprinted in *Dialogues avec l'incensé*, 157.

80 Lantéri-Laura, *Psychiatrie et connaissance*, 76.

81 Paul Bercherie points out that, in the early twentieth century, "Janet had … replaced Charcot (who had died in 1893) in the elaboration of theoretical models at la Salpêtrière. From that point on, the tendency would be to situate the occurrences of mental pathology in the analysis of personality disorders" (*Les fondements de la Clinique*, 180). On the pivotal role of Charcot in the genesis of the notion of personality via the memory, see Glasser, *Aux origines du cerveau moderne*.

82 Janet, *Les névroses*, 380. "With Pierre Janet," wrote Julien Rouart, "neurosis ceased to be the category into which everything that wasn't a well-documented mental illness was filed" ("Dépression," 463).

83 "At this point," Freud writes, "it might be useful to remark that the sense
   of guilt is fundamentally nothing other than a topical variety of anxiety;
   in its later phases it merges completely with fear of the super-ego ...
   It is present in some way behind all the symptoms" (*Civilization and Its
   Discontents*, 93). Janet writes: "I have tried to show that it [anxiety] occurs
   in depressed persons, who are incapable of accurately performing certain actions demanding a high psychological tension" (*Psychological
   Healing*, 1:629).

84 Freud, *Civilization and Its Discontents*, 91.

85 See Janet, *Les névroses*, 383–94.

86 Ibid., 386.

87 Janet, *Psychological Healing*, 1:693–4.

88 Janet, quoted in Andersson, *Freud avant Freud*, 173.

89 Janet, *La force et la faiblesse psychologiques*, 13. Janet refers to his book,
   Les obsessions et la psychasthénie (1903).

90 Janet, *Les névroses*, 365.

91 Janet, *Psychological Healing*, 2:1214.

92 Ibid., 1214.

93 Janet, *Psychological Healing*, 1:601.

94 Maître, *Une inconnue célèbre*, 140.

95 According to the famous expression in the preliminary communication:
   "The hysteric suffers mostly from reminiscences"(Breuer and Freud,
   Studies on Hysteria, 4).

96 Ibid., 179. As we know, Freud's "economic" viewpoint is thought of in
   terms of excess energy. The conflict is the result of opposing forces
   clashing, wherein the wrong outcome is the neurotic disorder and
   the right outcome is sublimation.

97 Freud, "Sexuality in the Etiology of the Neuroses" (1898), in *The Complete
   Psychological Works*, 3:272.

98 Freud, "'Civilized' Sexual Morality and Modern Nervousness," 15.

99 Ibid., 14.

100 Freud, "'Civilized' Sexual Morality and Modern Nervousness," 14–15.

101 Starobinski, "Le mot reaction," 47.

102 Breuer and Freud, *Studies in Hysteria*, 232.

103 Freud, "Sexuality in the Etiology of the Neuroses," in *Complete
    Psychological Works*, 3:284.

104 Vincent Descombes demonstrates that the substantive "unconscious"
    used by Freud is really "a semantic expansion of its adverbial meaning"
    ("L'inconscient adverbial," 780). The substantive "unconscious" is the
    equivalent of: he/she did it unconsciously. The semantic expansion
    means that one can have an unconscious that *wants* something. It emits

messages (i.e., symptoms) to signal this. In this sense, the unconscious is intentional. This cannot be said of an unconscious conceived of as an automatism or disintegration.

105 Breuer and Freud, *Studies in Hysteria*, 201.

106 After restating that the starting point of neuroses is depression, Janet comes to the central issue in his criticism of Freud: "It is far more likely that a symptom is caused by the laws of the disease than by accidental memories. We must not interpret symptoms historically unless clinical observation makes such interpretation indispensable" (*Psychological Healing*, 1:651).

107 Freud, "'Civilized' Sexual Morality and Modern Nervousness," 19.

108 Janet, *Psychological Healing*, 1:15. Thus, things are quite clear from the onset of this 1,265–page work

109 Corbin writes: "Throughout the century specialists remained convinced of the fundamental importance of an 'unconscious,' by which they meant, again in Starobinski's words, 'the obscure rumor of the visceral functions out of which acts of consciousness intermittently emerged.' ... Freud's genius was not to discover that large areas of subjectivity escaped consciousness yet played a part in determining mental activity, but rather to deny connections among organic life, social life, and mental activity." See Corbin, "Backstage," 494.

110 Freud, *Civilization and Its Discontents*, 77.

111 We return to this theme in chapter 7.

112 Freud, *Civilization and Its Discontents*, 82

113 Starobinski, "Le remède dans le mal," 274. This article appears in an issue of *Nouvelle Revue de psychanalyse* dedicated to the idea of healing.

114 Le Rider, *Modernity and Crises of Identity*, 5.

115 Janet, *La force et la faiblesse pychologiques*, 12.

CHAPTER TWO

1 Janet, *La force et la faiblesse pychologiques*, 269.

2 Freud, *An Outline of Psycho-Analysis*, 62.

3 Quoted in Lantéri-Laura, "Introduction historique et critique," 15.

4 Freud, *Inhibitions, Symptoms and Anxiety*, 58.

5 Laboucarie, "Discussion," 571.

6 On this point, see (especially) Evans, *Fits and Starts*, chap. 3; and Micale, *Approaching Hysteria*, 169–75.

7 Montassut, *La Dépression constitutionelle*, XXX. We still refer to Montassut occasionally to define the "depressive personality." See Péron and Galinowski, "La Personnalité depressive."

8 de Fleury, *Les états dépressifs de la neurasthénie.*

9 Montassut, *La dépression constitutionelle,* 158.

10 Montassut, "La fatigue de la neurasthénie," 69.

11 Savy, *Traité de la thérapeutique clinique,* 2:1996.

12 Ibid., 2:2055.

13 Montassut, "Le Traitement physique de la dépression constitutionnelle," 71–2.

14 Savy, *Traité de la thérapeutique clinique,* 2:2058.

15 Montassut, "Le traitement physique de la dépression constitutionnelle," 95.

16 Savy, *Traité de la thérapeutique clinique,* 2:2005. Caffeine, Benzedrine (an amphetamine synthesized in 1931), strychnine, cola, and so on.

17 Ibid., 2:2059.

18 Ibid., 2:2060.

19 Ibid., 2:2064 (emphasis mine).

20 "The true debate on opium," writes historian Roselyne Rey, "was more concerned with its fundamental effects: was it a sedative, i.e. something to calm one down, or was it, on the contrary, a stimulant?" (*The History of Pain,* 126). "Consequently, opposing medical concepts cohabited within the therapeutics field and this particular medical practice, which viewed illnesses as being due to a lack of stimulation, contributed to the increased use of opium" (Rey, *The History of Pain,* 127). See also Jackson, *Melancholia and Depression,* 394.

21 Ey, "Système nerveux et troubles nerveux," 97.

22 Leiris, *Manhood,* 157.

23 Corbin, "Backstage"; Vincent, "A History of Secrets?"; and Lejeune, *Le moi des demoiselles.*

24 Foucault, *Discipline and Punish.*

25 See Becker and Berstein, *Victoire et frustrations;* Dubief and Bernard, *The Decline of the Third Republic;* N. Mayer, "L'atelier et la boutique, deux filières de mobilité sociale" and J.-F. Sirinelli, "Des boursiers conquérants? École et 'promotion républicaine' sous la IIIe république," both in S. Berstein and O. Rudelle, *Le modèle républicain;* Hoffman, *In Search of France.*

26 Freud, *Civilization and Its Discontents,* 101.

27 Donzelot, *L'invention du social,* 98.

28 Théry, "Vie privée et monde commun," 142.

29 Breuer and Freud, *Studies on Hysteria,* 185. Breuer stresses this point. In the nineteenth century, "the problem of premature ejaculation, so frustrating for women, was ignored, although frequent mention [by doctors] of involuntary loss of semen suggests that it was widespread" (Ibid., 591–2).

30 Freud, *An Outline of Psycho-Analysis*, 51.

31 In 1948, Henri Ey wrote: "To a degree, the broader notion of 'syndrome' softens the boundaries between these bodies. The processes described come with many rules and categories. Large pathological groups, such as dermatology, gastroenterology, cardiology or neurology, tend to replace particular ailments" (*Études psychiatriques*, 27).

32 Nietzsche, *The Genealogy of Morals*, 36.

33 See chapters 4 and 5.

34 Ey served as secretary general of the World Psychiatric Association until the mid-1960s.

35 Delay, " Aspects de la psychiatrie moderne: Discours d'ouverture du premier congrès mondial de psychiatrie," in *Aspects de la psychiatrie moderne*, 50. The congress of 1900 (which took place in Paris during the *Exposition universelle*) was overshadowed by "concerns about attendance" and was beset with "fatalism" (Delay, *Aspects de la psychiatrie moderne*, 49).

36 Jaeger, *Le désordre psychiatrique*, 122. On the prevailing therapeutic climate after the war, see Ayme, *Chroniques de la psychiatrie publique*. For an evaluation of the psychiatric *aggiornamento* and an explanation of the professional reasoning that came with it, see Castel, *La gestion de risques*, chap. 1.

37 See the ground-breaking work of Fourquet and Murard, "Histoire de la psychiatrie de secteur."

38 According to Marcel Jaeger, "no fundamental changes occurred between 1950 and 1970 with regards to the framework of hospitals, the destitution of the patients, the weight of hierarchy amongst the 'healers' … The feeble desire for change is soon quelled by the institution" (*Le désordre psychiatrique*, 141).

39 For instance, in 1996 Michel Marie-Cardine wrote, "Having reviewed the first World Congress of Psychiatry, it appears that therapeutic psychiatry was quite rudimentary" ("Pharmacothérapie et psychotherapies," 44).

40 U. Cerletti, "Résumé du rapport," in Ey, Marty, and Dublineau, *Thérapeutiques biologiques*, 15.

41 All of the leading figures in French psychoanalysis participated. See Roudinesco, *Jacques Lacan & Co*, 173.

42 Evaluating neuroleptics in 1975, Henri Ey regretted that "biological therapeutics were all too often systematically abandoned" ("Neuroleptiques et services de *psychiatrie* hospitaliers," 41). See also Balvet, "Ébauche pour une histoire de la thérapeutique psychiatrique contemporaine."

43 Kraepelin, *Manic-Depressive Insanity and Paranoia*. On the history of schizophrenia, see Garabé, *Histoire de la schizophrénie*, and Barrett, *The*

Psychiatric Team and the Social Definition of Schizophrenia, chaps. 7 and 8. We do not have, to my knowledge, a social and cultural history of schizophrenia.

44 Kraepelin, *Manic-Depressive Insanity and Paranoia,* 77 (emphasis in original). Kraepelin speaks of melancholia simplex and melancholia gravis.

45 Minkowski, *Lived Time,* 72. This paragraph builds on Minkowski's analysis (70–6). Minkowski was a student of Bleuler. He brought the phenomenological approach to psychiatry to France, participated in the creation of the French psychoanalytic movement, and was a founding member of *L'Évolution psychiatrique.*

46 Minkowski, *Lived Time,* 73.

47 This is a common complaint about phenomenology: it provides deft descriptions that do not translate into concrete results.

48 See André Roumieux's description of the psychiatric hospital of Rodez, where Antonin Artaud was interned (*Artaud et l'asile,* vol. 1). They were so successful that they used electroshock therapy ad nauseam. To my knowledge, the history of methods using shocks, especially electroshocks, has yet to be written. Though they are too factual, I'd like to mention two articles by G.E. Berrios: "Early Electroconvulsive Therapy in Britain, France and Germany" and "The Scientific Origins of Electroconvulsive Therapy." There is also a very anecdotal historical chapter in Endler and Persad, *Electroconvulsive Therapy.*

49 See Jean Delay, "L'œuvre de Henri Claude," in *Études de psychologie médicale.* André Breton uses Henri Claude as a character in *Nadja.*

50 *L'Évolution psychiatrique* 4 (1946), quoted in Roudinesco, *La Bataille de cent ans,* 416.

51 Quoted in Delay, *Aspects de la psychiatrie moderne,* 16.

52 See Goldstein, *Console and Classify;* and Dowbiggin, who analyzes Claude's professional and institutional motives in *La folie héréditaire.* The preeminent figure behind this theory was Valentin Magnan, who was dean of admissions at St-Anne for forty years. In "Back to the Future," Dowbiggin describes the waning of this theme in the first quarter of the twentieth century.

53 For the dawn of a "psychological era," see Bercherie, *Fondements de la clinique.*

54 On institutional psychotherapy, see Fourquet and Murard, "Histoire de la psychiatrie de secteur."

55 See Ey, "Neuroleptiques et techniques psychiatriques," 33–5. At the Centre de traitement et de réadaptation de Ville-Évard, chronic psychoses apparently dropped from 36 percent from 1921 to 1937 to 16 percent

from 1938 to 1954 (35). On the combining of the two methods, see Balvet, "Ébauche pour une histoire." He argues that insulinotherapy "proved that schizophrenia could be cured, and it nullified the notion of 'dementia praecox' that was still present in our minds, despite how long it had been since Bleuler's first publication" (7).

56 Baruk and Launay, *Actualités de Thérapeutique Psychiatrique et de Psycho-pharmacologie*, 4. However, functional problems can definitely create lesions. See Delay, *Études de psychologie médicale*, 233.

57 Baruk and Launay, *Actualités de Thérapeutique Psychiatrique et de Psycho-pharmacologie*. In the 1930s, they write, "the role of certain chemical mediators (like serotonin) involved in the reproduction of experimental psychoses" was brought to the fore (7).

58 Ibid., 4, 5.

59 All of this warrants a more detailed examination. This is not to mention the role played by electro-encephalography or experimental neuroses on animals, based on the work of Pavlov.

60 Gustave Roussy, Préface to *Les dérèglements de l'humeur* by Jean Delay, x. Like everyone else, Roussy attributes the connection between the two centres to "the use of shocks, whether they are comatogenic shocks or epileptogenic shocks" (ix).

61 Charles Feré, quoted in Sulloway, *Freud, Biologist of the Mind*, 259. Sulloway explains that, like all the neurologists of his time, Freud knew Feré's work and was well aware of Jackson's doctrine.

62 The French Jacksonian "manifest" (Delay's term) was a work by Constantin Von Monakow and R. Mourgue entitled *Intégration et désinté-gration de la function* and published in 1928. Its reception alone deserves to be studied. Instinctive dynamism plays an important role in distinguishing the functions of the organism. See Delay, "Le jacksonisme et l'oeuvre de Ribot," in *Études de psychologie médicale*. See also Guiraud, *Psychiatrie générale*, chap. 5. "Here, for the first time," he writes, "we find a neuropsychiatric system studied in a biological light" (Ibid., 164). Henri Ey demonstrated this doctrine many times

63 Roussy points out the connection for Delay: "It is precisely with the perspective of Jackson's doctrine that Jean Delay examines mood disorders" (Préface to Delay, *Les dérèglements de l'humeur*, x).

64 Ey, *Études psychiatriques*, 163. In Ey's opinion, "Janet is the greatest French psychiatrist of this century" (158).

65 Ibid., 150.

66 Ibid., 149 (emphasis in original).

67 Ey, "Les limites de la psychiatrie et le problème de la psychogenèse," 13–4 (emphasis in original). The disagreement between Ey and Lacan over psychic causality is at the heart of this treatise.

68 Ibid., 12.

69 Ey, "Les limites de la psychiatrie et le problème de la psychogenèse," 19–20.

70 Ey, "Système nerveux et troubles nerveux," 104.

71 Guiraud, *Psychiatrie générale*, 184. "Why does Freud call the conflict 'psychogenic'? Because we only know how to analyze it in psychological terms. However, that does not prove that the conflict has no physiopathological aspect" (199).

72 Ibid., 200.

73 Ibid., 581, 586, 600, 606. At the first World Congress of Psychiatry in 1950, Guiraud declared, "the contribution of psychoanalysis to the pathogenesis of delirium has been invaluable" (Ey, Marty, Dublineau, *Psychopathologie générale*, 22). Until the end of the 1950s, his abstract on psychiatry (in collaboration with Maurice Dide, first published in 1922) was the key text not only for psychiatrists and students of psychiatry but for all doctors who wished to learn about psychiatry

74 Lacan, "Propos sur la causalité psychique," 25.

75 Ibid., 41.

76 Delay, *Les dérèglements de l'humeur*, 5.

77 Ibid., 73. Delmas-Marsalet confirms the numbers on melancholia at the 1950 congress in Ey, Marty, and Dublineau, *Psychopathologie générale*, 100. He published a large tome on electroshock therapy, wherein he described a different interpretation of the effects of the shocks. See Delmas-Marsalet, *Électrochoques et thérapeutiques nouvelles en neuropsychiatrie*. The humoral syndrome results neither from the diencephalon or any other region of the nervous system but, rather, from muscular exertion. And the healing derives more from the dissolving of the conscience than from an emotional shock.

78 Delay, *Les dérèglements de l'humeur*, 11 (emphasis Delay's). Ey describes the melancholic conscience: "Those who know about melancholic conscience but have not developed their own think it obvious that this morbid conscience, humane and moral though it may be, presents us with a (sinister and pathetic) caricature and therefore the situation is not really one of sin" ("Contribution à l'étude des relations des crises," 542).

79 Delay, *Les dérèglements de l'humeur*, 77. See also Daumézon, "Nosographie et thérapeutiques de choc," 247, 249, 252.

80 We know that Henri Ey called his notion of psychiatry "organo-dynamism." He writes: "In our minds, this organization is a movement and its history is a place from which the spirit emerges, commensurate to its organization. It is not the duality of the two entities that defines the clash between spirit and matter, but rather this bipolarity of structure. It is because I give meaning and reality to the psychic pole that I also give meaning and reality to the organic pole" ("Discussion du rapport de Lacan," in Bonnafé et al., *Le problème de la psychogenèse*, 56). Among the leaders in the field of psychiatry at the time, Jacques Lacan was alone in eschewing this movement.

81 Delay, *Études de la psychologie médicale*, 72. At the 1950 congress, Cerletti explained that Delay's work taught him that it is not the epileptic shock that heals but, rather, "humoral reaction itself." One of Delay's students pointed out that Cerletti's humoral research gave the biological effects a solid foundation. See "Rapport des discussions qui ont eu lieu dans les divers pays avant le congrès," in Ey, Marty, Dublineau, *Thérapeutiques biologiques*.

82 Delay, *Les dérèglements de l'humeur*, 9.

83 Wallez, "Limitation de la sismothérapie," 21.

84 According to Julien Rouart, "to psychiatrists, state of depression = melancholia. In its typical form, the body language associated with it is so distinctive that this condition can be recognized at a glance" ("Dépression et problèmes de psychiatrie générale," 460). Thirty years later, Arthur Tatossian added: "Even in medical terms, much time elapsed before the word took on its current meaning and it became possible to regroup different types of sadness under the umbrella term 'depressive states.' Until WWII, treatises and manuals tended to temper or denigrate the word melancholia with various epithets" (Tatossian, "Les pratiques de la dépression," 264). This is no doubt the most complete French document I consulted.

85 Le Mappian, "Aspects cliniques des états dépressifs." At the 1949 symposium on depressive states, Dr Jean Laboucarie assessed findings from studies involving two thousand cases of "melancholic states and neurotic depressions" that were conducted first in a controlled environment and then in a non-controlled environment. These states make up 15 percent of the patients of the first study and 47 percent of the latter. See Laboucarie, "Discussion," 564.

86 Wallez, "Limitation de la sismothérapie," 21–2.

87 Delay, *Les dérèglements de l'humeur*, 29.

88 Daumézon, "Nosographie et thérapeutiques de choc," 254.

89 Ibid.

90 Martin and Crémieux in Ey, Marty, Dublineau, *Psychopathologie générale*, 289. Delmas-Marsalet draws the opposite conclusion: "Without a doubt, it is easier to abolish a purely imaginary delirium than to erase the loss of a loved one, the loss of social situation, or defamatory social sanctions based on false accusations" (Ibid., 99–100). Similarly, Sargant argues that, "like the body, the brain is unrelenting in its demands that the proper, well-defined therapeutic agents be applied to equally well-defined mental illnesses" ("Indications et mécanisme de l'abréaction," 614.

91 Martin and Crémieux in Ey, Marty, Dublineau, *Psychopathologie générale*, 295.

92 Delay, *Les dérèglements de l'humeur*, 297.

93 Rouart, "Dépression et problèmes de psychopathologie générale," 459.

94 Mallet, "La dépression névrotique," 483. He adds: "Astonishing as it may seem, Freud was aware of melancholic depressions, yet he never dwelled on the matter" (485). According to Freud, an attack of melancholia can occur in an obsessional or hysterical neurosis: "The range of catalysts includes any situation involving prejudice, humiliation, or disappoint-ment" (*Métapsychologie*, 161).

95 Mallet, "La dépression névrotique," 487. According to Mallet, "From the very fact of their residual narcissism (that makes them attach exagger-ated importance to their psychical actions), neurotics react to their own desires like healthy people react to their own actions. Guilt gives way to dependence in the hysterical structure just as it gives way to self-tormenting in the obsessional" (490–1).

96 Ibid., 483.

97 Freud, *Inhibitions, Symptoms and Anxiety*, 97.

98 Ey, "Contribution à l'étude des relations des crises de mélancolie et des crises de dépression névrotique," 547.

99 "Endogeneity in depression appears as a significant factor in both cases" (Ey, "Contribution à l'étude des relations des crises," 535). This "founda-tion of depression makes this sufferer into the neurasthenic, 'anxiety-ridden,' 'depressed,' 'asthenic' person whose state of mind is completely mired in anxiety" (Ibid., 548).

100 Laboucarie, "Discussion," 565. Based on his experience with two thou-sand cases, Laboucarie deemed electroshock therapy effective in all instances of depression. Hence, according to him, "the artificial charac-ter of opposing melancholic and neurotic depression. There are marked differences in the rate and extent of the results, exactly in accordance

with the make-up of the underlying personality. It can be said that although the electroshocks act upon the disorders of the depressive mind, they have no effect on personality disorders" (568).

101 Le Mappian, "Aspects cliniques des états dépressifs," 222.

102 Ey sees the "multiple effects observed due to the use of electroshocks in *shock treatment therapeutics* on the evolution of the psychoses" as confirmation of his Jacksonian doctrine. "What we have here is a non-specific therapeutic that completely alters the clinical picture" (*Études psychiatriques*, 54, emphasis in original).

103 P. Delmas-Marsalet speaks of "depressive reactive psychoses that are only exaggerations of normal affective reactions. We could happily designate them as 'legitimate psychoses,' emphasizing that their greater resistance to electroshock therapy simply means that they walk the line between normal and morbid" (Ey, Marty, Dublineau, *Psychopathologie générale*, 99–100). "Shock treatment was used when the patients' agitation, depression, or delirium was such that they were beyond psychotherapy alone, could no longer be productive members of society and their thoughts and reactions made them a threat to themselves and to others" (Rickles and Polan, *Archives of Neurology and Psychiatry* 59 [1948]: 337, quoted in Daumézon, "Nosographie et thérapeutiques de choc," 250).

CHAPTER THREE

1 Previously, there were only barbiturates. For more on the strategies of the businesses in the depression industry, see Healy, *The Antidepressant Era*. Healy uses both psychiatric literature and a number of interviews with researchers and clinicians involved in psychopharmacology since the 1950s. See his collection of interviews in Healy, *The Psychopharmacologists*. A second volume was published in 1998. Pierre Pichot and Thérèse Lempérière are the only French interviewees included.

2 This theme is developed in the next chapter.

3 In a 1965 report on psychiatry, Henri Ey writes: "The practitioner has become more aware of psychopathology and the psychical 'element' of illnesses" ("Perspectives actuelles," 72).

4 Lacan, *L'angoisse*, 85.

5 Laplane, "Avant-propos."

6 Deniker, *La psychopharmacologie*, 98. Twenty-five years later, two psychiatrists consider that it is a "relatively new term." See Lôo and Lôo, *La dépression*, 6.

7 Moussaoui, "Biochimie de la dépression," 212.

8 Scotto et al., "Stratégie thérapeutique," 1633. In his introduction to the
   same issue, Daniel Widlöcher explains that "what makes epidemiological
   analysis difficult in the field of depression is that (more so than in other
   types of pathology) the definition of a 'case' is a particularly sensitive
   matter," ("Introduction," 1613).

9 Scotto, "Éditorial," 1.

10 Kendall, "The Classification of Depressions," 15.

11 Ibid., 16.

12 What is at stake in this transformation is discussed in chapter 5.

13 van Praag, "The DSM-IV (depression) classification," 148–9. The article
   appeared while preparations for the fourth edition of the *Diagnostic and
   Statistic Manual of Mental Disorders*, which was published in 1994, were
   being made. In general medical journals, we find the same difficulty.

14 Micale, *Approaching Hysteria*; and Evans, *Fits and Starts*.

15 "They are without a doubt among the most common psychiatric disorders," writes Heinz Lehmann, "Epidemiology of nervous disorders," 21.

16 Klein, "La physiologie et les troubles anxieux," 95.

17 Klein's argument links therapeutic testing and pharmacological dissection:
   "Many pathological symptoms are completely stopped by the appropriate
   treatments, while ordinary fear and social sensitivity remain unaffected"
   (Ibid., 98–9). In 1964, Klein demonstrated that one type of anxiety, the
   panic attack, was very responsive to imipramine (the first antidepressant).
   Based on his findings, he divided Freud's anxiety neurosis into two syndromes: the panic attack and the general anxiety disorder. Klein noted
   that some studies confused general anxiety with depression (Ibid., 107).

18 Lehmann, "Epidemiology of Nervous Disorders," 22. The depressive syndrome is more feared as a cause of suicide than is the anxiety syndrome.

19 The fact that the protagonist of Camus' *The Stranger* felt nothing when
   his mother died would be used against him during his trial. Here, the
   absence of sorrow and mental suffering are precisely pathological signs.

20 Delay and Deniker, *Méthodes chimiothérapiques en psychiatrie*, 317.

21 Green, "Chimiothérapiques et psychotherapies," 32.

22 I will not concern myself with anxiolytics since they are universally
   regarded as symptomatic medications. See, among others, Delay and
   Deniker, *Méthodes chimiothérapiques en psychiatrie*, 432.

23 Caldwell, *Origins of psychopharmacology*. Unfortunately, the test does not
   touch upon the institutional context. See Swazey, *Chlorpromazine in
   Psychiatry*. This work dwells on the early uses of neuroleptics in psychiatry.
   A second series of neuroleptics, derived from reserpine, was issued in
   1954. Given the objectives of this book, their history is not explored here.

24 Caldwell, *Origins of Psychopharmacology*, 21. Paul Guiraud reported on this
   in the 1950 publication *Psychiatrie générale*; however, he did not mention
   it at the World Congress, which took place that same year.

25 This synthesis was written by chemist Paul Charpentier. Simone
   Courvoisier then performed the pharmacological tests and presented
   her findings at a 1955 conference in a paper entitled "Sur les propriétés
   pharmaco-dynamiques de la chlorpromazine." She described the conditioned reflexes that the team sought to create by testing the molecule on
   animals: the experiments proved its "psychical deconditioning" function
   (1255) by "adhering as closely as possible to the guidelines put forth by
   Pavlov" (1249).

26 H. Laborit, P. Huguenard, R. Alliaume, "Un nouveau stabilisateur végéta-
   tif (le 4560 RP)," cited in Caldwell, *Origins of Psychopharmacology*, 135
   (emphasis mine).

27 Caldwell, *Origins of psychopharmacology*, 41; H. Laborit, *La vie antérieure*,
   106.

28 For a description of this "spectacular effect," see, for instance, Zirkle,
   "To Tranquilizers and Antidepressant." T. Kammerer, R. Ebtinger, and
   J.P. Bauer were less impressed, arguing that its advantages over electroshock were barely discernible ("Approche phénoménologique et psychodynamique des psychoses délirantes aiguës traitées par neuroleptiques
   majeurs," in Lambert, *La relation médecin-malade*, 33). Many reports at the
   Premier Colloque international sur la chlorpromazine et les médicaments
   neuroleptiques en thérapeutique psychiatrique expressed lukewarm
   enthusiasm. See, for instance, Rance, Jurquet, and Roger, "Remarques
   sur la thérapeutique des affections psychiatriques par la chlorpromazine
   et la réserpine."

29 J. Delay, P. Deniker, and J.-M. Harl, quoted in Delay and Deniker,
   Méthodes chimiothérapiques en psychiatrie, 21.

30 Overholser remarks: "Although barbiturates calmed the patient, they
   did so at the expense of the conscience and put the patient in a stupor"
   ("La chlorpromazine," 313).

31 Lehmann, "L'arrivée de la chlorpromazine," 58.

32 Deniker, "Qui a inventé les neuroleptiques?" 12.

33 Ibid., 12.

34 See R. Kuhn's thoughts on his tests with chlorpromazine, in Caldwell,
   Origins of Psychopharmacology, 191.

35 Delay, "Introduction au colloque international," 305. One hundred and
   forty-seven reports were proffered.

36 Delay, "Allocution finale," 1184.

37 Delay and Deniker mentioned this several times in *Méthodes chimiothéra-piques en psychiatrie.*

38 Kuhn, "The Imipramine Story," 207–8.

39 Ibid., 210. We know that neuroleptics were given to melancholics, with negative results. Certain studies show that, when anxiety is predominant in a case of depression, "the patients must be calmed … and then sub-mitted to electric shock treatment" (Staehelin and Labhard, "Les résul-tats obtenus par les neuroplégiques," 516). As for neurotics, Staehelin and Labhard mention that, "along with the failures, there were some very positive results" (517), for example, hiccups or asthma due to neu-roses. They also saw positive results with regard to drug addictions. Staehelin is the head of Basel's Psychiatric University Clinic.

40 Kuhn, "The Imipramine Story," 210.

41 Ibid., 211.

42 Ibid.

43 Ey stated in his report on the congress that "R. Kuhn (almost peripher-ally to the congress) reported irregular, yet noteworthy effects from a derivative of iminodibenzyl on depression-tinged schizophrenic out-bursts" (*Schizophrénie,* 363). Ey did not consider whether it might not be something else altogether.

44 Kuhn, "The Imipramine Story," 212.

45 Ibid. (emphasis in original).

46 This was partially confirmed by the assessment of patients in a number of articles. In an experiment conducted by Delay, Deniker, and Lempérière upon 137 patients, "the best results were achieved with the clear-cut mel-ancholic syndromes (74%), where the numbers drop to 54% for straight-forward depressions" (Lereboullet and Escourolle, "La neuropsychiatrie en 1960," 2913). Nevertheless, thirty years later, Kuhn wrote that "anti-depressants acted favourably on reactive depressions. We particularly wish to dwell on this point" ("Psychopharmacologie et analyse existen-tielle," 46).

47 Kuhn, "The Imipramine Story," 215–6.

48 Ibid., 216 (emphasis mine).

49 Ibid., 215–6, (emphasis in original).

50 Broadhurst, interview with Healy in Healy, *The Psychopharmacologists,* 1:119.

51 Guyotat, "Remarques sur les relations entre chimiothérapie et psychothé-rapie," 92. This work was published by the Comité lyonnais de thérapeu-tique psychiatrique. This group, which gathers pharmacologists and psychiatrists, is known for its focus on the role of psychotropes in dealing

with mental illnesses. Its first collected work was published in 1956 and entitled *La thérapeutique par la chlorpromazine en psychiatrie.*

52 Kline, "Monoamine oxidase inhibitors," in Ayd and Blackwell, *Discoveries in Biological Psychiatry.* The following cited passages are all from this article.

53 Kline, "Monoamine oxidase inhibitors," 196, (emphasis in original).

54 Ibid., 198.

55 Ibid., 197.

56 Ibid., 198.

57 Ibid., 200.

58 Ibid., 204.

59 Kline, quoted in Albert, *Psychanalyse et pharmacologie,* 52. French works point out that iproniazide "seems especially promising with regard to apathy, lack of initiative, asthenia ... We also observed positive results with hysterical depressions where the dominant aspects are emotional dependency, the need for gratification, and often, on the physical side, hypersomnia" (Guyotat, "Iproniazide et inhibiteurs de la monoamine oxydase," 295–6). In Green's opinion, the main problem with this molecule is that of "the patient's excessive euphorization" ("Chimiothérapies et psychothérapies," 71).

60 In 1974, Nathan Kline's *From Sad to Glad* was published. On the cover, the following slogan appeared: "Depression: You can conquer it without analysis!"

61 See chapter 6.

62 At the Second World Congress of Psychiatry in Zurich (1957), it was decided that an international collective would be formed to bring together all the fields that might have an interest in psychotropes. Known as the *Collegium International Neuro-Pharmacologicum,* it organizes conferences at which all the key figures from around the globe gather.

63 Healy, *The Antidepressant Era,* 111.

64 Delphaut, *Pharmacologie et psychologie,* 175.

65 Brisset, "La psychopharmacologie," 639–40. Records of the proceedings of the annual reunion of *L'Évolution psychiatrique* of 12 December 1965, devoted to psychopharmacology and psychotherapy. Brisset, with Ey and Bernard, is the author of the famous *Manuel de psychiatrie,* of which the sixth edition was published in 1989.

66 The biochemical aspects are described in chapter 6, where we discuss SSRIs.

67 Delay, "Adresse présidentielle," xv.

68 Delay and Deniker, *Méthodes chimiothérapiques en psychiatrie,* 377.

69 Ibid., 357 (emphasis in original).

70 Guyotat, "Remarques sur les relations entre chimiothérapie et psychothérapie," 91.

71 Ibid., 96. Guyotat finds it odd that "certain psychiatrists resist the common notion that a chemical substance can affect psychological balance. They concede that there may be minor effects on the symptoms, but not an overall psychological effect" (Ibid., 84). Green writes that "one of the significant advantages [of thymoanaleptics] is the possible association with psychotherapy, as pointed out by several authors. Most (Azima and Racamier, for instance) realize that with medication, the patient is more responsive to psychotherapy" ("Chimiothérapies et psychothérapies," 69–71). Among the psychoanalysts working with chemotherapy, Green could also have mentioned Nacht, Stein, Male, Bouvet, and the group from Lyon.

72 Sarradon, "Assises départementales de médecine sur les états dépressifs," 541.

73 Delay and Deniker, *Méthodes chimiothérapiques en psychiatrie*, 423.

74 Cf. Guyotat, "Remarques sur les relations entre chimiothérapie et psychothérapie"; and Kammerer, Israël, and Noel, "Une dépression guérie par l'imipramine."

75 Guyotat, Remarques sur les relations entre chimiothérapie et psychothérapie," 94.

76 Blanc, "La psychopharmacologie," 722.

77 Delay, "Adresse présidentielle," xx.

78 Blanc, "Conscience et inconscient dans la pensée neurobiologique actuelle," 213.

79 Kammerer, Ebtinger, and Bauer, "Approche phénoménologique et psychodynamique des psychoses délirantes," 17.

80 Green, "La psychopharmacologie."

81 Green, "Les portes de l'inconscient," 20.

82 Ibid., 22.

83 "The effect of stimulation is instantaneous; the organism responds with a motor reaction in order to expend the surplus of energy. This is, according to Freud, what we see with the reflex" (Lebovici and Diatkine, "Quelques notes sur l'inconscient," 57, 59).

84 Green, "Chimiothérapiques et psychothérapies," 89. To cite some contemporary writers, we can mention, among others, Nacht, Racamier, Stein, and Male.

85 Delay, "Adresse présidentielle," xxii.

86 Ey, "Neuroleptiques et services psychiatriques hospitaliers."

87 Delay, *Études de psychologie médicale*, 227. The citation pertains to narco-analysis.

88 Fouks, Lainé, and Périvier, "Les inhibiteurs de la monoamine oxydase," 150–1.

89 Blanc, "La psychopharmacologie," 716.

90 Chemotherapy "increases greatly the number of patients who can be treated with psychotherapy" (Delay and Deniker, *Méthodes chimiothérapiques en psychiatrie*, 422).

91 Marchais, "Essai d'approche clinique des états dépressifs névrotiques," 85.

92 According to Paul Balvet, "Along with nursing, insulinotherapy brought forward a psychotherapeutic element … For nearly all French hospital psychiatrists, this was a revelation" ("Ébauche pour une histoire de la thérapeutique psychiatrique contemporaine," 7). See also Roumieux, *Artaud et l'asile*.

93 Blavet, "Ébauche pour une histoire de la thérapeutique psychiatrique contemporaine," 9.

94 Daumézon, "Modification de la symptomatologie des troubles mentaux."

95 Delay, *Études de psychologie médicale*, 297.

96 Le Guillant et al., "Quelques remarques méthodologiques sur l'action des neuroleptiques" 1129.

97 "In the future, psychiatry will not be able to function out in the middle of nowhere, where the only possible institutions will be hospices and group homes" (Fouks, "Bilan actuel de la thérapeutique chimique en psychiatrie," 7).

98 Dr. C.-H. Nodet during the round table discussion at the end of the conference (Schneider et al.,"Table Ronde," 194). With great intuition, Professor Schneider, who led the discussion, commented: "I often have the feeling that we are in a type of honeymoon phase after this coming together, and I wonder how long it will last" (Schneider et al., "Table Ronde," 185).

99 These are Rümke's words. See Rümke, "Quelques remarques concernant la pharmacologie et la psychiatrie," 341. These were neuroses, according to Rümke, and, as such, were disorders that had to be separated "at once" from the conflicts that afflicted humanity. He was, let us remember, a pupil of Kraepelin. There would also be cause to take a closer look at the assessment of the biology of the disorders that are psychogenetic and those that are not.

100 Kielholz, "État actuel du traitement pharmacologique des dépressions," 398–9.

101 Brisset, "La psychopharmacologie," 649.

102 Cole, "The Future of Psychopharmacology," 82.

103 Kielholz, "État actuel du traitement pharmacologique des dépressions," 398.

104 M. Magdelaine, C. Magdelaine, and Portos, quoted in Péquignot and Van Amerongen, "Prescription et utilisation de neuroleptiques," 206.

105 Ibid.,

106 Laplane, "Avant-propos,"

107 Sempé, "Pratiques et institutions privées," 141.

108 Blanc, "La psychopharmacologie," 709.

109 Henne, "Besoins nationaux et nombre de médecins psychiatriques," 787.

110 Ey, "Perspectives actuelles de la psychiatrie," 73.

111 Guyotat, "Perspectives actuelles de la psychiatrie," 111.

112 Sempé, "Pratiques et institutions privées," 142.

113 Bertherat, "Enquête sur l'exercice de la psychiatrie en France," 223.

114 Sempé, "Pratiques et institutions privées," 148.

115 Daumézon, quoted in Bertherat, "Enquête sur l'exercice de la psychiatrie en France," 234.

116 Balvet, "Ébauche pour une histoire de la thérapeutique psychiatrique contemporaine," 11 and 13.

117 According to Élisabeth Roudinesco, "after Bonneval, interns would head towards (preferably Lacanian) couches, while reading *L'histoire de la folie*" (*La Bataille de cent ans*, 309).

118 R. Castel, *La gestion des risques*, 94.

119 Sempé, "Pratiques et institutions privées," 148.

120 Ey, "Perspectives actuelles de la psychiatrie," 71.

121 Ibid., 72.

122 Delmas-Marsalet, *Précis de bio-psychologie*; Delay and Pichot, *Abrégé de psychologie à l'usage de l'étudiant*; Nayrac, *Éléments de psychologie*; Koupernik, *Les médications du psychisme*.

123 Procacci, "Médecins en quête d'auteur ou les ruses de la médecine de sujet," in Carpentier et al., *Résistance à la médecine et démultiplication du concept de santé*.

124 Schneider et al., "Table Ronde," 204.

125 Perrault, "La thérapeutique en 1958," 3761. See also Claude Legrand's analysis of the content in *Médecine et malheur moral*.

126 Perrault, "La thérapeutique en 1958," 3753.

127 Ibid., 3754.

128 Ibid. (emphasis mine).

129 Coirault, "Introduction au problème des états dépressifs," in Baruk and Launey, *Les annales Moreau de tours*, 2:69.

130 Laplane, "Avant-propos," 2979.

131 Bertagna, "La chimiothérapie des états dépressifs," 2313.

132 Perrault, "La thérapeutique en 1958," 3758. Energizers give "the patient
the balance necessary for the fulfillment of the self" (Laplane, "Avant-
propos," 3761).

133 Bertagna, "La chimiothérapie des états dépressifs," 2313.

134 Ibid.

135 "Improvements by [trademark of imipramine] can be significant so long
as removing inhibitions or indecision leads to the elimination of fundamental pessimism" (Ibid., 2314).

136 Laplane, "L'utilisation pratique des médicaments anti-dépressifs," 184.

137 Laplane, "Avant-propos," 2979.

138 Follin, "Sémiologie des états dépressifs," 2987. Thérèse Lempérière
writes, "What's pathological is when sorrow overtakes the patient to the
extent that the patient can no longer rid him/herself of it" ("Les dépressions psychogènes," 3021).

139 Lereboullet, "Nouveaux neuroleptiques et tranquillisants," 122.

140 Ibid.

141 Bergouigan, "Les dépressions symptomatiques," 3033.

142 des Lauriers, "Le risque de suicide chez les déprimés," 3055. Pierre
Deniker, in the same issue, reminds us once again that "diagnosing depression is far from easy. Moreover, the term 'depression' is often accepted
in too vague a way and contains various clinical facts, both for doctors
and in modern language" ("Traitements des états dépressifs," 3063).

143 See Guyotat's comments on the absence of anxiogenic effects in chlori-
mipramine, which was the main molecule before Prozac, in "Perspectives
actuelles de la psychiatrie," 117. Lereboullet, Desrouesné, and Klein
speak of a new molecule that has the opposite effect: it energizes ("La
neuropsychiatrie en 1967," 2707).

144 This theme became commonplace. See, for instance, Fouks et al. at the
June 1962 symposium on MAOIS: "Antidepressants often lead to therapy
sessions where the patient's symptomology is less common and requires
more refined diagnostics" (Villeneuve, "Aspects modernes des troubles
de l'humeur," 431).

145 Delay, "Adresse présidentielle," xix.

146 Lambert, "Sur quelques perspectives de la pharmacologie," 238.

147 Fougère, Les médicaments du bien-être, 8.

148 Ibid., 169–70. According to Dr Paul Chauchard, the industry is searching for "chemical components that are free of toxicity … and effective in
every case … Generalists would then have at their disposal a medication

that is both active and versatile, which they could prescribe 'without
second thoughts' to patients deemed nervous and who have all the right
symptoms along with a propensity for developing psychosomatic troubles. Patients mired in situations of conflict could benefit from these
treatments, patients with 'emotional adaptation, familial, professional,
or social disorders' … Future research will no doubt move in this direction … Medications that will truly bring about well-being are still to
come" (*La Fatigue*, 55). In 1962, Dr Coirault's repeated outcries against
the toxicity of antidepressants led to the leitmotif of that era: "We believe
without current reserve that research will lead to new substances that will
be versatile and free of toxicity … We will soon have at our disposal
products that are effective and harmless" (Coirault, "Introduction au
problème des états dépressifs," in Baruk and Launey, *Les annales Moreau
de tours*, 2:70). "The large number of side effects and the absence of a
causal agent clearly illustrates how far we are from an ideal antidepressant" (Kielholz, "État actuel du traitement pharmacologique des dépressions," 401).

149 Delay, "Allocution Finale," 1181.
150 Perrault, "La thérapeutique en 1958," 3753 and 3762. In 1963, pharma-
    cologist Delphaut wrote: "we describe this medication [iproniazide] that
    seemingly brings back the will to live as a 'happy pill'" (*Pharmacologie et
    psychologie*).
151 Coirault, "Introduction au problèmes des états dépressifs," in Baruk and
    Launey, *Les annales Moreau de tours*, 2:69.
152 Deniker,"Traitements des états dépressifs," 3064.
153 Bertagna, "La chimiothérapie des états dépressifs," 2322.
154 Lambert, "Sur quelques perspectives de la pharmacologie," 238.
155 Porot, "Assises départementales de médecine sur les états dépressifs," 468.
156 "Due to excessive use, the term 'depression' has lost all meaning. The
    chronically delirious will tell their doctors that they have been institu-
    tionalized for 'depression'" (Laxenaire, quote in Porot, "Assises départe-
    mentales de médecine sur les états dépressifs." 467.

CHAPTER FOUR

1 Endogenous or exogenous, depending on the approach.
2 Pichot, "Conclusions," *L'Encéphale*, 567.
3 Israël, *L'hystérique*, 31.
4 "Analysis does not set out to prevent morbid reactions, but should give
  the patient's ego freedom to decide one way or another," *The Ego and the*

Id, in the Standard Edition of the Complete Psychological Works of Sigmund Freud, vol. 19 (1923–25), quoted in Gay, *Reading Freud,* 91.

5 Lehmann, "Epidemiology of Depressive Disorders," 22.

6 In 1975, *L'Express* published an article on this pathology, citing the same figure. It would be used repeatedly ("Les trucs anti-déprime," *Elle,* no. 1931 [1983]). See also Eisenberg's synthesis, "La dépression nerveuse."

7 Reigner, "La dépression ... une mode?" 3.

8 Ragot, "La dépression," 657. In 1973, at an international symposium on masked depression, several speakers brought up the theme of depressing civilization. See Kielholz, *Masked Depression.*

9 Bergeret, "Dépressivité et dépression," 1019.

10 Depoutot, "Névrose et dépression," 869.

11 Rieff, *The Triumph of the Therapeutic,* xi.

12 Schwartz, *Le monde privée des ouvriers,* 76.

13 Lin Tsung-Yi, "The Epidemiological Study of Medical Disorders," 511.

14 Sartorius, "Épidémiologie de la dépression," 465. Sartorius cites the same figures as Lehmann. This number does not seem to have been verified by any WHO studies. In 1981, Sartorius mentions these figures once again, believing that they will increase ("La dépression," 530).

15 Klerman and Weissman, "Increasing Rates of Depression." These studies used the clinical syndromes defined by the profession. They were conducted in developed Western countries (Sweden, New Zealand, United States, etc), with the exception of Korea and Puerto Rico. Klerman is perhaps the greatest American authority on the epidemiology of depression. For more on Klerman, see the interview with Mirna Weissman in Healy, *The Psychopharmacologists,* vol. 2.

16 In chapter 6, we see that – taking male alcoholism into account – the numbers are the same for men and women. For men, alcoholism is a defence mechanism against depression. See Führer and Lovell, "Troubles de la santé mentale," in Savrel-Cubizolles and Blondel, *La santé des femmes.*

17 Cross-National Collaborative Group, "The Changing Rate of Major Depression," 3098.

18 Except in the articles and studies devoted specifically to exhaustion or to psychosomatics, which started cropping up in France in the 1950s. It appears obvious here that exhaustion and depression were used interchangeably.

19 Auclair, "L'abus de tranquillisants," *Marie-Claire,* February 1963.

20 Auclair, "Cette peur qui nous fatigue," *Marie-Claire,* October 1963.

21 Grégoire, "Être une femme équilibrée," *Marie-Claire,* March 1970. The article was accompanied by the story of a woman who "explored her inner self" entitled "I Was Psychoanalyzed."

22 From 1955 to 1976, *Elle* magazine classified articles about neuroses and depressions under the heading "Nerves"; from 1976 to 1983, such articles were classified under "Illnesses/Nervous System." The heading "Fatigue" (from 1955 on) included psychic and related nervous disorders. In 1977, the "Stress" category came into being.

23 Dr O.P., "Docteur, répondez-moi," *Elle*, no. 508, 1955.

24 Ibid., no. 614, 1957.

25 "Les malades refusent de se considérer comme tels," *Elle*, no. 671, 1958.

26 *Elle*, nos. 740–5.

27 See: "La maîtrise de soi," *Elle*, no. 795, 1961. On physical excercises as a means to fight depression see "Étirez-vous: toujours, lorsqu'on se sent déprimé ou triste, on a tendance à se replier," *Elle*, no. 903, 1963; on ways to recover from violent emotions see "Dépressions nerveuses, crises de tachycardie, ulcères d'estomac et crise de foie, voilà la note que vous paierez tôt ou tard," *Elle*, no. 904, 1963; on preparing for an interview see *Elle*, no. 905, 1963; on relaxation for the "high-strung" see *Elle*, no. 906, 1963; on the depressed see "Comment apprendre le calme" *Elle*, no. 908, 1963; and on insomniacs see "Comment faire si la hantise de ne pas dormir vous ôte le sommeil," *Elle*, no. 911, 1963.

28 *Elle*, no. 1009, 1965.

29 "Le psychiatre soigne aussi bien les grandes fatigues que les grands désordres mentaux," *Elle*, no. 1057, 1966; "Comment vivre sans se fatiguer ni se tuer les nerfs" (*Elle*, no. 1050, 1966); "Si votre cafard est chronique, et si ces recettes ne peuvent en venir à bout, c'est qu'il s'agit de dépression ou d'asthénie: Consultez un médecin" (*Elle*, no. 1060, 1966); "Ayez les moyens de combattre la dépression" (*Elle*, no. 1082, 1966).

30 *L'Express*, no. 778, 16–22 May 1966.

31 Jacqueline Michel, *Marie-Claire*, September 1972, excerpt from *La Déprime. Marie-Claire* and *Elle* devoted many articles to this book in 1972 and 1973. Pierre Daninos is himself a proselyte in the last chapter of his *Le 36e dessous.*

32 "It's the medication for psychotic neuroses. They [antidepressants] act upon the very centres of the brain. ... They change dejection into euphoria, apathy into drive. But they cannot be used without strict supervision (which often means hospitalizing the patient)" (*Elle*, no. 1040, 1965).

33 Bugard, *Stress, fatigue et dépression.*

34 Ibid., 1:12.

35 "The very excess of choices is as traumatic as the lack of choice" (Ibid., 1:163.)

36 For some, the increasing number of depressions (essentially psychogenic) is due to the added pressures that industrialization puts on the

individual. For others, the instability of life – divorce, the dissolution of the family, changing jobs, and so on – forces them into a world without permanence. Still others would argue that we demand more from life than did our ancestors. Some also mention the materialism of our time. According to W. Walcher, "mention should be made in particular of ever-increasing chronic stress factors inherent in our modern way of life, stress factors which are due to our insistence on performance as the be-all and end-all of existence and which are liable to affect our behaviour both at work and in the home" ("Psychogenic Factors Responsible," 180).

37 *L'Express*, 3–9 January 1981.

38 Ibid., 2–8 June 1969.

39 *Marie-Claire*, February 1976.

40 *L'Express*, 2–8 June 1969. By and large, *L'Express* educated its readers about "nervous exhaustion and its complications, nervous depressions and neuroses," "relaxation," "the great outdoors," and "anti-fatigue medication," "psychotonic drugs" (i.e., doping), "tranquilizers, neuroleptics and nervous sedatives, metabolic correctors," and so on (7–14 May 1964). Not a word on antidepressants. The 11–17 November 1968 issue describes the roundtable discussion on anxiety at the Entretiens de Bichat; the 10–16 May 1969 issue discusses exhaustion and psychosomatic medicine; and so on.

41 See also "Quand la dépression vous guette," *Marie-Claire*, September 1969; and "Tension nerveuse," *Marie-Claire*, November 1969.

42 All these points were developed in A. Ehrenberg, *L'idividu incertain*.

43 Jacqueline Michel examines the enormous number of letters she received since her book was published. "Most readers can very much relate to my case: 'When I read your story, I thought I was reading my own,' or, 'It's me you're writing about, not you!' … The main point was to not be the only one suffering from an illness no one wanted to recognize, let alone heal" ("Comment, où guérir de la dépression? La question que l'on m'a posée 2,597 fois," *Marie-Claire*, March 1973).

44 Ibid.

45 A. Ehrenberg, *Le culte de la performance*, part 2, chap. 3; and *L'individu incertain*, chaps. 2 and 5.

46 Théry, *Le démariage*, chap. 2.

47 Haynal, "Le sens du désespoir," 96.

48 Rieff, *The Triumph of the Therapeutic*, 249.

49 Ibid., 242–3.

50 Ibid., 256. This is what Robert Castel called "the new psychological culture" in *La gestion des risques*, a work that takes stock of the 1970s. For a

psychoanalysis of the United States in that same era, see Lasch, *The Culture of Narcissism*; as well as Castel, Castel, and Lovell, *The Psychiatric Society*, part 3.

51 Rieff, *The Triumph of the Therapeutic*, 252.

52 Jean-Marie Lacrosse speaks of "a-normative conditions" ("Enquête sur le mouvement du potentiel humain," in Carpentier et al., *Résistance à la médecine*, 126).

53 See chapter 5.

54 Janov, *The Primal Scream*.

55 "Crier pour guérir," interview with M. Kohler, *Elle*, no. 1414, 1973. The magazine devoted another issue to primal scream therapy in 1975 ("Crier pour guérir," no. 1548, 1975), when Janov's book was first translated into French.

56 Lowen, *Depression and the Body*.

57 Ibid., 12.

58 Ibid., 11.

59 Cohen, "Revitalisation, décomposition ou redéfinition du catholicisme," 24.

60 "The idea of health (and healing), expanding into new psychic expectations, created new religious notions that took these needs into account, even as these notions integrated a wide range of knowledge and psychotherapeutic practices" (Cohen, "Revitalisation, décomposition ou redéfinition du catholicisme.")

61 Lovell, "Paroles de cure et énergies en société," in Carpentier et al., *Résistance à la médecine*, 85.

62 Ibid., 89.

63 Robert Castel took it upon himself to review this crucial period. He showed how the "techno-psychology," a new regulating device, came into being. Its purpose was not to bring a patient to a state of perfect psychological balance but, rather, to favour a "psychic growth" that would grant her a sense of personal well-being and promote openness towards others. Here, I modify Castel's hypothesis and state that the device leads less to the development of a new psychological culture that is "outside the normal and the pathological" (Castel, *La Gestion des riques*, 9) than to this new system of norms. Castel's hypothesis was beneficial. It helped demonstrate that the conditions of the illness led to mental medicine. It became a sociological dogma that defined what was "normal" and what was "pathological." This hearkens back to the double theme of the psychologizing of social interaction and the medicalization of the ill being. The result is that contemporary mental pathology remains in the unthought.

64 Rieff, *The Triumph of the Therapeutic*, 239.

65 Haynal, Introduction to "Le sens du désespoir," 10.

66 Bergeret, "Dépressivité et dépression," 915. Christopher Lasch based his notion of a culture of narcissism on the work of American psychoanalysts who perceived an increase in narcissistic pathologies among their clientele. One of the main references is Kernberg, *Borderline Conditions and Pathological Narcissism*. Sennett describes the writings of psychologists and psychoanalysts on the subject of narcissism "as veritable social descriptions" (*The Hidden Injuries of Class*, 261). He saw this as the decline of public culture.

67 For the history of this concept, see Timsit, "Les états-limites."

68 Lambert, "Sur quelques aspects psychanalytique," 558.

69 Fossi, "La psychanalyse de la dépression," in Bergeret and Reid, *Narcissisme et états-limites*, 54. Haynal writes that, "for many years, [depression's] role did not get the recognition it deserved. It was as if the importance properly accorded anxiety overshadowed it, as if any attention given one member of the anxiety-depression pair spelled the neglect of the other. This status of 'poor relation,' about which Karl Abraham complained as early as 1911 ..., was assigned by Freud from the onset" (*Depression and Creativity*, xi). Haynal cites Abraham (1911): "Whereas the states of morbid anxiety have been dealt with in detail in literature of psycho-analysis, depressive states have hitherto received less attention" (Ibid., 14).

70 Preface to "L'humeur et son changement," 5.

71 According to Timsit.

72 Bergeret, "La dépression dite 'névrotique' et le praticien," 2218. Highlighted by the author, who does not provide the source of these studies.

73 Dujarier, "Considérations psychanalytiques sur la dépression," 47. "The field of psychoanalysis has given a great deal of attention to affect disorders over the last dozen years or so" (Villeneuve, "Aspects modernes des troubles de l'humeur," 436). See also Lambert, "Sur quelques aspects psychanalytique," 3. In 1975, in the first article of the issue of *Nouvelle Revue de psychoanalyse*, entitled "Figures du vide," Guy Rosolato writes, "Depression seems to be more frequent in today's nosology" ("L'axe narcissique des dépressions," 5.)

74 Fédida, "L'agir dépressif," 48.

75 Kuhn, "Dépression endogène et dépression réactionelle," 15.

76 The work traditionally cited by psychoanalysts is "Mourning and Melancholia" by Freud.

77 Freud, "Mourning and Melancholia," 584.

78 Freud, *Inhibitions, Symptoms and Anxiety*, 95 and 96. The notion of affect was the subject of a report by André Green at the thirty-third congrès des psychanalystes de langue romane, "L'affect."

79 Jean Laplanche and Jean-Bertran Pontalis use the term "initial helplessness." See Lapalnce and Pontalis, *The Language of Psycho-Analysis*, 156.

80 Freud, *Inhibitions, Symptoms and Anxiety*, 97.

81 Haynal, *Depression and Creativity*, xxvii.

82 The key article on the matter is by Kernberg, "Borderline Personality Orgaization."

83 See the entry entitled "Ego-Ideal" in Laplanche and Pontalis, *The Language of Psycho-Analysis*, 144.

84 In 1973, Michel de M'uzan wrote that, "unlike the Super-ego, which requires a *not-doing*, the ideal of the Ego, as we know, demands a doing. Hence the idea of hope and project attached to it" (*De l'art à la mort*, 108).

85 Haynal writes: "Many cases labelled as evolving chronic depression are on the periphery of borderline personality disorder" ("Le sens du désespoir," 38).

86 Dujarier, 47. Emphasis mine.

87 Israël, *L'hystérique, le sexe et le médecin*, 157.

88 Haynal, " Le sens du désespoir," 37. Dujarier: "We often speak of neurotic depression. We would do better to describe it as depression with shades of narcissism … It is nearly always a case of *hysterical neurosis*" ("Considérations psychanalytiques sur la dépression," 40 [emphasis in original]). "Today", writes an Austrian psychiatrist in 1973, "hysteria has virtually disappeared as a diagnosis; neuroses are tending more and more to assume a depressive character … At the same time, persons enjoying good health are demanding an ever-increasing ration of pleasure as a motivation for the work they perform, whereas the notion of 'duty' is relegated to the limbo of outmoded ideas" (Demel, "Observations on the Clinical Nature of Masked Depression from the Standpoint of Practical Social Psychiatry," 248).

89 McDougall, *Plea for a Measure of Abnormality*, 478.

90 Widlöcher, "Le psychanalyste devant les problèmes de classification," 145.

91 A "vague suffering with some overtones of depression," writes Jean-François Narot ("Pour une psychopathologie historique," 169). "We find ourselves dealing … with an ever-increasing number of depressive cases whose depressivity cannot be written off as a passing phase in the course of a neurotic or psychotic type of structural evolution" (Bergeret and Reid, *Narcissisme et états-limites*, 162).

92 Narot, "Pour une psychopathologie historique," 166.

93 Daumézon refers to "the promoting of requests for help and especially of help for day-to-day living" in a discussion with Kammerer (Kammerer, "Les limites de la psychiatrie," 17). Henri Sztulman points out that "psychosis puts our freedom in doubt while neurosis does the same to our happiness" (Ibid., 18).

94 Freud, *The Origins of Psycho-Analysis*, 109.

95 In 1959, Nacht and Racamier describe depressives as "insatiable and unappeasable" ("Les états dépressifs.").

96 Haynal, "Le sens du désespoir," 102.

97 Dujarier, "Considérations psychanalytiques sur la dépression," 36–7. "Guilt can also be found in depressive cases, though it is much less specific than shame" (Ibid., 37). Dujarier discusses Bergeret's report at the thirty-sixth Congrès in clear terms. He notes, among other things, that "we run the risk of being fooled by the absence of conscious guilt, that the Oedipal level has not been reached, and to speak erroneously of a purely narcissistic or pre-Oedipal set of problems" ("États-limites et dépression," 1093).

98 Barazer, "Honte, vergogne, ironie."

99 Dujarier writes that, "for the patient, feeling guilty means moving away from the immutability of depression" ("Considérations psychanalytiques sur la dépression," 37).

100 Bergeret, "Dépressivité et dépression," 1022. See the numerous intercessions in Bergeret and Reid, *Narcissisme et états-limites*.

101 Bergeret, "Dépressivité et dépression," 830–1. See also Jeanneau, "Les risques d'une époque ou le narcissisme du dehors," in Bergeret and Reid, *Narcissisme et états-limites*. "Guilt without an instruction manual" is borrowed from Jeanneau.

102 Haynal, "Le sens du désespoir," 113. In his introductions, he points out that he "did not touch upon the 'equivalents' (toxicomania, anorexia)" (21).

103 Dujarier: "These patients seem to be shielding themselves from the risk of depression" ("Considérations psychanalytiques sur la dépression," 46). "Resorting to tranquilizers and barbiturates often leads to minor addictions"(Ibid., 41). For a synthesis of texts on alcoholism, see de Mijolla and Shentoub, *Pour une psychanalyse de l'alcoolisme*.

104 Akers, "Addiction," 780.

105 This is demonstrated in the first half of the 1970s by the work of Lee Robbins on Vietnam veterans ("Depression and Drug Addiction") and, particularly, by Norman Zinberg (*Drug, Set and Setting*). Zinberg depicts

the broad range of reactions heroin users have to the drug through his own clinical studies as well as through the findings of American ethnologists and sociologists.

106 See Alexander and Schweighofer, "Defining Addiction."

107 Peele, *The Meaning of Addiction*, 134. In 1989, Peele published a pamphlet entitled *Diseasing of America.*

108 Following a study of the American Psychological Society in January 1996, this now qualifies as a genuine addiction. The internet's biggest users meet all the psychiatric criteria set for alcohol and drug dependency. They have lost control of their internet use and cannot curb it despite the negative impact it is having on their lives. In most cases, they are middle-aged adults who "look high-functioning, but there are serious problems just under the surface," according to Kimberly Young of the University of Pittsburgh-Bradford (quoted in Elias, "Net Overuse Called 'True Addiction'").

109 Timsit, "Les états-limites," 703.

110 Painchaud and Montgrain, "Limites et états-limites," in Bergeret and Reid, *Narcissisme et états-limites*, 29.

111 Radó, "La psychanalyse des pharmacothymies," 606 and 609.

112 Ibid., 618.

113 Lebovici, 513. Bergeret: "These days, many turn to *drugs* – be they 'pharmaceutical' or 'stupefacient' – as a defence mechanisms. Moreover, they are often tied to group activity as a means for its individual members to stave off the effects of depression" ("Dépressivité et dépression," 916 [emphasis in original]).

114 Bergeret, "Dépressivité et dépression," 907.

115 Robbins, "Depression and Drug Addiction." The study focuses on 114 heroin addicts at the Veterans Hospital in Washington. For a recent synthesis of drug and alcohol addiction, see the special issue of *European Addiction Research* (1996).

116 Deglon, "Dépression et héroïnomanie," 793. Ten years later, Laqueille and Spadone concluded their article, "Les troubles dépressifs dans la prise à charge des toxicomanies," by pointing out that "depression among drug addicts is a key problem" (14).

117 Deglon, "Dépression et héroïnomanie," 793. The effects of zimelidine (an early antidepressant and serotoninergic) on the patients' mood were astounding: "the selective action of zimelidine on serotonin is the likeliest reason for the positive results" (Ibid., 795). For more on this molecule, see chapter 7.

118 Bailly, "Recherche épidémiologique," 290.
119 Flournoy, "Le moi-idéal," 45.
120 On the rivalry between psychoanalysis and the new psychological techniques, see R. Castel, *La gestion des risques*.

CHAPTER FIVE

1 Pichot, *Les voies nouvelles de la dépression*. In his introduction, he gives a perfect description of the new categories of depression that have replaced the classic tripartition.
2 Villeneuve, "Aspects modernes des troubles de l'humeur," 436.
3 Israël, *L'hystérique, le sexe et le médecin*, 156 (emphasis in original).
4 Still, on the cover of a book, taking up a quarter of the front, was the slogan: "Depression is neither madness nor weakness." See Lôo and Gallarda, *La maladie depressive*.
5 "The word 'depression' is but a common denominator for many clinical bodies. Furthermore, clear parameters for what is obviously little more than a way of reacting, or a syndrome, need to be established" (Pichot, "Conclusions.")
6 Kristeva, *Black Sun*, 21. In this case, the author is taking a position as she is aware of psychiatrists' research into the psychomotor aspects of depression.
7 Colvez, Michel, and Quemada, "Les maladies mentales et psychosociales." The first study was actually published in 1973, but it was on a village in Vaucluse. See Brunetti, "Prévalence des troubles mentaux."
8 Colvez et al., "Les maladies mentales et psychosociales," 12. It is a recurring theme. See Bendjilali, "Place de la toxicomanie dans la dépression masque,"; Rochette and Brassinne, "La toxicomanie." This theme comes up frequently in Kielholz, *Masked Depression*.
9 Eighty-seven point one percent of general practitioners and 52.2 percent of psychiatrists prescribe medication. Only 14.4 percent of the first recommend a follow-up appointment, while 51.6 percent of the latter did so: "Medication is very often prescribed by general practitioners, much more than other pathologies" (Colvez et al., "Les maladies mentales et psychosociales," 22). According to Arthur Tatossian, the number of psychical disorders dealt with by general practitioners varies (depending on the study and the criteria used), making up between 10 percent and 25 percent of their cases ("Les pratiques de la dépression," 273).
I borrowed the expression "triad" from Tatossian.
10 Aiach, Aiach and Colvez, "Motifs de consultations et diagnostics médicaux," 552.

11 Ibid., 554.

12 Lasvigne, *La dépression vue par les médecins généralistes du 11ᵉ arrondissement de Paris*, thèse de médecine, Paris-VI, 1978, quoted in Lempérière and Adès, "Problèmes posés au médecin praticien par la dépression," 484–5. Mineau and Boyer, "La notion de dépression en médecine générale," 632. See also Cremniter et al., "Une enquête sur les états dépressifs en médecine générale."

13 Mineau and Boyer, "La notion de dépression en médecine générale," 632.

14 The theme of exhaustion is ever-present. For instance, among many other articles, *Elle* featured a major article on the subject in 1976 ("La fatigue, mal du siècle," no. 1267): "Stimulants/sedatives are increasingly used to counter this tension/frustration. In the long run, they add to the exhaustion" (97). It featured another in 1977 (no. 1650), and so on. Exhaustion and stress have thus become themes one must address at least once a year.

15 Totossian, "Les pratiques de la dépression," 277.

16 Kielholz, "Opening Address: Psychosomatic aspects of Depressive Illness," 12.

17 He is one of the main advocates of the serotonergic hypothesis of depression, a hypothesis upon which he has been working since the end of the 1960s. See chapter 6.

18 Lempérière, "Les algies psychogènes." Also present at Entretiens de Bichat: Psychiatrie, 1973, was G. Hakim, also from Sainte-Anne, who spoke about masked depression in a report entitled, "Aspects modernes de la dépression." See also Gourévitch, "Les psychalgies"; and Burner, "Thérapeutique des états de fatigue."

19 Hole, "La dépression masquée et sa mise en évidence," 847.

20 See also Sutter, "Problèmes posés en médecine générale."

21 Tatossian, "Les pratiques de la dépression," 276.

22 Lempérière and Adès acknowledge this in the conclusion of their study of depression in general medicine: "If general practitioners struggle to find their way through the complexities of depression, is it not partly because we the psychiatrists have yet to clearly define depression for ourselves?" ("Problèmes posés au médecin praticien par la dépression," 489).

23 Lempérière and Adès, "Problèmes posés au médecin praticien par la dépression," 487.

24 "Patients' complaints about the secondary effects are inversely proportional to the severity of their condition," writes Hamilton ("Méthodologie d'appréciation de l'efficacité des antidépresseurs," 653).

25 Godard and Regnauld, "Consommation des psychotropes." The use of
    BZDS increased by 60 percent between 1978 and 1984 (from forty-five pills
    per adult per year to seventy-five).

26 Anxiolytics: amitriptyline, maprotiline, dosulepine. Stimulants: nomifen-
    sine, viloxazine, amineptine.

27 Besides the molecules discussed in the preceding note, psychiatrists are
    debating trazodone, fluvoxamine (an SSRI that was launched in 1988),
    fluoxetine (also known as Prozac), and fenfluramine. They were not
    on the market yet. In 1979, Ronald Fieve believed that viloxazine was
    "harmless, even in heavy doses." He added that "tricyclic antidepressant
    poisoning ha[d] become one of Western medicine's leading causes of
    self-poisoning" ("La recherche pour de nouveaux antidépresseurs," 674).
    "Though they are usually not as strong, the new antidepressants are
    nearly free of harmful side effects. Hence they are favoured by many
    general practitioners" (Scotto, Bougerol, and Arnaud-Castel-Castiglioni,
    "Stratégies thérapeutiques devant une dépression," 1634).

28 Tatossian, "Les pratiques de la dépression," 280.

29 Godard and Regnauld, "Consommation des psychotropes."

30 Maruani, "Antidépresseur," 638–9.

31 Telling anxiety and depression apart is a "major diagnostic difficulty,"
    according to Guelfi and Olivier-Martin, "Modalités d'appréciations de
    l'anxiété," 1926. It is a recurring theme in every colloquium on depression.

32 Tatossian, "Les pratiques de la dépression," 289.

33 J.-P. Boulenger and D. Moussaoui, "Perspectives pharmacologiques
    en psychiatrie biologique," 115 (emphasis mine). This special issue
    examines biological psychiatry since it came into being in the 1950s.

34 Lôo and Cuche, "Classification des antidépresseurs," 599 (emphasis mine).

35 Maruani, "Antidépresseurs," 639. "These first eight days are crucial
    for the patient, due to the risk of suicide, the level of discomfort, the
    temptation to stop taking the medication. The sufferer usually endures
    an additional pressure from his peers to put an end to the therapy"
    (Bertagna et al., "Commentaires de 'Les Dépressions' de C. Koupernik.")

36 Depression as pathology of action is examined in chapter 6.

37 Scotto et al., "Stratégies thérapeutiques devant une dépression," 1637.

38 Poignant, "Revue pharmacologique sur l'amineptine," 709. During clini-
    cal tests on forty patients, the authors observed that amineptine was
    effective against reactionary and neurotic depressions, that it "seemed to
    favour relationships and allowed for a better therapeutic relationship."
    Also, on a "semiological level, amineptine ... appeared to counter inhibi-
    tions, both physically and psychically" (Laxenaire and Marchand, "Essais
    cliniques de l'amineptine," 1731).

39 Guelfi, "Implication pratiques," 808. Godard and Regnauld observe that the "antidepressive elements are sometimes minimal and that some are more akin to psychostimulants" ("Consommation des psychotropes," 7). According to Fieve, nomifensine is more like an amphetamine ("La recherche pour de nouveaux antidépresseurs", 679). Porot (in 1973) urged caution in the use of fortifiers and psychostimulants: "The proper categorization of amphetamines helps prevent an error that (until recently) was all too common: prescribing a medication that has an anxiogenic effect instead of a healing effect" ("Principes généraux de la thérapeutique des états dépressifs," 575)

40 Colonna and Petit, "Sémiologie dépressive," 642.

41 Fieve, introduction to *Depression in the* 1970s, 2.

42 Introductory argument made in *La dépression*, Actes des VIIes Journées nationales de la psychiatrie privée, *Psychiatries* 36 (1979): 7.

43 "The complexity of the problem derives from the heterogeneity of depressions as well as the antidepressants" (Moussaoui, "Place respective des différents antidépresseurs en thérapeutique," 703).

44 "The group's use of various medications over an extended period of time can blur the initial, more typical reactions" (Ballus and Gasto "Le role du généraliste dans l'assistance psychiatrique," 74).

45 "Though there have been some exceptions, most published works have confirmed this general statement" (Hamilton, "Le pronostic dans les dépressions," 142). At the 1970 colloquium in New York, a psychophar- macologist presented a synthesis of the research organized under the supervision of the NIHM and directed by Jonathan Cole on how depres- sion is dealt with in hospitals. This research compared patients having received chlorpromazine, imipramine, a BZD, and a placebo. According to Raskin: "Neurotic depressions get the same results with a placebo as with any other active substance. These last results are consistent with studies showing that imipramine is particularly beneficial with endog- enous depressions and of little use with neurotic depressions. On the whole, I hope that these results will incite researchers to continue search- ing for an antidepressant drug that is more effective and has a broader spectrum" ("Drugs and Depression Subtypes," 94–5).

46 Kuhn, "Dépression endogène et dépression réactionnelle," 16.

47 Kuhn, "The Treatment of Masked Depression," 190.

48 "The effectiveness criteria currently being studied do not allow us to 'personalize' each compound, the only key symptoms singled out being the anxioletic effect, sedative, of stimulant" (Colonna and Petit, "Sémiologie depressive," 642).

49 Fieve, "La recherche pour de nouveaux antidépresseurs," 675.

50 I discuss serotonin in greater detail in the next chapter.

51 In particular, by Van Praag and Bruinvels, *Neurotransmission and Disturbed Behavior*. Essman, *Serotonin in Health and Disease*, assesses the situation twenty years later.

52 Lingjaerde, "Le rôle de la sérotonine dans les troubles de l'humeur," 500.

53 Amineptine, nomifensine, mianserin, piribedil, bromocriptine.

54 Boulenger and Massaoui, "Perspectives pharmacologiques en psychiatrie biologique," 117.

55 Lingjaerde: "However, reducing a psychopathological symptom in the dysfunctionality of a monoaminergic system does seem dangerous" ("Le rôle de la sérotonine dans les troubles de l'humeur," 116). Lôo and Cuche: "The monoaminergic theory in the genesis of the depression seems far too reductionist" ("Classification des antidépresseurs," 596).

56 Zarifian and H. Lôo, *Les antidépresseurs*, 89. In 1983, Pierre Deniker and Édouard Zarifian concluded that depression was "a heterogenous entity on the biochemical level, depite its univocal clinical aspect" ("Perspectives d'utilisation de la L. Dopa en psychiatrie," 339). L. Dopa is a precursor to dopamine

57 Tissot, "Indicateurs biologiques et prises de décision thérapeutiques," 621

58 Widlöcher and Delcros, "De la pychologie du deuil à la biochimie de la dépression," 2963. "These days, everything is labelled as depression by patients and sometimes even by doctors. The term is not only assigned to any form of sadness or tension due to everyday life, but also to a broad spectrum of mental disorders" (Widlöcher and F. Binoux, "La clinique de la dépression," 2953).

59 Scotto et al., "Stratégies thérapeutiques devant une dépression," 1633 (emphasis mine).

60 The DSM-I dates back to 1952. It was created to help diagnose forms of mental pathology that were less severe than psychoses. During the Second World War, the nomenclature of the day was of little use to military psychiatrists since it could not be used to diagnose psychopathologies caused by combat. DSM-I used the nomenclature employed by veteran administrations. It became a tool for a type of psychiatry that was starting to work with a non-hospitalized population that suffered from milder mental pathologies. DSM-II was based on the section in the eighth revision of the International Classification of Diseases (WHO) dedicated to Mental Disorders. They were both published in 1968. The expression "affective disorders" was used for the first time in the military administration's nomenclature. It is used again in the DSM-I. See Kirk and Kutchins, *The Selling of DSM*; Jackson, *Melancholia and Depression*; and Young, *The Harmony of Illusion*, 94–107.

61 Grob, *Mental Illness and American Society*; and F. Castel, R. Castel, and Lovell, *The Psychiatric Society*.

62 On Adolf Meyer, see Grob, *Mental Illness and American Society*, 112ff.

63 On the specificity of the French "subject" throughout hexagonal psychoanalysis, see chapter 7.

64 See Kirk and Kutchins, *The Selling of DSM*; Wilson, "DSM-III and the Transformations of American Psychiatry"; and Freedman, "American Viewpoints on Classification."

65 For cases of depression, see N. Sartorius, "Description and Classification of Depressive Disorders," 76.

66 See Healy, *The Antidepressant Era*, chap., 3.

67 Generally, broader polemics are more common in France than are meticulously constructed arguments. See Descombey, "Subjectivité, scientificité, objectivité, objectivation." In it, the author sees the death of psychiatry. *Confrontations psychiatriques* published an issue of reflections and descriptions in 1984. The editorial of Bailly-Salin expressed fear that "the essence of psychiatry would be ... eliminated" ("Éditorial," 7) and emphasized the importance of "rethinking current views on classification, or rather, on classifications" (8). In his article, "Classification et connaissance. Remarques sur l'art de diviser et l'institution du sujet," Pierre Legendre, law professor and psychoanalyst, wrote how he saw the DSM as an enterprise of desubjectivation in the name of typically American management.

68 There had been a demand for these methods since the 1960s. Here are two examples. First, in a bid to provide structure to the diagnostic chaos, Paul Kielholz concluded in 1962 that "it would be necessary to create a nomenclature and international diagnostical definitions for the different depressive symptoms" ("État actuel du traitement pharmacologique des dépressions," 403). Second, at the 1966 edition of the CINP Congress in Washington, Jean Delay declared that "as psychotropic drugs grow in number and variety, and as the scope of their uses reaches nearly every form of mental pathology, it becomes critical that we have better resources at our disposal. This is vital to our establishing relevant statistics – that is to say, homogenous statistics pertaining to diagnostics and to the evaluation of treatments" ("Adresse présidentielle," xix). "Experience," he adds, "has taught us that the surest way for all clinicians to reach a consensus is with the basic symptoms: to simply acknowledge their presence (or absence) without offering any pathogenic interpretation" (xx).

69 We find some history of the relations between psychology and psychoanalysis in France in Anzieu, "La psychanalyse au service de la psychologie."

70 Zarifian points out that psychopathology is now taught only in psychology (*Le Prix du bien-être*, 119). He also mentions that, in 1996 in France,
one hundred psychiatrists were working in teaching hospitals, four thousand in public health services, and six thousand in private practices. The
first are the elite, with most working at Sainte-Anne, which is known to
be "vitalist" (Ibid., 113). In the public health services we find pluralism
is prevalent in the working methods of the non-academic psychiatrists

71 Barazer and C. Ehrenberg, "La folie perdue de vue."

72 Quoted in Kirk and Kutchins, *The Selling of DSM*, 6. Donald W. Goodwin
recounts how he started his career in the late 1950s as an "ardent
Freudian." Then, he worked at Washington University in St Louis with
some of the future advocates of DSM-III: "I liked the way physicians acted
like physicians and not like swami and they had a practical approach to
psychiatry I felt was also scientific" (quoted in Edwards, *Addictions*, 145).

73 F. Castel, R. Castel, and Lovell, *The Psychiatric Society*, 159ff.

74 Robins and Regier, *Psychiatric Disorders in America*.

75 The introductions to the two following versions provide only slight differences from the point of view of psychiatric reasoning.

76 Spitzer, "Introduction" to DSM-III, 6.

77 Pierre Pichot, who supervised the translation of the DSM-III into French,
writes, "This is one of the most widely distributed psychiatric works in the
world ... It has quickly become a reference that all psychiatrists must be
aware of, similar to Kraepelin's *Treatise* at the end of the 19th century"
(Foreword to the French translation of *DSM-III*, vi).

78 Spitzer writes, "Because DSM-III is generally atheoretical with regard to
etiology, it attempts to describe comprehensively what the manifestations
of the mental disorders are, and only rarely attempts to account for *how*
the disturbances come about ... This approach can be said to be 'descriptive' in that the definitions of the disorders generally consist of descriptions
of the clinical features of the disorders" ("Introduction" to DSM-III, 7).

79 The original articles by Feighner et al. ("Diagnostic Criteria for Use in
Psychiatric Research," 1972) and by Spitzer et al., ("Research Diagnostic
Citeria," 1978) are seen as the most cited articles in international psychi-
atric literature.

80 "DSM-III and DSM-III-R reflect an increased commitment in our field to
reliance on data as the basis for understanding mental disorders"
(Spitzer, "Introduction" to DSM-III-R, xxvii).

81 APA, DSM-III, 305.

82 Ibid., app. C, 378.

83 Spitzer, "Introduction" to DSM-III-R, xxv.

84 Zero point thirty-seven for depression, 0.50 for schizophrenia. See G.L.
   Klerman et al., "Neurotic Depressions," quoted in Haynal, "Problèmes
   cliniques de la dépression," 610; and Pichot, "Actualisation du concept
   de dépression," 310. Klerman's study is very well known in psychiatry for
   it is the basis for the suppression of neurotic depression in the DSM-III.

85 In DSM-III, as in the two following versions, the symptoms have to manifest themselves for two weeks.

86 I will not elaborate on psychiatric casuistry. It has been pointed out that,
   in the DSM-III-R, affect is replaced by mood and that, in DSM-IV, new
   subdivisions appear. For a synthesis, see C.B. Pull, "Critères diagnostiques,"
   247ff.

87 Spitzer, "Introduction" to DSM-III, 9. Emphasis in original.

88 Interview with Wilson, "DSM-III and the Transformations of American
   Psychiatry," 407.

89 Spitzer, "Introduction" to DSM-III, 10

90 APA, DSM-III, app. C, 376.

91 Hence, in 1978, F. Amiel-Lebigre writes about the WHO's classifications:
   "The importance currently given to the range of thymic disorders is
   apparent in the evolution of the *Classification of Mental and Behavioural
   Disorders*. Whereas the eighth revision of the document featured five
   headings pertaining to depression, in the ninth version – on which specialists from thirty-five countries collaborated – there are now ten headings dealing with depression" ("Épidémiologie des dépressions," 21).

92 Pichot: "Neurotic depression ... is the most common diagnosis in psychiatry" ("Actualisation du concept de dépression," 310).

93 Amiel-Lebigre writes that "the main difficulty with evaluating depressions
   is that of neurotic depression" ("Épidémiologie des dépressions," 21).
   Haynal's comments are similar ("Problèmes cliniques de la dépression,"
   610). According to Sir M. Roth and T.-A. Kerr, "Eliminating neurotic
   depression has raised questions and contradictions, and has created ...
   several problems" ("Le concept dépression névrotique," in Pichot and
   Rein, *L'approche clinique*, 207).

94 Glas, "A Conceptual History of Anxiety and Depression," in den Boer Ad
   Sitsen, *Handbook of Depression and Anxiety*, 36. Arthur Tatossian stresses this
   point as well: "The prevalence of depressive disorders over anxious disorders is apparent in the DSM-III" ("Les pratiques de la dépression," 289).

95 In the introduction to the WHO's ICD-10, the authors write: "'Disorder' is
   not an exact term, but it is used here to imply the existence of a clinically recognizable set of symptoms or behaviour associated in most cases
   with distress and with interference with personal functions" (5).

96 Wilson, "DSM-III and the Transformations of American Psychiatry," 408.

97 Amiel-Lebigre,"Épidémiologie des dépressions," 21.

98 Éric Fombonne and Rebecca Führeer write: "The current absence of
    criteria for the validation of psychopathological phenomena or of formal
    proof of psychiatric illnesses does not prevent the precise measuring of
    well-defined clinical phenomena ... In the end, confusion often enters
    between, on one hand, the validity and, on the other, the definition of
    entities. Recently developed methods for epidemiological research have
    consisted of new proposed definitions of clinical phenomena in hopes
    of improving the accuracy of their measurement. These methods have
    been criticized in the name of validity, which is another issue" ("Épidé-
    miologie et psychiatrie," 111). See also Fombonne, "La contribution
    de l'épidémiologie."

99 Haynal, "Problèmes cliniques de la dépression," 612 (emphsis in original).

100 Tatossian, "Les pratiques de la dépression," 296 (emphasis mine).

101 Israël, "Fin des hystéries, fin d'une psychiatrie?" 1986, reprinted in
    Israël, Boiter n'est pas pécher, 208.

102 Bergeret, "Dépressivité et dépression," 919. "See, for instance, the cur-
    rent success we are having with psychotropes, which we use to regulate
    our moods and which create new ones. On the other hand, there is the
    drug, and addiction. Indeed, it is destructive in the long run, but what
    if initially it produced a burning desire for a change of state? What if
    it produced an immediate desire to transform the 'inner world?'"
    ("Présentation," 7).

103 Demel, "Observations on the Clinical Nature of Masked Depression from
    the Standpoint of Practical Social Psychiatry," 248–9.

104 Legendre, L'inestimable objet de la transmission, 362.

CHAPTER SIX

1 Self-affirmation is in itself quite a task; it has many demands and requires
   a special set of skills that may differ from those of the body, which have
   become well honed over time.

2 Jouvent and Pellet, "Les dépressions résistantes et leurs traitements," 1647.

3 Widlöcher and Colonna, "L'évaluation quantitative du ralentissement
   psychomoteur"; and Widlöcher, "L'échelle de ralentissement dépressif."
   According to Darcourt: "Certainly, psychomotor slowing was traditionally
   deemed to be a symptom of depression. Before this research, however,
   it was not considered to play a major role" ("Place du ralentissement,"
   61).

4 Widlöcher, "Fatigue et dépression," 349. This volume contains the proceedings of the colloquium entitled "Confrontation multidisciplinaire
européenne sur la dépression," held in Monte Carlo in December 1980.

5 Ibid., 349–50. Widlöcher sees there a "syndrome common to all clinical
forms of depression" ("L'échelle de ralentissement dépressif," 53).

6 Widlöcher, "L'échelle de ralentissement dépressif," 56.

7 Widlöcher, *Les logiques de la dépression*, 235.

8 Ibid., 255.

9 See Colonna, H. Lôo, and Zarifian, "Chimiothérapie des dépressions,"
4437.

10 See, for instance, Spadone and Vanelle "Les nouveaux antidépresseurs";
or Bourin, "Quel avenir pour les antidépresseurs?"

11 See Heninger, "Indoleamines," 479.

12 Lemoine, "Bien prescrire les psychotropes," 1413.

13 Ginestet, Chauchot, and Olive, "Existe-t-il des classifications pratiques
de psychotropes?" 38.

14 H. Lôo, "Préface" to "La dépression," 619.

15 See Rapoport, one of the leading authorities on this pathology, *The Boy
Who Couldn't Stop Washing*. There is an enormous amount of psychiatric
literature on OCDs. This category was brought to the fore when Geigy
launched clomipramine in 1964. See Georges Beaumont in Healy, *The
Psychopharmacologists*, 1:311; and Healy, "The History of British Psychopharmacology," 74. OCDs are included in the DSM-*III*.

16 Bourin, "Quel avenir pour les antidépresseurs?" 102. See also Champoux,
"Antidépresseur: Un terme trompeur," *Quotidien du médecin*, 12 June 1989,
28; Spadone, "Le big bang de la chimiothérapie psychotrope"; and
Peyré, "Les antidépresseurs en dehors de la dépression," 2300.

17 Decombe, Bentué-Ferrer, and Allain, "Le point sur la neurotransmission
dans les dépressions," 574.

18 Brown and van Praag, *The Role of Serotonin in Psychiatric Disorders*. See
especially the Introduction (3–7). See also Serena-Lynn Brown, Avraham
Bleich, and Herman M. van Praag, "The Monoamine Hypothesis of
Depression" (Ibid., 91–128).

19 See Herman M. van Praag, in Healy, *The Psychopharmacologists*, 1:370–2.

20 Cf. chap. 5. As Arthur Tatossian states: "It would seem that the very structure of the general practice as well as the often minor nature of the psychical pathology of its clientele needs to correspond to a proportionate
model" ("Les pratiques de la dépression.") See also Cremniter, "Aspects
épidémiologiques de la dépression."

21 Dufour, "Les inhibitions dépressives," 435.

22 Pélicier, "Séméiologie de l'inhibition," 403, introduction to the semiological part of the colloquium.

23 Widlöcher, "L'échelle du ralentissement dépressif," 55.

24 "We can hardly mention one of the two words, anxiety or inhibition, without mentioning the other," writes Colonna ("Les inhibitions anxieuses," 439). "If the psychomotoral inhibition is lifted, anxiety increases. Inhibition is therefore described as a defense mechanism against anxiety," writes Guyotat ("Inhibitions et antidépresseurs," 533).

25 Ginestet, Chauchot, and Olive, "Existe-t-il des classifications pratiques de psychotropes?" 40.

26 Martin, "L'inhibition en psychopathologie," 25.

27 Multidimensional study on 813 general practitioners who had diagnosed 15,076 patients. See Le Quotidien du médecin, 13 October 1997; and Pfizer, "Zoloft: une étude multicentrique française confirme son efficacité chez huit patients sur dix."

28 Bourin and Cerlebaud, "La dépression et les antidépresseurs en médecine générale," 2301. Study based on questionnaires sent to all the general practitioners in Loire-Atlantique (690 doctors).

29 Tignol and Bourgeois, "La désinhibition et ses risques," 460.

30 Guyotat, "Inhibitions et antidépresseurs," 537.

31 The substitution of guilt with asthenia is always emphasized, particularly in general medicine. See Cremniter, "Aspects épidémiologiques de la dépression vue en medicine"; Mockers, "Anxiété et dépression souvent associées." See also Gazette médicale, "Les états anxiodépressifs."

32 It is designated by the word "dysthymia," which I discuss in chapter 7. Pichot elaborates on the matter: "Under 'Neurasthenia,' both the indexes of the DSM-III and the DSM-III-R indicate to 'See Dysthymia'" ("La neurasthénie," 545).

33 Pichot, "La neurasthénie," 548. See also, in the same issue, Lecubrier and Weiller, "La neurasthénie et la thymasthénie," with thymia replacing nerves.

34 Wessely, "Le syndrome de fatigue chronique," 581. Also in the same issue, see L. Crocq, "Les recherches sur la fatigue en France."

35 On this topic, see Mulhern, "À la recherche du trauma perdu"; Mulhern, "L'inceste." See also Hacking, Rewriting the Soul.

36 Lempérière, "Les algies psychogènes," 285.

37 In 1978, Daniel Widlöcher wrote: "Cases of conversion disorder shy away from psychoanalysts and generally, from psychiatrists as well. In order to fulfill their needs, which are usually medical, they tend towards general practitioners and neurologists" ("L'hystérie dépossédée," 75).

38 According to Lucien Israël, "this is why the hysterical forms [of depression] are more common" (*L'hystérique*, 161). For Michel Patris, a service director at the UHC-Strasbourg, "an ever increasing number of cases of hysteria are adding depression to their traditional array of ailments, thus creating the illusion that their disorders can be treated with antidepressants" ("Dépression et suggestion hypnotique," 271).

39 Drs Garoux and Ranty, "L'asthénie en psychiatrie," 2539. This entire issue is devoted to exhaustion.

40 Gold, *The Good News about Depression*, vii.

41 Ibid., x,

42 Ibid., xi.

43 Spitzer, Introduction to the DSM-III, 5–6.

44 Frances, Introduction to the DSM-IV, xxi.

45 René Tissot, whose psycho-pharmacological qualifications are well established, writes: "A monoaminergic unbalance will never solely account for a melancholic's remorse" ("Quelques aspects biochimiques," 516).

46 Dowling, *You Mean I Don't Have to Feel This Way?* 23. The front matter features a quote by Nathan Kline: "Psychiatry has labored too long under the delusion that every emotional malfunction requires an endless talking out of everything the patient ever experienced" (vi).

47 The release of Olié, Poirier, and Lôo, *Les maladies dépressives*, is an example of this fragmenting. See also Lôo and Gallarda, *La maladie dépressive*. Nevertheless, Widlöcher, *Traité de psychopathologie*, is an exception.

48 Widlöcher, Introduction to the special issue of *La Revue du praticien*, entitled "La dépression," 1613. This was the generally accepted thesis in psychiatry. Experiments with imipramine (esp. those by Goodman and Gillman in 1970, which are frequently cited) on healthy volunteers have proven it: imipramine "does not cause euphoria in healthy subjects, but rather, fatigue" (Lambert, "Les effets indésirables," 271).

49 Jacobs and Fornal, "Serotonin and Behavior," 461. See also Heninger, "Indoleamines," 471.

50 See Norden, *Beyond Prozac*; Wurtzel, *Prozac Nation*; and Whybrow, *A Mood Apart*.

51 Colonna and Petit, "Sémiologie dépressive," 648. See also L. Colonna et al., "États dépressifs."

52 Glowinski, Julou, and Scatton, "Effets des neuroleptiques." Jacques Glowinski collaborated with Julius Axelrod in a bid to discover the noradrenaline receptors as well as their reuptake mechanism. Axelrod received the Nobel Prize for medicine for this discovery in 1970.

53 Snyder, "Molecular Strategies in Neuropharmacology," 17.

54 For more on these matters, see the interviews David Healy conducted with researchers who worked in pharmacology from the 1950s on in *The Psychopharmacologists*. For more on the monoaminergic hypothesis, see also Healy, *The Antidepressant Era*, 155–79.

55 On all these points, see Snyder, *Drugs and the Brain*, esp. chapters 3 and 4. Snyder worked on his doctorate in the 1960s in Axelrod's laboratory at the faculty of medicine in Bethesda, Maryland. See also Arvid Carlsson, "Monoamines of the Central Nervous System."

56 Tissot, "Monoamines et régulations thymiques," 122. One of the first studies on serotonin published in 1959 remains dubious (Mendes and Lopes do Rosario, "Signification et importance de la sérotonine en psychiatrie," 503).

57 Lôo and Colonna, "Abord critique," 364.

58 See, among dozens of articles on the subject, Boyer, "États dépressifs et marqueurs biologiques"; and Deniker, "Dépressions résistantes."

59 Dalery and Lôo, "Editorial," 179.

60 "In spite of 35 to 40 years of intensive biological research, there is no single biological variable with any diagnostic significance" (H. van Praag in Healy, *The Psychopharmacologists*, 1:367). See also the remarks of Alan Broadhurst, in ibid., 129; and Gram, "Concepts d'antidépresseurs," 115. In the introduction to DSM-IV, Allen Frances writes that the "clinical features ... were insufficiently sensitive or specific to be included in the final criteria set" (8). See also Cussey et al., "Sérotonine et dépression," 76.

61 Brown and van Praag, *The Role of Serotonin in Psychiatric Disorders*, 4. See also Hollister, "Strategies for Research in Clinical Psychopharmacology," 35. Snyder: "Receptor research made possible an understanding of drug side effects" ("Molecular Strategies in Neuropharmacology," 18).

62 "It was a rarity in the annals of medicine and pharmacy: we started with a biochemical hypothesis in order to create a medication whose primary purpose is to correct the specific flaw researchers brought to light" (Robert, "Études cliniques d'un sérotonergique," 881). It is a theme that recurs often.

63 Uzan, "Agents prosérotonininergiques et dépressions," 274. Marie Åsberg, et al. published the first decisive work, "Serotonin depression," in 1976, in which she succeeded in proving that 70 percent of patients suffering from depression are lacking in serotonin.

64 "This is what struck observers most: we were accustomed to seeing psychomotric inhibitions go before depressive moods" (Robert, "Études cliniques d'un sérotonergique," 883).

65 Ibid., 884.
66 Ibid., 883–4.
67 Wauters, "Les troubles de l'humeur," 83.
68 Prigent, "Psychodynamique des chimiothérapies antidépressives," 841.
69 *Elle*, no.1974, 1983.
70 Let us remember that Healy, in *The Antidepressant Era,* does not mention the existence of indalpine. It would seem that, in the Anglo-Saxon world, only zimelidine had an impact.
71 Phase II trials contrasted the molecule with amitriptyline. The side effects were relatively minor in comparison. Moreover, while patients given amitriptyline gained weight, those on zimelidine remained the same (Coppen et al., "Zimelidine," 201). It is worth mentioning that amitriptyline is one of the rare products to have been improved since 1957 (Lôo and Zarifian, *Limites de l'efficacité des chimiothérapies psychotropes,* 68).
72 See Healy, *The Antidepressant Era.* Brian B. Malloy, Ray W. Fuller, and David T. Wong are the three inventors of this antidepressant.
73 Ibid., 16.
74 For more on all these points, see the collection of interviews by Healy (*The Psychopharmacologists*). See also Healy, *The Antidepressant Era* and See also Medawar, "The Antidepressant Web," 86–8.
75 Gold, *The Good News about Depression,* x.
76 Snyder, "Molecular Strategies in Neuropharmacology," 21.
77 And for each type of dopaminergic receptor for schizophrenia, see D. Coleman, "Move Over Prozac: New Drugs," *International Herald Tribune,* 21 November 1996.
78 Stora and Peretti, "À déprimés divers," 20.
79 "Les inhibiteurs de la recapture de la sérotonine," 27.
80 Zarifian, *Le prix du bien-être,* 200.
81 Coignard, "Les prodiges de l'effet placebo," *Le Point,* 29 June 1996. Prozac is the only psychotrope among the twenty medications.
82 See the articles by B. Jönsson and P. Bebbington, J.-S. MacComb and M.-B. Nichol, and W.-F. Boyer and J.-P. Feighner in Jönsson and Rosenbaum, *Health Economics of Depression.* See also, among others, Stewart, "Revisiting the Relative Cost-Effectiveness of Selective Serotonin Reuptake Inhibitors and Tricyclic Antidepressants"; Wilde and Whittington, "Paroxetine"; Guze, "Selective Serotonin Reuptake Inhibitors"; and Davis and Wilde, "Sertraline." A report by the National Mental Health Association, an association sponsored by the pharmaceutical industry, estimates that the annual cost of depression for employers is $23.8 billion

(loss in work days and productivity). For the total savings to insurance companies due to the new antidepressants, see "New Approvals Change Depression Market," *Marketletter*, 17 January 1994.

83 It should have an optimal effectiveness on a clinical level, as long as it has a total therapeutic effectiveness (healing depression). The antidepressant effects take hold quickly and continue to be effective with repeat and resistant patients. See Gérard, Dagens, and Deslandes, "1960–2000."

84 "Mise au point de molécules de en plus sélectives," *Impact médecin hebdo*, no. 370, 13 June 1997. See also *Impact quotidien*, no. 941, 26 September 1996; *Le Quotidien du médecin*, 8 October 1996.

85 Dagognet, *La raison et les remèdes*, Paris, PUF, 1964, p. 330

86 Le Pape and Lecomte, *Aspects socioéconomiques de la dépression*, 49. The rate for those sixty and older has doubled but has remained stable in the twenty-to-twenty-nine category. Paris and its surroundings has a 5.4 percent depression rate, and the national average is 4.7 percent.

87 Findings by France's NIHMR conclude that the probability that people will face a depressive episode in their lives is at 10.7 percent for men and 22.4 percent for women. See Lepine et al., "L'épidémiologie des troubles anxieux."

88 Martineau, "Dépression en Europe," 8.

89 Le Pape and Lecomte, *Aspects socioéconomiques de la dépression*, 25.

90 Expenses doubled in ten years for the first and went up by 58 percent only for the latter.(Le Pape and Lecomte, *Aspects socioéconomiques de la dépression*, 8).

91 Michele Aulagnon, "La Conférence nationale de la santé met l'accent sur l'éducation sanitaire," *Le Monde*, 18 July 1997.

92 "Deuxième conférence national de santé," *Le Quotidien du médecin*, 23 Jul 1997,8. The French Economic and Social Council estimate that "nearly 20% of French citizens suffer from psychical and behavioural disorders"(Pierre Joly [reporter], *Prévention et soins des maladies mentales*, 35).

93 Lazarus (pres.), *Une souffrance qu'on ne peut plus cacher*, report by the Groupe du travail ville, santé mentale, précarité et exclusion sociale, February 1995, 15.

94 Commissariat général au plan, *Chômage: Le cas français*, quoted in P. Krémer, "Les sociologues redécouvrent les liens entre suicide et crise économique," *Le Monde*, 4 February 1998.

95 See Paugam, Zoyem, and Charbonnel, *Précarité et risque d'exclusion en France*.

96 Michele Aulagnon, "Les consultations et le soutien psychologique de L'Élan retrouvé," *Le Monde*, 4 June 1997.

97 Quoted in Laurence Folléa, "Des experts s'alarment des dégats de l'exclusion sur la santé," *Le Monde*, 22–23 February 1998.

98 For more on these, see: Lazarus, *Une souffrance qu'on ne peut plus cacher*, Kovess et al., "La psychiatrie face aux problèmes sociaux"; Roelandt, "Exclusion, insertion"; and Merceuil and Letout, "Précarité et troubles psychiques."

99 Merceuil and Letout, "Précarité et troubles psychiques," 3.

100 It is therefore significant that a psychiatrist/psychoanalyst such as Christophe Demers – one of the few researchers to have been studying work psychopathology for the past twenty years – should suddenly receive more press coverage for his latest work, *Souffrance en France*.

101 A. Ehrenberg, *Le culte de la performance*, 270–3.

102 Cohen, *Richesses du monde*, 78.

103 Ibid., 79.

104 Bourdieu and Passeron, *Reproduction in Education*.

105 Fatela, "Crise de l'école et fragilités adolescentes," 96.

106 See Dubet, *Les lycéens*. D. Goux and E. Maurin write: "Not long ago, children of humble origins were not stigmatized for their poor results in school because said results reflected the nature of the institution. Today, their mediocre scores are seen as the result of a competition they were allowed to participate in, but failed" ("L'égalité des chances," in Fondation Saint-Simon, *Pour une nouvelle république sociale*, 18–19).

107 J.-L. Donnet, "Une évolution de la demande au Centre Jean Favreau," 23. He notes the fact that a significant number of parents born during this time had incestuous relationships, sometimes lasting many years, in households that appeared wholesome from the outside (23).

108 See Ehrenberg, "Le harcèlement sexuel"; and Théry, "Vie privée et monde commun."

109 Jacques Donzelot's expression. On the path of progress to change and its implications regarding the notion of resposability, see Donzelot, *L'invention du social*.

110 Zarifian, "Médicaments anxiolytiques et inhibition." See also Amar and Barazer, "Tranquilité sur ordonnance."

111 Cuche and Gérard, "Antidépresseurs," 206.

112 Barazer and Cadoret, "Liminaire," 7–9.

113 Kramer, *Listening to Prozac*, 297.

114 Cuche and Gérard, "Antidépresseurs," 206. See Peter Kramer's many comments on this topic in *Listening to Prozac*. See also the works of Édouard Zarifian.

115 Dufour, "Les inhibitions dépressives," 433. Lucien Israël dwells on the "peculiar relationship with time most depressives have ... Time slows to a crawl, becomes endless" (*L'hystérique*, 161). We find the old correlation between boredom and melancholia. See Starobinski, *La mélancolie au miroir*, and Huguet, *L'ennui et ses discours*.

116 Carlsson, "Monoamines of the Central Nervous System."

117 Interviews with Jonathan Cole and Donald F. Klein, in Healy, *The Psychopharmacologists*, 1:258 and 351–2. Researchers conclude that the quest for more effective antidepressants is inhibited by the monoaminergic hypothesis, which steers creativity down the beaten paths. See in particular Leo E. Hollister, "Strategies for Research in Clinical Psychopharmacology," 34–5.

118 Karp, "Taking Anti-Depressant Medications." To my knowledge, this is the only work on the uses of antidepressants. On the patients' ambivalence towards their psychotropic medications, see the ethnologic study by Haxaire et al., "'C'était pas comme une drogue.'" Claudie Haxaire is also a pharmacologist.

119 Dagognet, *La raison et les remèdes*, 328.

CHAPTER SEVEN

1 Comité de Rédaction, "Editorial," 3. In 1994, an article on SSRIs in *La Revue du praticien* deemed that psychotherapies must be applied in cases of "complicated depressions combined with a pathological personality or chronic depressions. Conversely, the depression of the 'everyman' should be treated with antidepressants without hesitation"(Bougerol, "Antidépresseurs de génération récente," 2293).

2 Möller and Volz, "Drug Treatment of Depression in the 1990s," 625. This is a recurring theme.

3 An independent group of American experts analyzed the results of double-blind tests comparing a molecule with a placebo. The results show that "there is good reason to believe that most studies on antidepressants are not conducted under true double-blind conditions" (Fischer and Greenberg, "Examining Antidepressant and Effectiveness," 10). The use of inactive placebos that give the patient no unpleasant sensation is inadequate. The authors deem that "these molecules are lacking an adequate scientific evaluation" (29). The conclusion of the nine studies collected in this work (on anxiety, electroshocks, Ritalin, schizophrenia, etc.) is that there is no fair and rational assessment in biological psychology. The greatest obstacles are "the failure in the use

of inactive placebos, the extreme selectiveness of the samples, and the miasmic wave of definitions for what a level of 'therapeutic' effect means" (Fischer and Greenberg, "A Second Opinion," 322).

4 Reports from the international colloquium, "Les dépressions résistantes aux traitements antidépresseurs," Paris, 17 January 1986, *L'Encéphale* 12 spec. issue (October 1986).

5 Chignon and Abbar, "Traitement du déprimé," 195. See also Bougerol and Scotto, "Le déprimé."

6 Cuche and Gérard, "Antidépresseurs," 210. Of the APA's, "Practice Guideline for Major Depressive Disorder in Adults," Vanelle and Féline, write: "it only retains arguments in favour of the pursuit of antidepressors with a prophylactic purpose ("Arrêt du traitement médicamenteux dans la dépression," 225).

7 Bougerol and Scotto, "Le déprimé," 233. "For most patients, depression is a recidivist disorder, if not a lifelong problem" (Stokes, "La fluoxetine.").

8 Cardot and Rouillon, "Évolution à long terme des dépressions."

9 Bougerol and Scotto, "Le déprimé," 232.

10 Ibid., 232.

11 "Declaring patients cured of their depressions is declaring them cured of their episodes, not of the disorders themselves" (Poirier, "Critères psychobiologiques de guérison," 451).

12 Olivier-Martin, "Facteurs psychologiques," 198.

13 Hardy, "Notion de dépression résistante," 192.

14 See Montgomery and Rouillon, *Long-Term Treatment of Depression.*

15 "The actual length of the treatment remains unclear" (Dalery and Sechter, "Traitement prolongé d'antidépresseurs," 209). See also Sechter, "Les effets cliniques à long terme des antidépresseurs."

16 In Vanelle and Féline, "Arrêt du traitement médicamenteux dans la dépression." According to H.-S. Akiskal, "Studies conducted on the general public have shown that a third of depressions are chronic and that most of the others are recurring" ("Personnalité pathologique," 47). The authoritative work on long-term treatment is by Kupfer et al., "Five Year Outcome for Maintenance Therapy in Recurring Depressions." See also Cassano, Maggini and Longo, "Les dépressions chroniques."

17 Pringuey et al., "L'efficacité des antidépresseurs," 61.

18 Ibid., 69. Which confirms the enormous study overseen by Fischer and Greenberg, *The Limits of Biological Treatments for Psychological Distress.*

19 Cuche and Gérard, "Antidépresseurs," 206.

20 Ibid., 205 and 211.

21 Sechter, "Les effets cliniques à long terme des antidépresseurs," 36.

22 See Scotto, introduction to "La durée des traitements de dépression," 1.

23 Sechter, "Les effets cliniques à long terme des antidépresseurs," 38. Reference to Montgomery et al., "Impact of Neuropsychology in the 1990s."

24 Dalery and Sechter, "Traitment prolongé d'antidépresseurs," 212.

25 Vanelle and Féline, "Arrêt du traitement médicamenteux dans la dépression," 226. René Tissot believes that "MAOIs are the only antidepressants proven … to raise the spirits of those who are not depressed" ("Indicateurs biologiques," 623). For a synthesis aimed at general practitioners, see Giraud, Lemonnier, and Bigot, who write: "Several factors attest to the fact that psychological dependence appears to be one of the dominant reasons for chronic intoxication and pharmacodependence" ("Pharmacodépendence et psychotropes," 2229).

26 Poirier and Ginestet, "Médicaments détournés à des fins toxicomaniaques," 1365. SSRIs are not said to cause any withdrawal symptoms.

27 Cardot and Rouillon, "Évolution à long terme des dépressions," 51.

28 In 1978, Tissot could still claim that "the difference between treating melancholia successfully with antidepressants and transforming schizophrenics with neuroleptics is similar to the difference between treating pneumonia with antibiotics and correcting cardiac deficiencies with digital technology" ("Quelques aspects biochimiques," 517).

29 Deniker, "Dépressions résistantes," 188. "Neurotic personality traits had a negative impact on development" (Cardot and Rouillon, "L'évolution à long terme des dépressions," 55). "Some of the neurotic disorders formerly tagged as anxious are now referred to as chronic mild depressions" (Lecrubier and Jourdain, "Description de troubles dépressifs," 656).

30 Bougerol and Scotto, "Le déprimé," 233.

31 J.-P. Boulenger and Y.-J. Lavallée, "Attaques de panique," 73 (emphasis mine). See also Boulenger, L'attaque de panique; and Martinot, Raffaitin, and Olié, "Attaques de panique et dépressions anxieuses."

32 Herman van Praag, in Healy, The Psychopharmacologists, 1: 364.

33 Thomas Ban, in Healy, The Psychopharmacologists, 1:617. Also in Healy, see Arvid Carlsson (76–7), Heinz Lehmann, (184–5), J. Angst (302), Donald F. Klein, (351–2), and M. Lader (480).

34 Édouard Zarifian mentions that "much effort was made so the concept of anxious depression would be included in the WHO classifications, and now it is" (Le prix du bien-être, 220).

35 Chignon, "Le syndrome anxiodépressif," 1275. For a synthesis, see Hardy, "L'anxiété dans ses rapports avec la dépression."

36 Boulenger and Lavallée, "Anxiété ou dépression."

37 For a French study, see Lépine et al., "L'épidémiologie des troubles anxieux." For an international synthesis, see, among others, Jean-Pierre Lépine and Jean-Michel Chignon, "Épidémiologie des troubles anxieux et névrotiques," in Rouillon, Lépine, and Terra, *Épidémiologie psychiatrique*.

38 If his definition changes between DSM-III, III-R, and IV, "the chronic character of evolution remains a constant in dysthemic disorders" (Hardy, "Le traitement de consolidation," 40).

39 Debray, Interview with Hagop Akiksal, 13. According to Julien-Daniel Guelfi: "The realm of personality disorders and subsyndromic depressive disorders is in all likelihood where the relationships between antidepressants and diagnostic classifications will advance most in the years to come. Studies on the connections between mood and personality are increasing in number. Recent findings show that antidepressants could modify certain aspects of the personality" (Guelfi et al., "Antidépresseurs et classifications diagnostiques chez l'adulte," 10).

40 In his interview with David Healy, Herman van Praag stated, "dysthemia responds very well to serotoninergics. I think that Prozac's success has a lot to do with this" (*The Psychopharmacologists*, 1:20).

41 According to Péron-Magnan, temperament has made a comeback because of the notion of depressive personality ("Tempérament et dépression," 184). "For depressive personalities, the psychical life is composed of depressive feelings that are *infinite*, temporally" (Péron-Magnan and Galinowski, "La personnalité dépressive," 95 [emphasis in original]). Allen Frances deems that, "for the moment, the boundaries between the depressive personality and the existing categories of mood disorders are not clearly established" (Interview in *Psychiatrie internationale*, 8).

42 Hardy, "Le traitement de consolidation," 41.

43 Patrick Lemoine, "Qualité de vie et psychose," in Terra, *Qualité de vie subjective et santé mentale*, 45.

44 P. Gérin, M. Sali, A. Dazord, "Propositions pour une définition de la 'qualité de vie subjective,'" in Terra, *Qualité de vie subjective et santé mentale*, 87. See also Besançon, "La qualité de vie."

45 P. Gérin, M. Sali, A. Dazord, "Propositions pour une définition de la 'qualité de vie subjective,'" in Terra, *Qualité de vie subjective et santé mentale*, 87–8.

46 P. Lemoine, "Qualité de vie et psychose," in Terra, *Qualité de vie subjective et santé mentale*, 46. "In fact, any study on the quality of living raises the issue of happiness" (Ibid., 47).

47 P. Martin, "Le concept de qualité de vie," 22. The author is a neuropharmacologist. Also on the same topic, see C. Seulin and P. Gérin,

"Évaluation de la qualité de vie en santé mentale"; and C. Martin and
J. Tignol, "Évaluation de la satisfaction du client en psychiatrie," in
Rouillon, Lépine, and Terra, *Épidémiologie psychiatrique*.

48 See Herzlich, *Illness in Self and Society*.

49 P. Lemoine, "Qualité de vie et psychose," in Terra, *Qualité de vie subjective et santé mentale*, 29. See also P. Martin, "Le concept de qualité de vie," 73.

50 Olivier-Martin, "Facteurs psychologiques," 199.

51 To see this type of analysis applied to all chronic illnesses, refer to
J.-F. d'Ivernois, "Apprendre au patient à se soigner," *Le Monde*,
27 April 1994. For patients suffering from chronic physical illnesses,
see Baszanger, *Inventing Pain Medicine*. Baszanger notes the importance
of cognitive behavioural therapies in dealing with chronic pain. The pain
is not just an objective state but also a behaviour (190).

52 Dalery and Lôo, Éditorial in *L'Encéphale*, 179.

53 Lambert, *Psychanalyse et psychopharmacologie*, 56. See, among others,
Zarifian, *Les jardiniers de la folie*, 198; and Peele, *Diseasing of America*.

54 Cuche and Gérard, "Antidépresseurs," 206 and 207.

55 Péron-Magnan and Galinowski write about the "feeling of powerlessness,
of biological inferiority" experienced by the depressive personality
("La personnalité depressive," 97) as well as the "psychology of the
defeated"(105).

56 Widlöcher, introduction to a special issue of *La Revue du praticien*,
1613–14.

57 Pierre Pichot, in Healy, *The Psychopharmacologists*, 1:17 and 22. Jean-
Claude Scotto, introducing a colloquium, held in January 1994 in
Marseille, on the length of treatments, writes once again that depression
remains a "vast realm with vague parameters." He says that "empiricism
still rules: unclear concepts and rudimentary models. The criteria for the
choice of medicine and its dosage have very little, if any, scientific basis"
(Introduction to "La durée des traitements de dépression," 1).

58 Haynal, "Le sens du désespoir," 119.

59 Canguilhem, "Une pédagogie de la guérison est-elle possible?" 25.

60 Ibid., 25–6 (emphasis mine).

61 Israël, *Boiter n'est pas pécher*, 35. He writes, "desire and happiness are not
compatible" (31).

62 Roustang, *Influence*, 11.

63 Ibid., 111.

64 Roustang, *How to Make a Paranoid Laugh*, 84.

65 Ibid., 114.

66 McDougall, *Plea for a Measure of Abnormality*, 479.

67 See, for example, the issues "Figures du vide," *Nouvelle Revue de psychoanalyse*, 11, 1975; and "Les cas difficiles," *Revue française de psychoanalyse*, 54, no.2, 1990.

68 Donnet, "Une évolution de la demande au centre Jean Favreau," 17 (emphasis mine). Because the treatment is free, the clientele is not quite representative of those who go to private practices.

69 Ibid., 18.

70 Ibid., 19.

71 Ibid., 19–20.

72 Ibid., 23 (emphasis in original).

73 Legendre, *Le crime du caporal*, 155n8.

74 Legendre, *L'inestimable objet de la transmission*, 364.

75 Kramer, *Listening to Prozac*, 322.

76 Ibid., 265.

77 Kramer goes on to say: "Clinically, doctors no longer consider remission of acute symptoms to be a marker of adequate treatment; they expect to see personality change as well ... I will remind myself a more limited result – relief from tearfulness, insomnia, and grief – was understood as complete resonse (Ibid., 319–20).

78 Healy, *The Antidepressant Era*, 261.

79 Ibid., 264.

80 Kramer, *Listening to Prozac*, 407. Peter Whybrow develops a similar argument in *A Mood Apart*. He believes that "hypomania ... is good for the individual and for the social group" (256).

81 Bonnafé, et al., *Le problème de la psychogenèse*, 9 (emphasis in original).

82 Janet, *Psychological Healing*, 1:335.

83 Dagognet, *La raison et les remèdes*, 329.

84 See, for example, Jeannerod, *De la physiologie mentale*. Widlöcher writes: "Although they do not say so, a number of 'scientists' believe that once we know which neuronal mechanisms are in question, as well as what the problems and the corrections are, that adjusting the brain's chemical state will be enough to solve the problem. When will this be possible and for what 'illnesses?'" (*Les nouvelles cartes de la psychanalyse*, 269).

85 Kramer, *Listening to Prozac*, 409–10.

86 I refer here to Claude Lefort's political analysis, "Reversability." The invention of the social alludes to the work by Jacques Donzelot, *L'invention du social*.

87 Legendre, *L'inestimable objet de la transmission*, 101. The final sentence is italicized in the original.

88 In a tribute to Hesnard, Henri Ey writes (in 1971), "he was obsessed with this idea his entire life" ("A. Hesnard – Biologiste, psychiatre, psychanalyste," 304). In a well-documented article, psychoanalyst Victor N. Smirnoff writes: "It will surprise no one to read Pichon's statement [in 1938] that the psychoanalytic field in France 'has always paid close attention to vital matters like psychoanalysis and morality.' He calls to mind the keen interest French writers like Laforgue, Hesnard, and Odier have in the need for punishment" ("De Vienne à Paris," 44). A substantial part of Lacan's thesis on paranoia (published in 1932) is devoted to self-punishment.

89 Hesnard, *Freud dans la société d'après guerre*, 25. Hesnard's first work on psychoanalysis was written in collaboration with his "boss," Emmanuel Régis, and is entitled *La psycho-analyse des névroses et des psychoses*. The third edition, published in 1929, was greatly edited. Most notably, the numerous criticisms of Freud were removed.

90 Lacan, *Ethics of Psychoanalysis: 1959–1960*, 13.

91 *Ibid.*, 307. The cited sentence was repeated in the concluding session of July 1960. Lacan continues, sating that the distinction between the "castrating father" and "the father as origin of the superego" is "basic to everything Freud articulated" (307).

92 See Garapon, *Le gardien des promesses*, 68–9.

93 Gore Vidal's *Duluth* depicts this democratization with great humour.

94 Musil, *The Man without Qualities*, 1:174. The story takes place in 1913–14.

95 Nietzsche, *The Genealogy of Morals*, 36.

96 Ibid., 36

97 A third theme has recently emerged: the new continent of sexual violence.

98 See A. Ehrenberg, *L'individu incertain*, chap. 2.

99 Vernant and Vidal-Naquet, *Myth and Tragedy in Ancient Greece*, 49.

100 Deitch, *Post-Human*, Lausanne, Musée d'Art contemporain de Lausanne. Reshaping oneself is one of the main features of the virtual world's ideology. See A. Ehrenberg, "Cyberespaces, New Age électronique," in *L'individu incertain*, 274–94.

101 Héritier, *Two Sisters and Their Mother*, 62.

102 For more on this view, see Anatrella, *Non à la société dépressive*.

103 "The *raison d'être* of politics is freedom, and its field of experience is action," writes Hannah Arendt (*Between Past and Future*, 146).

104 On the decline of the character of the enemy, see Bergougnioux and Manin, *La social-démocratie ou le compromis*.

105 Jacques Donzelot has defended this thesis since *L'invention du social* in 1984.

106 Wyvekins, "Délinquences des mineurs," 168.

107 Astier, "RMI," 144.

108 Lazarus, *Une souffrance qu'on ne peut plus cacher*, 14.

109 "The social individual as the always impossible and always realized coexistence of a private world (*kosmos idios*) and of a common or public world" (Castoriadis, *The Imaginary Institution of Society*, 300).

110 Quoted in Descombes, *Les institutions du sens*, 296.

CONCLUSION

1 "The main 'fact' of the 20th century is the concept of the *unlimited possibility*," writes James G. Ballard, in the introduction to the 1974 French edition of his novel, *Crash*, 8 (emphasis in original). Hence, the mission he attaches to science fiction: "Given this immense continent of possibility, few literatures would seem better equipped to deal with their subject matter than science fiction" (Ibid., 8)

2 S. Toubiana, "L'homme tout bête," 8–9. Woody Allen appears to represent the other side of interior cinema. He recently declared: "I'm the product of television and psychological problems. I'm more interested in interior movements ... The setting for comedy has shifted from the exterior to the interior. We're no longer battling locomotives. It's up to me to make these new conflicts exciting" (interview conducted by Marcus Rothe in *Libération*, 21 January 1988, 33).

3 Tresson, "Voyage au bout de l'envers," 9.

4 C. Desbarat cited by Mongin, *La violence des images*, 11. Olivier Mongin shows that, in contemporary cinema, "violence teeters between a repressive interiorization and explosive acting out ... [When the conflict] can no longer be translated or symbolized, the resulting violence can be formidable and extreme" (Ibid., 67–8).

5 Ballard, *Crash!* 9–10.

6 Arendt, *The Human Condition*, 190.

7 Title of the segment Lefort devotes to political theology in *Democracy and Political Theory*.

8 Freud, *Civilization and Its Discontents*, 69.

Bibliography

Aiach, P., I. Aiach, and A. Colvez. "Motifs de consultations et diagnostics médicaux en matière de troubles mentaux: analyse de leur correspondance, approche critique sur le plan épidémiologique." *Psychologie médicale* 15, no. 4 (1983): 545–55.

Akers, R.L. "Addiction: the troublesome concept." *The Journal of Drug Issues* 21, no. 4 (1991): 777–93.

Akiskal, Hagop S. "Personnalité pathologique, tempérament et dépression." *L'Encéphale* 21, sp. 2 (March 1995): 47–9.

Albert, P.A. *Psychanalyse et pharmacologie.* Paris: Masson, 1990.

Alexander, B. and A-R-F. Schweighofer. "Defining Addiction." *Canadian Psychology,* 29 no. 2 (April 1988): 151–62.

Amar, Salomon and Claude Barazer. "La *tranquilité sur ordonnance,* ou la réponse 'BZD.'" Esprit no. 165 (Oct. 1990): 46–53.

American Psychiatric Association. "Practice Guideline for Major Depressive Disorder in Adults." *American Journal of Pyschiatry* 150, no. 4 (1993): 1–26.

American Psychiatric Association, Task Force on Nomenclature and Statistics. *DSM-III: Diagnostic and Statistical Manual of Mental Disorders.* 3rd ed. Washington: American Psychiatric Press, 1980.

American Psychiatric Association, Work Group to Revise *DSM-III. DSM-III-R: Diagnostic and Statistical Manual of Mental Disorders.* 3rd ed., rev. Washington: American Psychiatric Association, 1987.

Amiel-Lebigre, F. "Épidémiologie des dépressions." In Pichot, *Les Voies nouvelles de la dépression,* 19–30.

Anatrella, Tony. *Non à la société depressive.* Paris: Flammarion, 1993.

Andersson, Ola. *Freud Avant Freud: la préhistoire de la psychanalyse (1886–1896).* Paris: Les Empêcheurs de penser en rond, 1998.

Anzieu, Didier. "La psychanalyse au service de la psychologie." *Nouvelle revue de la psychanalyse, Regards sur la psychanalyse en France*, 20 (1979): 59–75.

Anonymous, "Why Having a Mental Illness is not like Having Diabetes" *Schizophrenia Bulletin* 33 no. 4 (2007): 846–47.

Arendt, Hannah. *Between Past and Future*. New York: Pengiun Classics, 1993.

– *The Human Condition*. Chicago: The University of Chicago Press, 1965.

– *On Revolution*. New York: Viking, 1965.

Åsberg, Marie, et al. "Serotonin depression – a biochemical subgroup within the affective disorders." *Science* 191, n° 4226 (1976): 478–80.

Astier, Isabelle. "RMI: du travail social à une politique des individus." Esprit, March-April 1998, 142–57.

Ayme, Jean. *Chroniques de la psychiatrie publique*. Ramonville Saint-Agne: Éres, 1995.

Bailly, D. "Recherche épidémiologique, troubles du comportement alimentaire et conduites de dépendence." *L'Encéphale* 19, no. 4 (1993): 285–92.

Bailly-Salin, P. "Éditorial." *Confrontations Psychiatriques* 24 (1984): 7–9.

Ballard, James Graham. *Crash!* Translated by Robert Louit. Paris: Calmann-Lévy, 1974.

Ballus, C., and C. Gasto. "Le rôle du généraliste dans l'assistance psychiatrique." In Pichot and Rein, *L'Approche Clinique en psychiatrie*, vol. 3, 71–95.

Balvet, Paul. "Ébauche pour une histoire de la thérapeutique psychiatrique contemporaine." In Lambert, *La Relation médecin-malade au cours des chimiothérapies psychiatriques*, 5–16.

Barazer, Claude and Michèle Cadoret. "Liminaire." *Psychanalystes, revue du collège des psychanalystes*, no. 39 (July 1991): 7–9.

– "Honte, vergogne, ironie." "Modernités, résonances psychiques." *Psychanalyses, traversées, anthropologie* 1–2 (1997).

Barazer, Claude and Corinne Ehrenberg. "La folie perdue de vue." *Esprit*, no. 205 (Oct.,1994): 29–39.

Barke, Megan. Rebecca Fribush and Peter N. Stearns. "Nervous Breakdown in 20th-Century America." *The Journal of Social History* 33, no. 3 (2000): 565–80.

Barrett, Robert J. *The Psychiatric Team and the Social Definition of Schizophrenia: An Anthropological Study of Person and Illness*. Cambridge: Cambridge University Press, 2006.

Baruk, Henri and Jacques Launay, eds. *Actualités de Thérapeutique Psychiatrique et de Psychopharmacologie*. Vol. 2, *Annales Moreau de Tours*. Paris: PUF, 1965.

Baszanger, I. *Inventing Pain Medicine: From the Laboratory to the Clinic.* New Brunswick, NJ: Rutgers University Press, 1998.

Baudelaire, Charles. *Artificial Paradise: On Hashish and Wine as a Means of Expanding Individuality.* Translated by Ellen Fox. New York: Herder and Herder, 1971.

Beard, George. *A Practical Treatise on Nervous Exhaustion.* New York: 1869.

Becker, Jean-Jacques, and Serge Berstein. *Victoire et Frustrations (1914–29). Vol. 12, Nouvelle histoire de la France contemporaine.* Paris: Seuil, 1990.

Bellah, Robert N., Richard Madsen, William M. Sullivan, Anne Swidler and Steven M. Tipton. *Habits of the Heart: Individualism and Commitment in American Life.* Updated edition. Berkeley, University of California Press, 1996.

Bendjilali, D. "Place de la toxicomanie dans la dépression masque: Valeur dépressive de certaines conduites pathologiques." *Actualités psychiatriques* no. 1 (1980): 89–96.

Bercherie, Paul. *Les Fondements de la Clinique: Histoire et structure du savoir psychiatrique.* Paris: Ornicar, 1980.

Bercovitch, Sacvan. *The Puritan Origins of the American Self.* New Haven: Yale University Press, 1975.

Bergeret, Jean. "La dépression dite 'névrotique' et le praticien." *Concours médical* no. 12 (1972): 2216–22.

– "Dépressivité et dépression dans le cadre de l'économie défensive," a presentation at the XXXVIe Congrès des psychanalystes de langues romanes, June 1976. *Revue française de psychanalyse* nos. 5–6, (Sept.-Dec. 1976): 809–1044.

Bergeret, Jean and Wilfred Reid, eds. *Narcissisme et états-limites.* Paris: Dunod, 1986.

Bergouigan, M. "Les dépressions symptomatiques." *La Revue du praticien* 13 (Oct. 1, 1963): 3033–43.

Bergougnioux Alain, and Bernard Manin. *La Social-Démocratie ou le Compromis.* Paris: PUF, 1979.

Berrios, German E. "Early electroconvulsive therapy in Britain, France and Germany: a conceptual history." In *The Aftermath.* Volume 2 of *150 Years of British Psychiatry,* edited by Hugh Freeman and German E. Berrios, 3–15. London: Athlone, 1996.

– "The scientific origins of electroconvulsive therapy: a conceptual history." *History of Psychiatry* 8 no. 29 (1997): 105–19.

Berstein, Serge and Odile Rudelle. *Le Modèle républicain.* Paris: PUF, 1992.

Bertagna, L. "La chimiothérapie des états dépressifs." *La Revue du praticien* 9, no. 21 (21 July 1959): 2313–14.

Bertagna, L., J.-P. Chartier, and C. Brisset. "Commentaires de 'Les Dépressions' de C. Koupernik. Stratégie de la thérapeutique prophylactique par le lithium " *Concours médical* no. 15 (1975): 2502–8.

Bertherat, Y. "Enquête sur l'exercice de la psychiatrie en France." *L'Information psychiatrique* 41, no. 3, (March 1965): 219–52.

Besançon, G. "La qualité de vie chez le malade somatique grave et chez le transplanté." *Synapse: Journal de psychiatrie et système nerveux central* no. 98 (July-Aug. 1993): 36–44.

Blanc, Claude. "Conscience et inconscient dans la pensée neurobiologique actuelle: Quelques réflexions sur les faits et les méthodes." In Ey, *L'Inconscient, 6e Colloque de Bonneval,* 1960, 181–229.

– "La psychopharmacologie: les mots, les drogues et l'esprit." *L'Évolution psychiatrique* 31, no. 4 (1966): 707–40.

Bloom, Floyd E. and David J. Kupfer, eds. *Psychopharmacology: The Fourth Generation of Progress.* Raven Press: New York, 1995.

den Boer, J.A. and J.M. Ad Sitsen, eds. *Handbook of Depression and Anxiety: A Biological Approach.* New York: Marcel Dekker Inc., 1994.

Bonnafé, Lucien, Henri Ey, Sven Follin, Jacques Lacan, and Julien Rouart, eds. *Le Problème de la psychogénèse des névroses et des psychoses.* Paris: Desclée de Brouwer, 1950.

Bonnefoy, Yves. Preface to *La Mélancholie au miroir,* by Jean Starobinski, 7–9. Paris, Julliard, 1989.

Bougerol, Thierry. "Antidépresseurs de génération récente." *La Revue du praticien* 44, no. 17, (Nov. 1, 1994): 2293–8.

Bougerol, Thierry, and Jean-Claude Scotto. "Le déprimé: rémission ou guérison?" *L'Encéphale,* 20, sp.no. 1 (April 1994): 231–6.

Bouin, Michel and C. Cerlebaud, "La dépression et les antidépresseurs en médecine générale." *Le Concours médical* 111 (July 8, 1989): 2299–302.

Boulenger, Jean-Pierre, ed. *L'Attaque de panique: un nouveau concept?* Paris: Édition Jean-Pierre Goureau, 1987.

Boulenger, Jean-Pierre and Y.-J. Lavallée. "Anxiété ou dépression: dilemme diagnostique ou thérapeutique?" *Concours médicale* 113, no. 21 (June 15, 1991): 1799–1804.

– "Attaques de panique, trouble panique et agoraphobie: Un modèle exemplaire de la plurifactorialité de la pathologie mentale." *Confrontations psychiatriques* 36 (1995): 53–77.

Boulenger, Jean-Pierre and Driss Moussaoui. "Perspectives pharmacologiques en psychiatrie biologique." *Perspectives psychiatriques* 2, no. 76 (1980): 115–25.

Bourdieu, Pierre and Jean-Claude Passeron. *Reproduction in Education, Society, and Culture.* Translated by Richard Nice. London: Sage Publications, 2000.

Bourin, Michel. "Quel avenir pour les antidépresseurs?" *La lettre du pharmacologue* 8, no. 4 (April 1994): 99–102.

Boyer, P. "États dépressifs et marqueurs biologiques." *La Revue du praticien* 35, no. 27 (May 11, 1985): 1627–32.

Brandom, Robert. "From a Critique of Cognitive Internalism to a Conception of Objective Spirit: Reflections on Descombes' Anthropological Holism." *Inquiry* 47, no. 3 (2004): 236–53.

Breton, André. *Nadja.* 1928. Translated by Richard Howard. New York: Grove Press: 1960.

Breuer, Joseph and Sigmund Freud. *Studies on Hysteria.* Translated by A.A. Brill. Boston: Beacon Press, 2007.

Brisset, Charles. "La psychopharmacologie: Étude de nos moyens de connaissance des médicaments en psychiatrie." *L'Évolution psychiatrique* 31, no. 4 (1966): 639–60.

Brown, Serena-Lynn, and Herman M. van Praag, eds. *The Role of Serotonin in Psychiatric Disorders.* New York: Brunner/Mazel, 1991.

Brunetti, P.M. "Prévalence des troubles mentaux dans une population rurale du Vaucluse: données nouvelles et récapitulatives." *L'Hygiène Mentale,* suppl. to *L'Encéphale,* no. 61 (1973): 1–15.

Bugard. P., ed. *Stress, fatigue et dépression: L'homme et les agressions de la vie quotidienne.* 2 vols. Paris: Doin, 1974.

Burner, M. "Thérapeutique des états de fatigue." *Psychologie médicale,* 18, no. 8 (1986): 1205–10.

Caldwell, Anne E. *Origins of psychopharmacology: From CPZ to LSD.* Springfield: Charles C. Thomas, 1970.

Canguilhem, Georges. *Études d'histoire et de philosophie des sciences,* 7th edition. Paris: Vrin, 1994.

– *La formation du concept de réflexe au XVIIe et XVIIIe siècles.* (1955) Paris: Vrin, 1977.

– "Une pédagogie de la guérison est-elle possible?" *Nouvelle revue de psychanalyse* no. 17 (Spring 1978): 13–26.

Cardot, H. and Frédéric Rouillon. "Évolution à long terme des dépressions (épidémiologique et clinique)." *L'Encéphale* 21, sp.no. 2 (March 1995): 51–9.

Carlsson, Arvid. "Monoamines of the Central Nervous System: A Historical Perspective." In Meltzer, *Psychopharmacology: The Third Generation of Progress,* 39–48.

Carpentier J., R. Castel, J. Donzelot, J.-M. Lacrosse, A. Lovell, and G. Procacci, eds. *Résistance à la médecine et démultiplication du concept de santé.* Collège de France/CORDES, Nov. 1980.

Carroy, Jacqueline. *Les Personnalités doubles et multiples: entre science et fiction.* Paris: PUF, 1993.

"Les cas difficiles." *Revue française de psychanalyse* 54, no. 2 (1990): 307–608.

Cassano, Giovanni B., C. Maggini and E. Longo. "Les dépressions chroniques." *L'Encéphale* 5 (1979): 449–58.

Castel, Robert. *La Gestion de risques.* Paris: Éditions de Minuit, 1981.

Castel, Françoise, Robert Castel, and Anne Lovell. The psychiatric society. Translated by Arthur Goldhammer. New York: Columbia University Press, 1982.

Castoriadis, Cornelius. *The Imaginary Institution of Society.* Translated by Kathleen Blamey. Cambridge, MA: MIT Press, 1998.

Cavell, Stanley. The Claim of Reason: Wittgenstein, Skepticism, Morality and Tragedy. New York: Oxford University Press, 1999.

Clarke, Edwin, and L.S. Jacyna. *Nineteenth Century Origins of Neuroscientific Concepts.* Berkley: University of California Press, 1987.

Champoux, S. "Antidépresseur: un terme trompeur," *Quotidien du médecin.* June 12, 1989: 28.

Chauchard, Paul. *La Fatigue.* 4th ed. Collection Que sais-je?. Paris: PUF, 1968.

Chignon, Jean-Michel. "Le syndrome anxiodépressif: une réalité clinique fréquente." *La Revue du praticien* 5, no. 139 (May 27, 1991): 1274–6.

Chignon, Jean-Michel, and M. Abbar. "Traitement du déprimé: moyens et étapes." *L'Encéphale* 20, sp.no. 1 (Jan. 1994): 195–202.

Coblence, Francoise. *Le dandysme, obligation d'incertitude.* Paris: Presses Universitaires de France, 1988.

Cohen, Daniel. *Richesses du monde, pauvreté des nations.* Paris: Flammarion, 1997.

Cohen, M. "Revitalisation, décomposition ou redéfinition du catholicisme: Le Renouveau charismatique français et salut religieux et psychothérapie." *Recherches sociologiques* 29, no. 22 (1997): 19–36.

Coignard, S. "Les prodiges de l'effet placebo." *Le Point* no. 1241 (June 29, 1996): 78–86.

Coirault, R. "Introduction au problème des états dépressifs." In Baruk and Launay, *Actualités de Thérapeutique Psychiatrique et de Psychopharmacologie,* 69–70.

Cole, Jonathan O. "The Future of Psychopharmacology." In Fieve, *Depression in the 1970's,* 81–6.

Colonna, Lucien. "Les inhibitions anxieuses." *L'Encéphale* 4, no. 5, supplement (1978): 439–42.

Colonna, Lucien, Henri Lôo, and Édouard Zarifian. "Chimiothérapie des dépressions." *La Revue du praticien* 22, no. 32 (Dec. 11, 1972): 4437–53.

Colonna, Lucien, and Michel Petit. "Sémiologie dépressive et orientation de la prescription." *L'Encéphale* 5, no. 5 (1979): 641–50.

Colonna, Lucien, Michel Petit, J.P. Lepine, and F. Boismare. "États dépressifs: symptômes cliniques et hypothèses monoaminergiques." *L'Encéphale* 4, no. 1 (1978): 5–17.

Colvez, A., E. Michel, and N. Quemada. "Les maladies mentales et psychosociales dans la pratique libérale: Approche épidémiologique." *Psychiatrie française* 10 no. 1 (1979): 13–24.

Comité de Rédaction. "Editorial." *Revue internationale de psychopathologie* no. 21, (1996): 3–5.

Coppen, A., V.A. Rama Rao, C. Swade and K. Wood. "Zimelidine: A Therapeutic and Pharmokinetic Study in Depression." *Psychopharmacology* 63 (1979): 199–202.

Corbin, Alain. "Backstage." In *A History of Private Life: From the Fires of Revolution to the Great War.* Edited by Michelle Perrot. Volume 4 of *A History of Private Life.* Edited by Phillippe Ariès and George Duby. Translated by Arthur Goldhammer, 451–668. Cambridge: Harvard University Press, 1990.

Courvoisier, Simone. "Sur les propriétés pharmaco-dynamiques de la chlorpromazine en rapport avec son emploi en psychiatrie." Paper presented at *Premier Colloque international sur la chlorpromazine et les médicaments neuroleptiques en thérapeutique psychiatrique. L'Encéphale* 45, no. 4 (1956): 1248–57.

Crabtree, Adam. *From Mesmer to Freud: Magnetic Sleep and the Roots of Psychological Healing.* New Haven and London: Yale University Press, 1993.

Cremniter, D. "Aspects épidémiologiques de la dépression vue en médecine: Généralistes et psychiatres ne voient pas les mêmes dépressions." *La Revue du praticien* 10, no. 325 (Jan. 22, 1996): 24–7.

Cremniter, D., J. Delcros, Julien-Daniel Guelfi, and J. Fermanian. "Une enquête sur les états dépressifs en médecine générale." *L'Encéphale* 8, no. 4 (1982): 523–37.

Crocq, L. "Les recherches sur la fatigue en France dans les vingt dernières années." *L'Encéphale* 20, no. 3, special issue(1994): 615–18.

Cross-National Collaborative Group. "The Changing Rate of Major Depression: Cross-National Comparisons." *JAMA* 268, no. 21 (Dec. 2, 1992): 3098–105.

Crozier, Michel. *Le phénomène bureaucratique*. Paris: Seuil, 1963.

Cuche, Henri and A. Gérard. "Antidépresseurs: bénéfices/risques." *L'Encéphale* 20, no. sp.1 (April 1994): 203–7.

Cussey, J., B. Bonin, S. Vandel, D. Sechter, and P. Bizouard. "Sérotonine et dépression: aspects méthodologiques." *Psychologie médicale* 21 no. 1 (1993): 73–8.

Dalery, J. and Henri Lôo. "Editorial." *L'Encéphale* 20 (April 1994): 179.

Dalery J. and D. Sechter. "Traitement prolongé d'antidépresseurs." *L'Encéphale* 20 (April 1994): 209–14.

Darcourt, G. "Place du ralentissement parmi les autres symptômes dépressifs." *Psychologie médicale* 13B (1981): 61–6.

Daumézon, Georges. "Lecture historique de *L'Histoire de la folie*." *L'Évolution psychiatrique* 36, no. 2 (1971): 227–42.

– "Modification de la symptomatologie des troubles mentaux et de la sémiologie psychiatrique au cours des cinquante dernières années." *Journal de psychologie* 74, no. 4 (1977): 389–407.

– "Nosographie et thérapeutiques de choc." *L'Évolution psychiatrique*, 15 no. 1 (1950): 247–52.

Davis, R., and M.I. Wilde. "Sertraline: A Pharmacoeconomic Evaluation of its Use in Depression." *Pharmacoeconomics* 10, no. 4 (1996): 409–31.

Debray, Quentin. Interview with Hagop Akiksal, conducted by Quentin Debray. *Synapse: Journal de psychiatrie et système nerveux central*, no. 125 (April, 1996): 13–20.

Decombe, R., D. Bentué-Ferrer, and H. Allain, "Le point sur la neuro-transmission dans les dépressions." *Neuro-psy* 6, no. 11 (Dec. 1991): 289–91.

– *Medicine and the Mind: (la Médecine de L'Esprit)*. Translated by Stacy B. Collins. London: Downey & Co, 1900.

Deglon, J-J. "Dépression et héroïnomanie." *Psychologie médicale* 16 no. 5 (1984): 793–6.

Deitch, Jeffrey. *Post-Human*. Pully/Lausanne: Musée d'Art contemporain de Lausanne, 1992–3.

Delay, Jean. "Adresse présidentielle." In *Neuro-Pharmacology: Proceedings of the Fifth International Congress of the Collegium Internationale Neuro-Pharmacologie*, edited by H. Brill, xv-xxiv. Amsterdam: Exerpta Medica Foundation, 1967.

– "Allocution finale." Speech given at the *Premier Colloque international sur la chlorpromazine et les médicaments neuroleptiques en thérapeutique psychiatrique. L'Encéphale*. 45, no. 5 (1956): 1181–4.

– *Aspects de la psychiatrie moderne*. Paris: PUF, 1956.

– *Les Dérèglements de l'humeur*. Paris: PUF, 1961.

– *Études de psychologie médicale*. Paris: PUF, 1953.

– "Introduction au colloque international." *Premier Colloque international sur la chlorpromazine et les médicaments neuroleptiques en thérapeutique psychiatrique. L'Encéphale*, no. 4 (1956): 303–6.

Delay, Jean and Pierre Deniker. *Méthodes chimiothérapiques en psychiatrie: les nouveaux médicaments psychotropes*. Paris: Masson, 1961.

Delay, Jean and Pierre Pichot. *Abrégé de psychologie à l'usage de l'étudiant*. Paris: Masson, 1962.

Delmas-Marsalet, Paul. *Électrochoques et thérapeutiques nouvelles en neuropsychiatrie*. Paris: Baillère, 1946.

– *Précis de Bio-Psychologie*. Paris: Maloine, 1961.

Delphaut, J. *Pharmacologie et psychologie*. Paris: Armand Colin, 1961.

Demazeux, Steeves. "Cachez cette tristesse que l'on ne saurait voir." http://www.nonfiction.fr/article-950-cachez_cette_tristesse_que_lon_ne_saurait_voir.htm. Accessed April 3, 2009.

– "Pour une critique constructive de la psychiatrie américaine: Entretien avec Jerome Wakefield." *PSN* 7, no. 1 (Feb. 2009): 15–22.

Demel, H. "Observations on the clinical nature of masked depression from the standpoint of practical social psychiatry." In Kielholz, *Masked Depression*, 247–52.

Demers, Christopher. *Souffrance en France – La banalisation de l'injustice sociale*. Paris: Le Seuil, 1998.

Deniker, Pierre. "Dépressions résistantes." *L'Encéphale* 12, special no. (Oct, 1986): 187–8.

– *La Psychopharmacologie*. Collection Que sais-je?. Paris: PUF, 1966.

– "Traitements des états dépressifs." *La Revue du praticien* 12, special issue, "Syndromes dépressifs" (Oct. 1, 1963): 3063–9.

– "Qui a inventé les neuroleptiques?" *Confrontations psychiatriques* no. 13 (1975): 7–19.

Deniker, Pierre, and Édouard Zarifian "Perspectives d'utilisation de la L. Dopa en psychiatrie." In *Entretiens de Bichat Psychiatrie*, 224–8. Paris: Expansion scientifique française, 1983.

Depoutot, J.C. "Névrose et dépression." *Annales médicales de Nancy* 12 (April 1973): 869–72.

De Quincey, Thomas. *Confessions of an English Opium Eater*. New York: Penguin Classics, 2003.

Descombes, Vincent. *Les Institutions du sens*. Paris: Éditions de Minuit, 1996.

– "L'inconscient adverbial." *Critique* 40, no. 449 (October 1984): 775–96.

– *The Mind's Provisions: A Critique of Cognitism.* Translated by Stephen Adam Schwartz. Princeton: Princeton University Press, 2001.

Descombey, J.P. "Subjectivité, scientificité, objectivité, objectivation: le DSM-III et ses retombées sur la pratique et la recherche." *L'Information psychiatrique* 61, no. 5 (1985): 681–9.

Donnet, Jean-Luc. "Une évolution de la demande au Centre Jean Favreau." *Revue française de psychanalyse*, coll. "Débats de psychanalyse" (Nov. 1997).

Donzelot, Jacques. *L'Invention du social.* Paris: Fayard, 1984.

Dowbiggin, Ian. "Back to the Future: Valentin Magnan, French Psychiatry, and the classification of mental diseases, 1885–1925." *Social History of Medicine* 9 no. 2 (1996): 383–408.

– *La Folie Héréditaire.* Paris: EPEL, 1993.

Dowling, Colette. *You Mean I Don't Have to Feel This Way?: New Help for Depression, Anxiety, Depression.* New York: Bantam Books, 1993.

Dagognet, François. *La Raison et les remèdes: essais sur l'imaginaire et le réel dans la thérapeutique contemporaine.* Paris: PUF, 1964.

Dubet, François. *Les Lycéens.* Paris: Le Seuil, 1991.

Dubief, Henri and Philippe Bernard. *The Decline of the Third Republic, 1914–1938.* Translated by Anthony Forster. Cambridge: Cambridge University Press, 1988.

Dufour, H. "Les inhibitions dépressives." *L'Encéphale* 4, no. 5, suppl., (1978): 431–7.

Dujarier, L. "Considérations psychanalytiques sur la dépression." *Psychiatres*, no. 36 (1979).

– "Etats-limites et dépression: critique des conceptions de J. Bergeret sur "une lignée dépressive limite." *Revue Française de Psychanalyse* 40, n° 5–6 (1976): 1092–6.

Dumont, Louis. *Essays on individualism: modern ideology in anthropological perspective.* Chicago: University of Chicago Press, 1986.

Durkheim, Émile. *On Suicide.* Translated by Robin Buss. London: Penguin, 2006.

Edwards, Griffith, ed. *Addictions: Personal Influences and Scientific Movements.* New Brunswick-London: Transaction Publishers, 1991.

Ehrenberg, Alain. *Le culte de la performance.* Paris: Calmann-Lévy, 1991.

– *La grande névrose.* Paris: Odile Jacob, forthcoming.

– "Le harcèlement sexuel, naissance d'un délit." *Esprit* no. 196 (Nov. 1993): 73–98.

– *L'Individu incertain.* Paris: Calmann-Lévy, 1995.

– "Le sujet cérébral." *Esprit* no. 309 (November 2004): 130–55.

Eisenberg, L., "La dépression nerveuse," *La Recherche*, no. 119, Feb., 1981, 160–72.

Elias, Marylin. "Net overuse called 'true addiction.'" *USA Today*, July 1, 1996, High Tech Section.

Endler, Norman S. and Emanuel Persad. *Electroconvulsive Therapy: The Myths and the Realities*. Vienne-Stuttgart-Berne: Hans Huber, 1986.

Essman, W.B., ed. *Serotonin in Health and Disease*. New York: Spectrum, 1997.

Evans, Martha Noel. *Fits and Starts: A Genealogy of Hysteria in Modern France*. Ithaca and London: Cornell University Press, 1991.

Ey, Henri. "A. Hesnard – Biologiste, psychiatre, psychanalyste." *L'Évolution psychiatrique* 36, no. 2 (1971): 303–7.

– "Commentaires critiques sur *L'Histoire de la folie* de Michel Foucault." *L'Évolution psychiatrique* 36, no. 2 (1971): 243–58.

– "Contribution à l'étude des relations des crises de mélancolie et des crises de dépression névrotique." *L'Évolution psychiatrique* 20 no. 3 (1955): 532–53.

– *L'Inconscient, 6e Colloque de Bonneval, 1960*. Paris: Desclée de Brouwer, 1966.

– *Études psychiatriques: Historique, méthodologie, psychopathologie générale*. Paris: Desclée de Brouwer, 1948.

– "Les limites de la psychiatrie et le problème de la psychogénèse." Introduction to Bonnafé, et al., *Le Problème de la psychogénèse des névroses et des psychoses*, 9–20.

– "Neuroleptiques et services de *psychiatrie* hospitaliers." *Confrontations Psychiatriques*, no. 13 (1975): 19–59.

– "Perspectives actuelles de la psychiatrie." *La Revue du praticien*, 15, spécial issue entitled *L'Année du praticien* (Dec. 7, 1965): 71–4.

– *Schizophrénie – Études cliniques et psychopathologiques*. Le Plessis-Robinson: Les Empêcheurs de penser en rond, 1996.

– "Système nerveux et troubles nerveux." *L'Évolution psychiatrique* 12, no. 1 (1947): 71–104.

Ey, Henri, Paul Bernard and Charles Brisset. *Manuel de Psychiatrie*. 6th ed. Paris: Masson, 1989.

Ey, Henri, P. Marty, and J. Dublineau. *Psychopathologie générale*. Volume I of *Premier Congrès mondiale de la psychiatrie*. Paris:Hermann, 1952.

– *Thérapeutiques biologiques*, Volume IV of *Premier Congrès mondiale de la psychiatrie*. Paris: Hermann, 1952.

Fatela, J. "Crise de l'école et fragilités adolescentes." In *Drogues, Politique et Société*, edited by Alain Ehrenberg and Patrick Mignon, 87–98. Paris: Le Monde Éd. and Éd. Descartes, 1992.

Fédida, P. "L'Agir dépressif: Contribution phénoménologique à une théorie psychanalytique de la dépression." *Psychiatres*, no. 28 (1976): 41–8.

Feighner, J.P., E. Robins, S.B. Guze, R.A. Woodruff, G. Winokur and R. Munoz. "Diagnostic criteria for use in psychiatric research." *Archives of General Psychiatry* 26 (1972): 57–63.

Fieve Ronald R., ed. *Depression in the 1970's: Modern Theory and Research*. Amsterdam: Exerpta Medica, 1971.

Fieve, Ronald R. "La recherche pour de nouveaux antidépresseurs: orientations actuelles." *L'Encéphale* 5, no. 5 (1979): 671–88.

"Figures du vide." *Nouvelle Revue de psychanalyse* 11 (1975).

Fischer, Seymour and Roger P. Greenberg. "Examining Antidepressant and Effectiveness: Findings, Ambiguities, and Some Vexing Puzzles." In Fischer and Greenberg, eds., *The Limits of Biological Treatments for Psychological Distress*, 1–38.

– eds. *The Limits of Biological Treatments for Psychological Distress: Comparisons with Psychotherapy and Placebo*. Hillsdale, NJ: LEA, 1989.

– "A Second Opinion: Rethinking the Claims of Biological Psychiatry" In Fischer and Greenberg, eds., *The Limits of Biological Treatments for Psychological Distress*, 309–36. Hillsdale, NJ: LEA, 1989.

Fischer-Homberg, Esther. *Die traumatische Neurose: Vom somatischen zum sozialen Leiden*. Berne: Huber, 1975.

de Fleury, Maurice. *Les États dépressifs de la neurasthénie*. Paris: Félix Alcan, 1924.

Flournoy, O. "Le Moi-idéal: vecteur de vide." "Figures du Vide," special issue, *Nouvelle Revue de psychanalyse* no. 11 (1975): 45–62.

Follin, Sven. "Sémiologie des états dépressifs." *La Revue du praticien* 13 (Oct. 1, 1963): 2987–98.

Fombonne, Éric. "La contribution de l'épidémiologie à la rercherche étiologique en psychiatrie: des facteurs de risque aux mécanismes de risqué." Revue d'épidémiologie et de santé publique 41, no. 4 (1993): 263–73.

Fombonne, Éric and Rebecca Führer. "Épidémiologie et psychiatrie: questions et méthodes." *Sciences sociales et santé* 4, no. 1 (1986): 97–117.

Fondation Saint-Simon. *Pour une nouvelle république sociale*. Paris: Calmann-Lévy, 1997.

Fougère, P. *Les médicaments du bien-être*. Collection On en parle. Paris: Hachette, 1970.

Fouks, L. "Bilan actuel de la thérapeutique chimique en psychiatrie et perspectives d'avenir." In Volume 3 of *Annales de thérapeutique psychiatrique*, edited by Henri Baruk and Jacques Launay, 3–7. Paris: PUF, 1967.

Fouks, L., T. Lainé, E. Périvier. "Les inhibiteurs de la monoamine oxydase." Paper presented at symposium on depressive states, June 1962. In Baruk and Launay *Actualités de Thérapeutique Psychiatrique et de Psychopharmacologie*, 148–52.

Foucault, Michel. *The Birth of the Clinic: An Archaeology of Medical Perception*. 3rd ed. Translated by A.M. Sheridan Smith. London: Routledge, 2003.

– *Discipline and Punish: the Birth of the Prison*. Translated by Alan Sheridan. New York: Vintage Books, 1995.

Fourquet, François and Lion Murard, eds. "Histoire de la psychiatrie de secteur ou le secteur impossible?" Special issue, *Recherches* no. 17 (1975).

France. Délégation interministérielle à la ville et au développement social urbain and Délégation interministérielle au revenu minimum d'insertion. *Une souffrance qu'on ne peut plus cacher*, by the work group Ville, santé mentale, précarité et exclusion sociale, Antoine Lazarus (president). February, 1995.

Frances, Allen. Interview in *Psychiatrie internationale*, no. 6 (1993): 8.

– Introduction to *DSM-IV: Diagnostic and Statistical Manual of Mental Disorders*. 4th ed. Prepared by the Task Force on DSM-IV and other committees and work groups of the American Psychiatric Association, xv–xxv. Washington: American Psychiatric Press, 1994.

Fraser, A. et al. "Intéractions de la sérotonine et de la noradrénaline dans la dépression." Paper presented at the 10th colloquium of the Collegium Internationale Neuro-Psychopharmacologicum, Melbourne, June, 1996.

Freedman, Alfred M. "American Viewpoints on Classification." *Integrative Psychiatry* 7 (1991): 11–15.

Freud, Sigmund. *The Complete Psychological Works of Sigmund Freud*. 24 vols. Translated by James Strachey. London: The Hogarth Press, 1966–74.

– *Civilization and its Discontents*. Revised Edition. Translated by David McLintock. London: Penguin UK, 2005.

– "'Civilized' Sexual Morality and Modern Nervousness." 1908. In *Sexuality and the Psychology of Love*, 10–30. New York: Touchstone, 1997.

– *Inhibitions, Symptoms and Anxiety*. Translated by A. Strachey. New York: W.W. Norton & Company, 1959.

– *Métapsychologie*. Paris: Gallimard, 1968.

– "Mourning and Melancholia." In *The Freud Reader*, edited by Peter Gay, 584–8. New York: W.W. Norton & Company, 1995.

– *The Origins of Psycho-Analysis.* Garden City, NY: Doubleday Anchor Books, 1957.

– *An Outline of Psycho-Analysis.* Translated by James Strachey. New York: W.W. Norton & Company, 1989.

Fumaroli, Marc. "'Nous serons guéri si nous le voulons': Classicisme français et maladie de l'âme." *Le Débat,* no. 29 (1984): 92–114.

Gauchet, Marcel. *L'Inconscient cérébral.* Paris: Le Seuil, 1992.

Garabé, Jean. *Histoire de la schizophrénie.* Paris: Seghers, 1992.

Garapon, Antoine. *Le gardien des promesses – justice et démocratie.* Paris: Odile Jacob, 1996.

Garoux, R. and Y. Ranty. "L'asthénie en psychiatrie et en pathologie-psychosomatique." *Psychologie médicale* 10, no. 12 (1978): 2533–40.

Gay, Peter. *Freud: A Life for Our Time.* New York: W.W. Norton and Company, 1998.

– *Reading Freud: Explorations and Entertainments.* New Haven: Yale University Press, 1990.

Gazette médicale in association with the office of Antoine Minkowski. "Les états anxiodépressifs: deux personnes sur dix sont concernées," *Gazette médicale* no. 24 (1991): 39–43.

Gérard, P.E., V. Dagens, and A. Deslandes. "1960–2000: 40 ans d'utilisation d'antidépresseurs." *Semaine des hôpitaux de Paris* 71, nos. 23–24 (1995): 727–34.

Ginestet, D., F. Chauchot, and D. Olive. "Existe-t-il des classifications pratiques de psychotropes?" *La Gazette médicale* 99, no. 21 (1992): 35–40.

Giraud, M.J., E. Lemonnier, and T. Bigot. "Pharmacodépendence et psychotropes." *La Revue du praticien* 44, no. 17 (Nov. 1, 1994): 2325–31.

Glaser, Hermann. *Sigmund Freud et l'âme du XXᵉ siècle.* Paris: PUF, 1995.

Glasser, J. *Aux origines du cerveau moderne: Localisations, langage et mémoire dans l'œuvre de Charcot.* Paris: Fayard, 1995.

Glowinski, J., L. Julou, and B. Scatton. "Effets des neuroleptiques sur les systèmes aminergiques centraux." *Confrontations psychiatriques* no. 13 (1975): 61–104.

Godard, A. and M.H. Regnauld, "Consommation des psychotropes." *Revue française de santé publique.* 33 (1986): 5–12.

Gold, Mark S. *The Good News About Depression: Cures and Treatments in the New Age of Psychiatry.* New York: Bantam Books, 1995.

Goldstein, Jan. *Console and Classify: The French Psychiatric Profession in the Nineteenth Century.* Cambridge: University Press, 1987.

Gosling, F.G. *Before Freud: Neurasthenia and the American Medical Community,* 1870–1910. Urbana and Chicago: University of Illinois Press, 1987.

Gourévitch, Michel. "La dépression, fille de l'art romantique." *Psychologie médicale* 16, no. 4, (1984): 705–6.

– "Esquirol et lypémanie. Naissance de la dépression mélancolique." In Pichot, *Les voies nouvelles de la dépression,* 12–18.

Gram, L.F. "Concepts d'antidépresseurs de seconde génération." *L'Encéphale* 17, no. 1, special issue (May-June, 1991): 115–16.

– "Les psychalgies." *Concours médical* 101 no. 45 (1979): 7359–71.

Green, André. "L'affect." *Revue française de psychanalyse* 34 nos. 5–6 (1971): 1171–215.

– "Chimiothérapiques et psychothérapies (Problèmes posés par les comparaisons des techniques chimiothérapeutiques et leur association en technique psychiatrique)." *L'Encéphale* 50, no. 1 (1961): 29–101.

– "Les portes de l'inconscient." In Ey, *L'Inconscient, 6e Colloque de Bonneval,* 1960, 17–44.

– "La psychopharmacologie: ouvertures, impasses, perspectives." *L'Évolution psychiatrique* 31, no. 4 (1966): 681–705.

Grob, Gerald N. *Mental Illness and American Society,* 1875–1940. Princeton: Princeton University Press, 1983.

Grünenberg, Serge. *David* Cronenberg. Paris: Cahiers du cinéma, 1992.

Guardian, The. "The creation of the Prozac myth." February 28, 2007. http://www.guardian.co.uk/society/2008/feb/27/mentalhealth. health1 (accessed April 3, 2009).

Guelfi, Julien-Daniel. "Implications pratiques des données modernes de la psychopharmacologie" *L'Évolution psychiatrique* 45 no. 4 (1980): 805–24.

Guelfi, Julien-Daniel, E. Corruble and C. Dure. "Antidépresseurs et classifications diagnostiques chez l'adulte." *Actualités médicales internationales Psychiatrie,* no. 193, suppl. (Oct. 1996): 8–10.

Guelfi, Julien-Daniel, and R. Olivier-Martin. "Modalités d'appréciations de l'anxiété: Conséquences thérapeutiques." *La Revue du praticien* 22, no. 12 (1972): 1925–38.

le Guillant, Louis, M. Bailly-Salin, P. Bequart, A. Corre, J. Kestenberg, M. Plichet and R. Roelins. "Quelques remarques méthodologiques sur l'action des neuroleptiques." *L'Encéphale,* 45, no. 4 (1956): 1128–35.

Guiraud, Paul. *Psychiatrie générale.* Paris: La François Éditeur, 1950.

Guyotat, J. "Inhibitions et antidépresseurs." *L'Encéphale* 4, no. 5, supplement (1978): 533–9.

– "Perspectives actuelles de la psychiatrie." *La Revue du praticien* 18 no. 31, *bis* (Dec. 7, 1968): 111–18.

– "Remarques sur les relations entre chimiothérapie et psychothérapie."
  In *Actualités de thérapeutique psychiatrique,* by the Comité lyonnais de
  recherches thérapeutiques en psychiatrie, 79–101. Paris: Masson,
  1963.

Guze, B.H. "Selective Serotonin Reuptake Inhibitors: Assessment for
  Formulary Inclusion." *Pharmacoeconomics* 9, no. 5 (May 1996): 430–2.

Hacking, Ian. *Rewriting the Soul: Multiple Personality and the Sciences of
  Memory.* Princeton: Princeton University Press, 1995.

Hakim, G. "Aspects modernes de la dépression." Paper presented at
  Entretiens de Bichat: Psychiatrie, Paris, France, October 3, 1973.

Hamilton, M. "Méthodologie d'appréciation de l'efficacité des antidépresseurs." *L'Encéphale* 5, (1979): 651–4.

– "Le pronostic dans les dépressions." *La Revue de médecine* no. 3–4
  (1980): 139–44.

Hardy, P. "L'anxiété dans ses rapports avec la dépression." *Confrontations
  psychiatriques,* special issue, (1989): 48–72.

– "Notion de dépression résistante." *L'Encéphale* 12, sp.no. Reports from
  the international colloquium, "Les dépressions résistantes aux traitements antidépresseurs" (Paris, Jan. 17, 1986). (Oct. 1986): 191–6.

– "Le traitement de consolidation: La situation des dysthymies."
  L'Encéphale 21, sp.no. 2 (March 1995): 39–42.

Haxaire, Claudie, Brabant-Hamonic, and J., E. Cambon. "'C'était pas
  comme une drogue, si vous voulez, mais enfin': Appropriation de
  la notion de dépendence et opportunité des psychotropes à travers
  l'étude de pharmacies familiales dans une région rurale de Basse-
  Normandie", *Drogues et médicaments psychotropes: Le trouble des frontières,*
  edited by Alain Ehrenberg, 171–208. Paris: Éditions Esprit, 1998.

Haynal, André. *Depression and Creativity.* New York: International Universities Press, 1985.

– Introduction to "Le sens du désespoir: la problématique de la dépression dans la théorie psychanalytique," by André Haynal. *Revue française
  de psychanalyse,* nos. 1–2 (Jan.-April 1977): 5–16.

– "Problèmes cliniques de la dépression." *Psychologie médicale* 16, no. 4
  (1984): 607–16.

– "Le sens du désespoir: la problématique de la dépression dans la
  théorie psychanalytique." Paper presented at the XXXVIe Congrès
  des psychanalystes de langues romance, June 1976. *Revue française
  de psychanalyse,* nos. 1–2, (Jan.-April 1977): 17–186.

Healy, David. *The Antidepressant Era.* Cambridge, Mass.: Harvard University Press, 1997.

– "The History of British Psychopharmacology." In *The Aftermath.* Volume 2 of 150 *Years of British Psychiatry,* edited by Hugh Freeman and German E. Berrios, 61–88. London: Athlone, 1996.

– *The Psychopharmacologists: Inverviews.* 3 vols. London: Arnold, 1998–.

Heninger, G.R. "Indoleamines: The role of serotonin in clinical disorders." In Bloom and Kupfer, eds., *Psychopharmacology: The Fourth Generation of Progress,* 471–82.

Henne, M. "Besoins nationaux et nombre de médecins psychiatriques nécessaires à l'exercice de la psychiatrie en secteur privé et en secteur publique." *La Revue du praticien* 32, no. 4 (1967): 783–9.

Héritier, Françoise. *Two Sisters and Their Mother: The Anthropology of Incest.* Translated by Jeanine Hermann. New York: Zone Books, 1999.

Herzlich, Claudine. *Illness in Self and Society.* Translated by Elborg Forster. Baltimore: Johns Hopkins University Press, 1987.

Hesnard, Angélo. *Freud dans la société d'après guerre.* Geneva: Éd. Du Mont-Blanc, 1946.

Hoffman, Stanley. *In Search of France: The Economy, Society, and Political System in the Twentieth Century.* Cambridge: Harvard University Press, 1963.

Hole, G. "La dépression masquée et sa mise en évidence." *Les Cahiers de médecine* no. 7, (1973).

Hollister, Leo E. "Strategies for Research in Clinical Psychopharmacology." In Meltzer, *Psychopharmacology: The Third Generation of Progress,* 31–8.

Horwitz, Alan V. and Wakefield, Jerome. *The Loss of Sadness: How Psychiatry Transformed Normal Sorrow into Depressive Disorder* (2007)

Huguet, M. *L'Ennui et ses discours.* Paris: PUF, 1984.

"Les inhibiteurs de la recapture de la sérotonine." *The Lancet,* Fr. Ed, no. 15 (1990): 27–8.

Israël, Lucien. *Boiter n'est pas pécher.* Paris: Denoël, 1989.

– *L'Hystérique, le sexe et le médecin.* Paris: Masson, 1976.

Jackson, Stanley W. *Melancholia and Depression: From Hippocratic Times to Modern Times.* New Haven and London: Yale University Press, 1986.

Jacobs B.L., and C.-A. Fornal. "Serotonin and Behavior: A General Hypothesis." In Bloom and Kupfer, eds., *Psychopharmacology: The Fourth Generation of Progress,* 461–70.

Jaeger, Marcel. *Le désordre psychiatrique.* Paris: Payot, 1988.

Janet, Pierre. *De l'angoisse à l'extase.* Vol. 2, *Les sentiments fondamentaux.* Paris: Odile Jacob, 1999.

– *La Force et la faiblesse psychologiques.* Paris: Maloine, 1932.

– *Les Névroses.* Paris: Flammarion, 1909.

– *Psychological Healing: A Historical and Clinical Study*. 2 vols. New York: Arno Press, 1976.

Janov, A. *The Primal Scream: Primal Therapy, The Cure For Neurosis*. New York: Dell, 1970.

Jeannerod, Marc. *De la physiologie mentale: histoire des relations entre biologie et psychologie*, Paris: Odile Jacob, 1996.

Joly, Pierre. *Prévention et soins des maladies mentales – Bilan et perspectives*. Journal Officiel de la République Française no. 14 (July 18, 1997): 1–130.

Jönsson, Bengt and J. Rosenbaum, eds. *Health Economics of Depression*. Perspectives in Psychiatry 4. Chichester: John Wiley and Sons Ltd., 1993

Jouvent R., and J. Pellet. "Les dépressions résistantes et leurs traitements." *La Revue du praticien* 35, no. 27 (May 11, 1985): 1647–53.

Kammerer, T. "Les limites de la psychiatrie." *Actualités psychiatriques*. No. 4 (1977): 14–20.

Kammerer, T., R. Ebtinger and J.P. Bauer. "Approche phénoménologique et psychodynamique des psychoses délirantes aiguës traitées par neuroleptiques majeurs." In Lambert, *La relation médecin-malade au cours des chimiothérapies psychiatriques*, 17–40.

Kammerer, T., Lucien Israël, and C. Noel. "Une dépression guérie par l'imipramine: Étude critique." *Cahiers de psychiatrie* no. 14 (1960): 61–75.

Karp, David A. "Taking Anti-Depressant Medications: Resistance, Trial Commitment, Conversion, Disenchantment." *Qualitative Sociology* 16, no. 4 (1993): 337–59.

– *Speaking of Sadness: Depression, Disconnection, and the Meanings of Illness*. Oxford: Oxford University Press, 1996

Kendall, R.E. "The Classification of Depressions: A Review of Contemporary Confusion," *British Journal of Psychiatry*, 129, (1976): 15–28.

Kernberg, Otto F. *Borderline Conditions and Pathological Narcissism*. New York: Jason Aronson, 1975.

– "Borderline Personality Orgaization," *Journal of American Pyschoanalysis Association*, # 15, 1967.

Kielholz, Paul. "État actuel du traitement pharmacologique des dépressions." *L'Encéphale* 5 (1962): 397–408.

– ed. *Masked Depression*. Bern: Hans Huber, 1973.

– "Opening Address: Psychosomatic aspects of depressive illness – masked depression and somatic equivalents." In Kielholz, *Masked Depression*, 11–3.

Kirk, Stuart A. and Herb Kutchins. *The Selling of* DSM: *The Rhetoric of Science in Psychiatry.* New York: Aldine de Gruyter, 1992.

Kirsch I., B.J. Deacon, T.B. Huedo-Medina, A. Scoboria, T.J. Moore, et al. (2008) "Initial Severity and Antidepressant Benefits: A Meta-Analysis of Data Submitted to the Food and Drug Administration." PLoS Med 5, no. 2 (2008): e45. doi:10.1371/journal.pmed.0050045 http://www.plosmedicine.org/article/info:doi/10.1371/journal.pmed.0050045. Accessed April 3, 2009.

Klein, Donald F. "La physiologie et les troubles anxieux." In *Stress et anxiété: les faux semblants,* edited by L. Chneiweiss and E. Albert, 93–114. Paris: Laboratoires Upjohn, 1993.

Klerman, Gerald L., and Mirna Weissman. "Increasing Rates of Depression." *JAMA* 261, no. 15 (April 21, 1989): 2229–35.

Klibansky, Raymond, Erwin Panofsky, and Fritz Saxl. *Saturn and Melancholy; Studies in the History of Natural Philosophy, Religion, and Art.* London: Thomas Nelson and Sons, 1964.

– *Saturne et la mélancholie,* Paris, Gallimard, 1989.

Kline, Nathan S. *From Sad to Glad.* New York: Putnam, 1974.

– "Monoamine oxidase inhibitors: an unfinished picaresque tale." In *Discoveries in Biological Psychiatry,* edited by Frank J. Ayd and Barry Blackwell, 194–204. Philadelphia: Lippincott, 1970.

Kohler, M., "Crier pour guérir," *Elle,* no. 1414, 1973.

Koupernik, C. *Les médications du psychisme.* Paris: Hachette, 1964.

Kovess, V., S. Gysens, R. Poinsard, and P.F. Chanoit. "La psychiatrie face aux problems sociaux: la prise en charge des RMistes à Paris." *L'Information psychiatrique* 71, no. 3 (March 1995): 273–85.

Kraepelin, Emil. *Manic-Depressive Insanity and Paranoia.* Translated by R. Mary Barclay. Edinburgh: E. & S. Livingstone, 1921.

Kramer, Peter D. *Listening to Prozac: The Landmark Book About Antidepressants and the Remaking of the Self.* Rev. ed. New York: Penguin, 1997

Krausz, M. ed. "Comorbidity of Severe Mental Illness and Addictive Behaviour." Special Issue. *European Addiction Research* 2, nos. 1–2 (1996).

Kristeva, Julia. *Black Sun: Depression and melancholia.* Translated by Leon S. Roudiez, New York: Columbia University Press, 1992.

Kuhn, R. "Dépression endogène et dépression réactionnelle." *Psychiatries* no. 36 (1979): 9–17.

– "The imipramine story." In *Discoveries in Biological Psychiatry,* edited by Frank J. Ayd and Barry Blackwell, 205–217. Philadelphia: Lippincott, 1970.

– "Psychopharmacologie et analyse existentielle." *Revue internationale de psychopathologie* no. 1 (1990): 43–67.

– "The treatment of masked depression." In Kielholz, *Masked Depression*, 188–94.

Kupfer, David J., Ellen Frank, James M. Perel, Cleon Cornes, Alan G. Mallinger, Michael E. Thase, Ann B. McEachran, and Victoria J. Grochocinski. "Five Year Outcome for Maintenance Therapy in Recurring Depressions." *Archives of General Psychiatry* 49, no. 10 (1992): 769–773.

Laborit, H. *La Vie antérieure*. Paris: Grasset, 1989.

Laboucarie, J. "Discussion." Procedings of the Symposium des états dépressifs, Paris, Nov. 1954. *L'Évolution psychiatrique* no. 3 (1955): 564–71.

Lacan, Jacques. *L'Angoisse:* 1962–1963. Book 10 of *Le Séminaire*. Paris: Seuil, 2004.

– *Ethics of Psychoanalysis:* 1959–1960. Edited by Jacques Alain-Miller. Book 7 of The Seminar of Jacques Lacan. translated by Dennis Porter. New York: W.W. Norton & Company, 1997.

– "Propos sur la causalité psychique." In Bonnafé, et al., *Le Problème de la psychogénèse des névroses et des psychoses*, 23–54.

Lambert, Pierre A. "Les effets indésirables des antidépresseurs tricycliques." *Thérapie* 28 no. 2 (1973): 269–305.

– *Psychanalyse et psychopharmacologie*. Paris: Masson, 1990.

– *La Relation médicin-malade au cours des chimiothérapies psychiatriques*. Paris: Masson, 1965.

– "Sur quelques aspects psychanalytiques des traitements de la psychose maniaco-dépressive." *L'Évolution psychiatrique* 41, no. 3 (1976): 557–82.

– "Sur quelques perspectives de la pharmacologie." *Confrontations psychiatriques*, no. 9 (1972): 229–43.

Lambotte, Marie-Claude. *Le Discours mélancolique de la phénoménologie à la métapsychologie*. Paris: Anthropos, 1993.

Lantéri-Laura, Georges. "La connaissance clinique: histoire et structure en médecine et en psychiatrie." *L'Évolution psychiatrique* 47 no. 2 (1987): 423–70.

– "Introduction historique et critique à la notion de douleur en psychiatrie." In *La Douleur Morale*, edited by Rémi Tevissen. Paris: Éditions du Temps, 1996.

– *Psychiatrie et connaissance*. Paris: Sciences en situation, 1991.

Laplanche, J. and Pontalis, J-B. *The Language of Psycho-Analysis.* Translated by Donald Nicholson-Smith. New York: W.W. Norton & Company, 1973.

Laplane, D. "L'utilisation pratique des médicaments anti-dépressifs." *La Revue du praticien* 14, suppl. issue (Dec. 9, 1964): 184–8.

– "Avant-propos." *La Revue du praticien* 13, no. 25 (Oct. 1, 1963): 2979–84.

Laqueille, X. and C. Spadone. "Les troubles dépressifs dans la prise à charge des toxicomanies." *L'Encéphale* 21, sp. no. 4 (1995) 11–4.

Lasch, C. *The culture of narcissism: American life in an age of diminishing expectations.* New York: W.W. Norton & Company, 1978.

des Lauriers, A. "Le risque de suicide chez les déprimés." *La Revue du praticien* 12, special issue, "Syndromes dépressifs" (Oct. 1, 1963): 3253–61.

Laxenaire, M. *Les Cahiers de médecine no. 7* (June 1973).

Laxenaire, M, and P. Marchand, "Essais cliniques de l'amineptine (à propos de 40 cas)." *Psychologie médicale* 11, no. 8, (1979): 1727–34.

Lazarus, Antoine. See France. Délégation interministérielle à la ville et au développement social urbain and Délégation interministérielle au revenu minimum d'insertion.

Lebovici, Serge. 1955.

Lebovici, Serge, and René Diatkine. "Quelques notes sur l'inconscient." In Ey, *L'Inconscient, 6e Colloque de Bonneval,* 1960, 47–76.

Lecrubier, Y. and G. Jourdain. "Despcription de troubles dépressifs légers chez 3 090 consultants de médecine générale." *Semaine des hôpitaux* 66, no. 12 (March 22, 1990): 655–8.

Lecrubier, Y., and E. Weiller. "La neurasthénie et la thymasthénie." *L'Encéphale* 20, no. 3, special issue, "Syndrome de fatigue, neurasthénie, psychasthénie, thymasthénie, dysthymies" (1994): 559–62.

Lefort, Claude. "Reversibility: Political Freedom and Freedom of the Original." In *Democracy and Political Theory,* 165–82. Translated by David Macey. Cambridge: Polity Press in association with Basil Blackwell, 1988.

Legendre, Pierre. "Classification et connaissance. Remarques sur l'art de diviser et l'institution du sujet." *Confrontations Psychiatriques* 24 (1984): 41–5.

– *Le Crime du caporal Lortie: Traité sur le père.* Paris: Fayard, 1989.

– *L'Inestimable objet de la transmission: Étude sur le principe généalologique en Occident.* Paris: Fayard, 1985.

Legrand, Claude. *Médecine et malheur moral – Les modes de prescription de psychotropes dans la presse professionnelle depuis* 1950. MIRELERS, November 1996.

Lehmann, Heinz. "L'Arrivée de la chlorpromazine sur le continent nord-américain." *L'Encéphale* 19, no. 1 (1993): 57–9.

– "Epidemiology of depressive disorders." In Fieve, *Depression in the 1970's,* 21–30.

Leiris, Michel. *Manhood: A Journey from Childhood into the Fierce Order of Virility.* Translated by Richard Howard. Chicago: University of Chicago Press, 1992.

Lejeune, Philippe. *Le Moi des demoiselles: Enquête sur le journal d'une jeune fille.* Paris: Le Seuil, 1993.

Le Mappian, M. "Aspects cliniques des états dépressifs." *L'Encéphale* 38 no. 5 (1949): 220–44.

Lemoine, P. "Bien prescrire les psychotropes, les antidépresseurs." *Le Concours médical* 113, no. 17 (May 18, 1991): 1411–9.

Lempérière, Thérèse. "Les algies psychogènes." In *Entretiens de Bichat: Psychiatrie,* 281–6. Paris: Expansion scientifique française, 1973.

– "Les dépressions psychogènes. Dépressions réactionnelles, dépressions d'épuisement, dépressions névrotiques." *La Revue du praticien* 13 (Oct. 1, 1963): 3021–31.

Lempérière, Thérèse, and J. Adès. "Problèmes posés au médecin praticien par la dépression." *L'Encéphale* no. 5 (1979): 483–90.

Le Pape, Annick and Thérèse Lecomte. *Aspects socioéconomiques de la dépression: Évolution* 1980–1981/1991–1992. Paris: CREDES, 1996.

Lépine, Jean-Pierre, J. Lellouch, A. Lovella, M. Teherani, and P. Pariente. "L'épidémiologie des troubles anxieux et dépressifs dans une population générale française." *Confrontations psychiatriques* no. 35 (1993): 139–61.

Lereboullet, J. "Nouveaux neuroleptiques et tranquillisants." *La Revue du praticien,* 12, special issue, (Dec. 7, 1962): 117–22.

Lereboullet, J., C. Desrouesné and J.P. Klein. "La neuropsychiatrie en 1967." *La Revue du praticien* 18, no. 18 (June 21, 1968): 2683–711.

Lereboullet, J. and R. Escourolle. "La neuropsychiatrie en 1960." *La Revue du praticien* 10 no. 27 (Oct. 27, 1960): 2889–919.

Le Rider, Jacques. *Modernity and Crises of Identity: Culture and Society in Fin-de-Siècle Vienna.* New York: Continuum, 1993.

Lin, Tsung-Yi. "The Epidemiological Study of Medical Disorders." *WHO Chronicle,* no. 21 (1967): 509–16.

Lingjaerde, O. "Le rôle de la sérotonine dans les troubles de l'humeur."
    L'Encéphale 5, suppl. to no. 5 (1979): 499–506.
Lôo, Henri. Preface to "La dépression: de la biologie à la pathologie."
    L'Encéphale 20, no. 4 (Dec. 1994): 619–20.
Lôo, Henri and Lucien Colonna. "Abord critique des recherches de
    perturbations monoaminergiques dans les dépressions." *Confrontations
    psychiatriques,* special issue "Autour de la dépression" (1989): 351–76.
Lôo, Henri and H. Cuche. "Classification des antidépresseurs." *L'Encéphale*
    5 suppl. to no. 5 (1979): 591–603.
Lôo, Henri and Pierre Deniker, eds. "La dépression: de la biologie à la
    pathologie." Special issue of *L'Encéphale* 20, no. 4 (Dec. 1994).
Lôo, Henri and Thierry Gallarda. *La Maladie dépressive.* Paris: Flammarion,
    1997.
Lôo, Henri, and P. Lôo. *La Dépression.* Collection Que sais-je?. Paris: PUF,
    1991.
Lovell, Anne M. "Mania and the Making of Contemporary US Culture,"
    Biosocieties 3 no. 3 (2007): 349–51.
Lôo, Henri, and Édouard Zarifian *Limites de l'efficacité des chimiothérapies
    psychotropes.* Paris: Masson, 1977.
Lovell, A., and R. Führer, R. "Troubles de la santé mentale – La plus grande
    'fragilité' des femmes remise en cause." In *La Santé des femmes,* by M.-J.
    Savrel-Cubizolles and B. Blondel, 258–83. Paris: Flammarion, 1996.
Lowen, Alexander. *Depression and the Body: The Biological Basis of Faith and
    Reality.* New York: Penguin, 1993.
Maître, Jacques. *Une inconnue célèbre: la Madeleine Lebouc de Janet.* Paris:
    Anthropos, 1993
Mallet, J. "La dépression névrotique." *L'Évolution psychiatrique,* 20 no. 3
    (1955): 483–501.
Marchais, P., "Essai d'approche clinique des états dépressifs névrotiques:
    Leurs indications chimiothérapiques actuelles." In Baruk and Launay,
    Actualités de Thérapeutique Psychiatrique et de Psychopharmacologie, 79–85.
Marie-Cardine, Michel. "Pharmacothérapie et psychotherapies: histo-
    rique des recherches." *Revue internationale de psychopathologie* no. 21
    (1996): 43–65.
Martin, A. "L'inhibition en psychopathologie: Historique de l'approche
    clinique." *Nervure,* special issue, "Psychasthénie et inhibition" 9
    (Jan. 1996): 25–34.
Martin, Emily. *Bipolar Expeditions: Mania and Depression in American
    Culture.* Princeton: Princeton University Press, 2007.

Martin, P. "Le concept de la qualité de vie: son évaluation en psychiatrie." *Synapse: Journal de psychiatrie et système nerveux central* no. 98 (July-Aug. 1993): 22–9.

Martineau, Caroline. "Dépression en Europe, la France est le pays le plus touché." *Quotidien du médecin*, no. 5727 (Nov. 8, 1995): 8.

Martinot, J.L., F. Raffaitin, and Jean-Pierre. Olié. "Attaques de panique et dépressions anxieuses." *L'Encéphale* 12, no. 6 (1986): 321–6.

Maruani, G. "Antidépresseurs: doping ou autolytique?" *Psychologie médicale* 16 (1984): 637–40.

Mauzi, Robert. *L'Idée du Bonheur dans la literature et la pensée française au XVIIIᵉ siécle*, Paris: Albin Michel, 1979.

McDougall, Joyce. *Plea for a Measure of Abnormality*. New York: Psychology Press, 1972.

Medawar, C. "The Antidepressant Web: Marketing Depression and Making Medicines Work." *International Journal of Risk and Safety in Medicine* 10 (1997): 75–126.

Meltzer, Herbert Y. *Psychopharmacology: The Third Generation of Progress*, New York, Raven Press, 1987.

Mendes, J.M. Fragoso and J.A. lopes do Rosario. "Signification et importance de la sérotonine en psychiatrie." *L'Encéphale* 48, no. 6 (1959): 501–9.

Merceuil Alain, and Brigitte Letout. "Précarité et troubles psychiques." *Nervure*, supplement FMC, 10, no. 7 (Oct. 1997): 1–4.

Micale, Mark S. *Approaching Hysteria: Disease and its Interpretations*. Princeton: Princeton University Press, 1994.

Michel, Jacqueline. *La Déprime*. Paris: Stock, 1972

Mijolla, A. de and S.A. Shentoub, *Pour une psychanalyse de l'alcoolisme*. Paris: Payot, 1973.

Mineau, P. and P. Boyer, "La notion de dépression en médecine générale; à propos d'une enquête statistique réalisée auprès de 59 médecins." *Annales médico-psychologiques* 137 (1979): 626–35.

Minkowski, Eugène. *Lived Time: Phenomenological and Psychopathological Studies*. Translated by Nancy Metzel. Evanston: Northwestern University Press: 1970.

Mockers, Christian. "Anxiété et dépression souvent associées." *Panorama du médecin* no. 3426 July 15, 1991.

Möller H.J., and H.-P. Volz, "Drug Treatment of Depression in the 1990s: An Overview of Achievemens and Future Possibilities." *Drugs* 52, no. 5 (Nov. 1996): 625–38.

von Monakow, Constantin, and R. Morgue. *Intégration et désintégration de la function*. Paris: Alcan, 1928.

Mongin, O. *La Violence des images*. Paris: Le Seuil, 1997.

Montassut, M. *La Dépression constitutionelle*. Paris: Masson, 1938.

– "La fatigue du neurasthénique." *L'Évolution psychiatrique* 11, no. 2 (1939): 55–80.

– "Le Traitement physique de la dépression constitutionnelle." *L'Évolution psychiatrique* 9, no. 1 (1937): 71–95.

Montgomery, Stuart A., G. Racagni, A. Coppen, W.E. Bunney, P. Carlsson, C. De Montigny, C. Giurgea, B. Hansen, F. Holsboer, L.L. Judd, S.Z. Langer, P. Leber, J. Mendlewicz, R. Post, T. Shibuya. Task Force of the CINP. "Impact of Neuropsychology in the 1990s: Strategies for the therapy of depressive illness." *European Neuropsychopharmacology* 3, no. 2 (1993): 153–6.

Montgomery, Stuart A., and Frédéric Rouillon, eds. *Long-term Treatment of Depression*. Chichester: John Wiley and Sons, 1992.

Montesquieu, Charles de Secondat, baron de. *Montesquieu: The Spirit of the Laws*. Translated by Anne M. Cohler, Basia C. Miller, Harold Stone. Cambridge: Cambridge University Press, 1989.

Moussaoui, Driss. "Biochimie de la dépression: Analyse de la litérature," *L'Encéphale* 4 (1978): 193–222.

– "Place respective des différents antidépresseurs en thérapeutique." *L'Encéphale* 5 (1979): 701–8.

Mulhern, Sherrill. "À la recherche du trauma perdu: le trouble de la personnalité multiple." *Chimères* no. 18 (Winter 1992–3): 53–85.

– "L'inceste, au carrefour des fantasmes et des fantômes." In *Incestes*, edited by Dana Castro, 71–105. Paris: L'Esprit du Temps, 1995.

Musil, Robert. *The Man Without Qualities*. 3 vols. New York: Coward-McCann, Inc., 1953.

M'uzan, M. de. *De l'art à la mort*. Collection Tel. Paris: Gallimard, 1977.

Naipal, V.S. *A Bend in the River*. New York: Vintage, 1989.

Nacht, S and P.C. Racamier. "Les états dépressifs: étude psychanalytique." *Revue française de psychanalyse* 23 no. 5 (1959): 567–605.

Narot, Jean-François. "Pour une psychopatholgie historique: Introduction à une enquête sur les patients d'aujourd'hui." *Le Débat* no. 61 (Sept.-Oct. 1990): 165–86.

Nayrac, P. *Éléments de psychologie*. Paris: Flammarion, 1962.

Nietzsche, Friedrich. *The Genealogy of Morals*. New York: Courier Dover Publications, 2003.

– *Twilight of the Idols, or How to Philosophize with a Hammer.* Translated by Duncan Large. Oxford, New York: Oxford University Press, 1988.

Norden, Michael J. *Beyond Prozac.* New York: Harper-Collins, 1995.

Nye, Robert. *Crime, Madness and Politics in Modern France: The Medical Concept of National Decline.* Princeton: Princeton University Press, 1984.

Office of the Surgeon General. *Mental Health: A Report of the Surgeon General.* Rockville, Md.: Dept. of Health and Human Services, U.S. Public Health Service, 1999.

Olié, Jean-Pierre, Marie-France Poirier, and Henri Lôo. *Les maladies dépressives.* Paris: Flammarion, 1995.

Olivier-Martin, R. "Facteurs psychologiques, observance et résistance aux traitements antidépresseurs." *L'Encéphale* 12, sp.no. Reports from the international colloquium, "Les dépressions résistantes aux traitements antidépresseurs" (Paris, Jan. 17, 1986). (Oct., 1986): 197–203.

Overholser, W., "La chlorpromazine ouvre-t-elle une ère nouvelle dans les hôpitaux psychiatriques?" *Premier Colloque international sur la chlorpromazine et les médicaments neuroleptiques en thérapeutique psychiatrique. L'Encéphale* no. 4 (1956): 313–19.

Pachet, Pierre. *Les Baromètres de l'âme – Naissance du journal intime.* Paris: Hatier, 1990.

– *Le Premier venu: Essai sur la politique baudelairienne.* Paris: Denoël, 1976.

Patris, Michel. "Dépression et suggestion hypnotique." *Confrontations psychiatriques,* special issue "Autour de la dépression" (1989): 267–73.

Paugam, S., J.-P. Zoyem, and J.-M. Charbonnel. *Précarité et risque d'exclusion en France.* Paris: La Documentation française, 1994.

Peele, Stanton. *Diseasing of America: Addiction Treatment Out of Control.* Lexington, Mass.: Lexington Books, 1989.

– *The Meaning of Addiction: Compulsive Experience and its Interpretation.* Lexington, Mass.: Lexington Books, 1985.

Pélicier, Y. "Séméiologie de l'inhibition: Introduction." *L'Encéphale* 4, no. 5, supplement, (1978): 403–4.

Péquignot, H. and P. Van Amerongen. "Prescription et utilisation de neuroleptiques en médecine générale." *Confrontations psychiatriques* no. 13 (1975): 205–24.

Péron-Magnan, P. "Tempérament et dépression." In Olié, Poirier and Lôo, *Les maladies dépressives,* 183–91.

Péron-Magnan, P. and A. Galinowski. "La Personnalité dépressive." In *La Dépression: Études.* Edited by A. Féline, P. Hardy, and M. de Bonis, 93–115. Paris: Masson, 1990.

Perrault, M. "La thérapeutique en 1958." *La Revue du praticien* 8, no. 33 (Dec. 21, 1958): 3753–78.

Pétillon, Pierre-Yves. *L'Europe aux anciens parapets*. Paris: Éditions du Seuil, 1986.

Peyré, F. "Les antidépresseurs en dehors de la dépression." *La Revue du praticien* 44, no. 17 (1994): 2299–301.

PfizerLaboratory. "Zoloft: une étude multicentrique française confirme son efficacité chez huit patients sur dix" L*'Information psychiatrique*, November 1998, 1056–7.

Pichot, Pierre. "Actualisation du concept de dépression." *L'Encéphale* 7 no. 4 (1981): 307–14.

– Foreword to the *DSM-III: manuel diagnostique et statistique des troubles mentaux*, by the American Psychiatric Association, Taskforce on Nomenclature and Statistics, v-vii. Translation co-ordinated by Pierre Pichot and Julien-Daniel Guelfi. Paris, Masson: 1983.

– "Conclusions." Conclusions resulting from the conference, *Confrontation multidisciplinaire européenne sur la dépression*, Monaco, Dec. 5–6, 1980. *L'Encéphale* 7, no. 4 suppl. (1981): 567–8.

– "La neurasthénie, hier et aujourd'hui." *L'Encéphale* 20, no. 3, special issue, "Syndrome de fatigue, neurasthénie, psychasthénie, thymasthénie, dysthymies" (1994): 545–9.

– ed. *Les Voies nouvelles de la dépression*. Paris: Masson, 1978.

Pichot, Pierre and Werner Rein, eds. *L'Approche Clinique en psychiatrie*. 3 vols. Paris: Delagrange, 1992–.

Poignant, Jean-Claude. "Revue pharmacologique sur l'amineptine." *L'Encéphale* 5 (1979): 709–20.

Poirier, Marie-France. "Critères psychobiologiques de guérison." *L'Encéphale* 19, sp. no. 3 (1993): 451–8.

Poirier, Marie-France and D. Ginestet. "Médicaments détournés à des fins toxicomaniaques." *La Revue du praticien* 45, no. 11 (1995): 1364–6.

Porot, M. "Assises départementales de médecine sur les états dépressifs." *Les Cahiers de médecine no. 7* (June 1973).

– "Principes généraux de la thérapeutique des états dépressifs." *Les Cahiers de médecine* no. 7, (June 1973).

van Praag, H.M. "The DSM-IV (depression) classification: to be or not to be?" *The Journal of Nervous and Mental Disease*. 78 no. 3 (March 1990): 147–9.

Preface to "L'humeur et son changement." Special Issue, *Nouvelle Revue de psychanalyse*, no. 32 (Autumn 1985) 5–8.

Prigent, Yves. "Psychodynamique des chimiothérapies antidépressives." *L'Information psychiatrique* 67, no. 9 (Nov. 1991): 837–44.

Pringuey, D., P. Robert, F. Giacomoni, L. Talichet, and G. Darcourt. "L'efficacité des antidépresseurs et des thymorégulateurs dans l'évolution à long terme des dépressions." *L'Encéphale* 21, sp.no. 2 (March 1995): 61–70.

Pull, C.B. "Critères diagnostiques." In Olié, Poirier and Lôo, *Les maladies dépressives*, 247–57.

Putnam, Hilary. *The Collapse of the Fact/Value Dichotomy and Other Essays.* Boston: Harvard University Press, 2002.

Putnam, Robert. *Bowling Alone: The Collapse and Revival of American Community*, Simon and Schuster, 2000.

Rabinbach, Anson. *The Human Motor: Energy, Fatigue and the Origins of Modernity.* Berkeley: University of California Press, 1990.

Radó, Sándor. "La psychanalyse des pharmacothymies." *Revue française de psychanalyse* 39, no. 4 (1975): 603–18.

Ragot, M. "La dépression, la civilisation moderne et les médicaments thymo-analeptiques." *Annales médicopsychologiques*, 7, no. 4 (April 1977): 654–60.

Rance, A.-M., A. Jurquet, and J. Roger. "Remarques sur la thérapeutique des affectations psychiatriques par la chlorpromazine et la réserpine." *L'Encéphale*, special issue, no. 5 (1956): 477–93.

Rapoport, Judith. *The Boy Who Couldn't Stop Washing: The Experience & Treatment of Obsessive-Compulsive Disorder.* New York: Dutton, 1989.

Raskin, Allen. "Drugs and Depression Subtypes." In Fieve, *Depression in the 1970's: Modern Theory and Research,* 87–96.

Régis, Emmanuel, and Angélo Hesnard. *La Psycho-Analyse des névroses et des psychoses.* Paris: Félix Alcan, 1913.

Reigner, A. "La dépression... une mode?" *La Vie médicale*, special issue, "Les dépressions", Editorial, Sept. 1979.

Rey, Roselyne. *The History of Pain.* Translated by Louise Elliott Wallace, J.A. Cadden, and S.W. Cadden. Cambridge: Harvard University Press, 1995.

Ricoeur, Paul. *Oneself as Another.* Translated by Kathleen Blamey. Chicago: University of Chicago Press 1992.

Rieff, Philip. *The Triumph of Therapeutic: Uses of Faith after Freud.* Chicago: University of Chicago Press, 1966.

Rigaud, A. and M.-M. Maquet. "Propos critiques sur les notions d'addiction et de conduits de dépendance: Entre lieux communs et chimères." In *Dépendance et conduites de dépendance*, edited by D. Baily and J.-L. Venisse, 38–60. Paris, Masson, 1994

Robins, L.N. and D.A. Regier, eds. *Psychiatric Disorders in America: The Epidemiological Catchment Area.* New York: Free Press, 1991.

Robbins, P.R. "Depression and Drug Addiction." *Psychiatric Quarterly* 48, no. 3 (1974): 374–86.

Robert, G. "Études cliniques d'un sérotonergique: Examen de ses caractères spécifiques." *Psychologie médicale* 16 no. 5 (1984): 881–4.

Rochette, E. and M. Brassinne. "La toxicomanie: un comportement antidépressif." *Concours médicale*, no. 41 (1980): 6263–7.

Roelandt, J.L. "Exclusion, insertion: les frontières de l'étrange." *Lettre de l'union syndicale de la psychiatrie* no. 1 (Jan. 1996): 116–36.

Rosolato, Guy. "L'axe narcissique des dépressions." *Nouvelle Revue de psychanalyse* no. 11 (1975): 5–33.

Roth M., Sir, and T.-A. Kerr. "Le concept dépression névrotique: plaidoyer pour une reintégration." In Pichot and Rein, *L'Approche Clinique en psychiatrie*, vol. 3, 207–54.

Rothe, Marcus. Interview with Woody Allen in *Libération* (Jan. 21, 1988): 33.

Rouart, Julien. "Dépression et problèmes de psychopathologie générale." *L'Évolution psychiatrique* 20 no. 3 (1955): 459–66.

Roudinesco, Élisabeth. *La Bataille de cent ans: Histoire de la psychosnalyse en France, 1885–1939.* Vol. 1. Paris: Ramsay, 1982.

– *Jacques Lacan & Co.: A History of psychoanalysis in France, 1925–1985.* Translated by Jeffrey Mehlman. Chicago: University of Chicago Press, 1990.

Rouillon, Frédéric, Jean-Pierre Lépine, and Jean-Louis Terra. *Épidémiologie psychiatrique.* Paris: Upjohn, 1995.

Roumieux, André. *Artaud et l'asile: Au-delà des murs, la mémoire.* 2 vols. Paris: Séguier, 1996.

Roustang, François. *How to Make a Paranoid Laugh, or, What is Psychoanalysis?* Translated by Anne C. Vila. Philadelphia: University of Pennsylvania Press, 2000.

– *Influence.* Paris: Éditions de Minuit, 1990.

Roussy, Gustave. Préface to *Les Dérèglements de l'humeur*, by Jean Delay, vii-xii. Paris: PUF, 1946.

Rümke, M. "Quelques remarques concernant la pharmacologie et la psychiatrie." *Premier Colloque international sur la chlorpromazine et les médicaments neuroleptiques en thérapeutique psychiatrique. L'Encéphale* 45, no. 4 (1956): 339–43.

Sacks, Oliver. "A Summer of Madness." The New York Review of Books 55, no. 14 (Sept. 25, 2008): 57–61.

Sargant, W. "Indications et mécanisme de l'abréaction et ses relations avec les thérapeutiques de choc." *L'Évolution psychiatrique* 15, no. 4 (1950): 607–18.

Sarradon, A. "Assises départementales de médecine sur les états dépressifs." 1972. *Les Cahiers de médecine* 7 (June 1973).

Sartorius, N. "La dépression: épidémiologie et priorités pour les recherches futures." *L'Encéphale* 7 (1981): 527–33.

– "Description and Classification of Depressive Disorders: Contribution for the Definition of the Therapy-Resistance and of the Therapy Resistant Depression." *Pharmakopsychiatrie, Neuro-Psychopharmakologie* 7 (1974): 76–80.

– "Épidémiologie de la dépression," *Chronique* OMS 29, no. 11 (1975): 464–8.

Savy, Paul. *Traité de la thérapeutique clinique.* 3 vols. Paris, Masson, 1948.

Schneider, M. et al. "Table Ronde." In Lambert, *La relation médecin-malade au cours des chimiothérapies psychiatriques,* 183–214.

Schorske, Carl. *Fin-de-siècle Vienna: politics and culture.* New York: Vintage Books, 1981.

Scotto, Jean-Claude. "Éditorial." Special issue containing the proceedings of "Les nouveaux champs de la dépression," Symposium Lilly France, Paris, Nov. 1995. *L'Encéphale* 22, sp.no. 1 (May 1996):1–2.

– Introduction to "La durée des traitements de dépression." *L'Encéphale* 21 sp.no. 2 (March 1995): 1–2.

Scotto, Jean-Claude, Thierry Bougerol, and R. Arnaud-Castel-Castiglioni, "Stratégies thérapeutiques devant une dépression." *La Revue du praticien* 35, no. 27 (May 11,1985): 1633–8.

Sechter, D. "Les effets cliniques à long terme des antidépresseurs." *L'Encéphale* 21, sp. no. 2 (March 1995): 35–8.

Séglas, Jules. "De la mélancholie sans délire." In *La Douleur Morale,* edited by Rémi Tevissen. Paris: Éditions du Temps, 1996.

Seigel, Jerrold. *Bohemian Paris: Culture, Politics, and the Boundaries of Bourgeois Life,* 1830–1930. New York: Penguin Books, 1987.

Sempé, J.-C. "Pratiques et institutions privées." *L'Évolution psychiatrique,* "Livre blanc de la psychiatrie française," 30 supplement to no. 3 (Nov., 1965): 137–57.

Sennett, Richard. *The Fall of Public Man.* New York: W.W. Norton & Company, 1992.

Sennett, Richard and Jonathan Cobb. *The Hidden Injuries of Class.* New York: W.W. Norton & Company, 1993.

Shawn, Allan. *Wish I Could Be There: Notes from a Phobic Life.* New York: Viking, 2007.

Shorter, Edward. *A History of Psychiatry: From the Era of the Asylum to the Age of Prozac.* New York: John Wiley and Sons, 1997.

Simmel, Georg. *Michel-Ange et Rodin*. Translated by Sabine Cornille and Phillippe Ivernel. Paris: Rivages, 1996.

Smirnoff, Victor N. "De Vienne à Paris – Sur les origines d'une psychanalyse 'à la française.'" *Nouvelle Revue de psychanalyse*, no. 20 (Fall 1979): 13–58.

Snyder, Solomon H. *Drugs and the Brain*. New York: W.H. Freeman and Co., 1986.

– "Molecular Strategies in Neuropharmacology: Old and New." In Meltzer, *Psychopharmacology: The Third Generation of Progress*, 17–21.

Solomon, Andrew. *Noonday Demon: An Atlas of Depression*. Touchstone, Simon and Schuster, 2001.

Soury, Jules. *Le système nerveux central: structure et fonctions; histoire critique des théories et des doctrines*. Paris: G. Carré et C. Naud, 1899.

Spadone, C. "Le big bang de la chimiothérapie psychotrope." *Abstract neuro & psy*, no. 100, (May 15–31, 1993): 7–11.

Spadone, C. and J.-M. Vanelle "Les nouveaux antidépresseurs." *La Revue du praticien* 8, no. 268 (Sept. 26, 1994): 13–15.

Speaker, Susan L. "From 'Happiness Pills' to 'National Nightmare': Changing Cultural Assesment of Minor Tranquilizers in America, 1955–1980." *Journal of the History of Medicine and Allied Sciences* 52, no. 3 (1997): 338–76.

Spitzer, Robert L. Introduction to *DSM-III: Diagnostic and Statistical Manual of Mental Disorders*. 3rd ed. Prepared by the Task Force on Nomenclature and Statistics of the American Psychiatric Association, 1–12. Washington: American Psychiatric Press, 1980.

– Introduction to *DSM-III-R: Diagnostic and Statistical Manual of Mental Disorders*. 3rd ed., rev. Prepared by the Work Group to Revise *DSM-III* of the American Psychiatric Association, xvii-xxvii. Washington: American Psychiatric Association, 1987.

Spitzer, Robert L., J. Endicott and E. Robins. "Research diagnostic criteria, rationale and reliability." *Archives of General Psychiatry* 35 (1978): 773–82.

Staehelin, J.-E., and F. Labhard. "Les résultats obtenus par les neuroplégiques dans le traitement des psychoses et des névroses." Paper presented at the *Premier Colloque international sur la chlorpromazine et les médicaments neuroleptiques en thérapeutique psychiatrique. L'Encéphale* 45, no. 4 (1956): 511–17.

Starobinski, Jean. *Histoire du traitement de la mélancolie des origines à 1900*. Basle: Geigy, 1960.

– *La Mélancolie au miroir – Trois lectures de Beaudelaire*. Paris: Julliard, 1989.

– "Le Mot réaction: de la physique à la psychiatrie." *Diogène* no. 93 (1976): 3–30.

– "Le Remède dans le mal." *Nouvelle Revue de psychanalyse,* no. 17 (1978): 251–74.

Stewart, A. "Revisiting the Relative Cost-Effectiveness of Selective Serotonin Reuptake Inhibitors and Tricyclic Antidepressants: What Price Inflation and Subtherapeutic Dosages?" *British Journal of Medical Economics* 10, no. 3 (1996): 203–16.

Stokes, P.E. "La fluoxetine: revue de cinq années d'utilisation." *Nervure* 4, no. 10 (Dec. 1993–Jan. 1994): 7–26.

Sulloway, Frank. J. *Freud, Biologist of the Mind: Beyond the Psychoanalytic Legend.* New York: Basic Books, 1979.

Sutter, J.M. "Problèmes posés en médecine générale par les formes atypiques des états dépressifs." *Les Cahiers de médecine,* no. 7 (1973).

Swain, Gladys. *Dialogue avec l'insensé: À la recherche d'une autre histoire de la folie.* Paris: Gallimard, 1994.

– *Le sujet de la folie: naissance de la psychiatrie.* Toulouse: Privat,1977.

Swain, Gladys and Marcel Gauchet. *Le sujet de la folie: naissance de la psychiatrie.* Paris: Calmann-Lévy, 1997.

Schwartz, Olivier. *Le monde privé des ouvriers: Hommes et femmes du Nord.* Paris: PUF, 1990.

Swazey, J.-P. *Chlorpromazine in Psychiatry: A Study of Therapeutic Innovation.* Cambridge, Mass.: MIT Press, 1974.

Tatossian, Arthur. "Les pratiques de la dépression: étude critique." *Psychiatrie Française* 16 (1985): 257–309.

Terra, Jean-Louis, ed. *Qualité de vie subjective et santé mentale.* Paris: Ellipses, 1994.

Théry, Irène. *Le démariage: Justice et vie privée.* Paris: Odile Jacob, 1993.

– "Vie Privée et monde commun – Réflexions sur l'enlisement gestionnaire du droit." *Le Débat* no. 85 (1995): 141–9.

Thompson, Tracy. *The Beast: A Journey Through Depression.* New York: Plume Books, 1996.

Tignol, J. and M. Bourgeois. "La désinhibition et ses risques." *L'Encéphale* 4, no. 5, supplement (1978): 459–63.

Timsit, M. "Les états-limites, Évolution des concepts." *L'Évolution psychiatrique,* 36, no. 4 (1971): 679–724.

Tissot, René. "Indicateurs biologiques et prises de décision thérapeutiques." *Psychologie médicale,* 16, no. 4 (1984): 621–31.

– "Monoamines et régulations thymiques." *Confrontations psychiatriques* no. 6 (1970): 87–152.

– "Quelques aspects biochimiques du concept d'inhibition en psychiatrie." *L'Encéphale* 4 no. 5, suppl. (1978): 513–20.

Toubiana, Serge. "L'Homme tout bête." *Cahiers du cinéma*, no. 453,
(March 1992): 8–9.

Tresson, Charles. "Voyage au bout de l'envers." *Cahiers du cinéma*,
no. 416, (Feb. 1989): 8–12.

Uzan, A. "Agents prosérotonininergiques et dépressions." *L'Encéphale* 8,
no. 2 (1982): 273–89.

Vanelle, J.M. and A. Féline. "Arrêt du traitement médicamenteux dans la
dépression." *L'Encéphale* 20, sp.no. 1 (1994): 223–9.

Van Praag, H.M, and J. Bruinvels, eds. *Neurotransmission and Disturbed
Behavior*. Amsterdam: Bohn BV, 1977.

Verhaegen, L. *Les psychiatres: Médecine de pointe ou d'assistance?* Louvain-la-
Neuve: Cabay, 1985.

Vernant, Jean-Pierre. "L'individu dans la cité." In *Sur L'individu*, edited by
Paul Veyne, 20–37. Fondation Royaument, Association dialogue entre
les cultures. Paris: Le Seuil, 1987.

Vernant, Jean-Pierre, and Pierre Vidal-Naquet. *Myth and Tragedy in
Ancient Greece*. Translated by Janet Lloyd. New York: Zone Books, 1990.

Vidal, Gore. *Duluth*. New York: Penguin Books, 1983.

Villeneuve, A. "Aspects modernes des troubles de l'humeur." *L'Encéphale*
5 (1979): 427–41.

Vincent, Gérard. "A History of Secrets?" In *A History of Private Life: Riddles
of Identity in Modern Times*. Edited by Antoine Prost and Gérard Vincent.
Volume 5 of *A History of Private Life*, edited by Phillippe Ariès and
George Duby, 145–282. Translated by Arthur Goldhammer. Cambridge:
Harvard University Press, 1991.

Wakefield, Jerome. "The Concept of Mental Disorder: On the Boundary
between Biological Facts and Social Values." *American Psychologist* 47
no. 3 (1992): 373–88.

Walcher, W., "Psychogenic factors responsible for triggering of masked
endogenous depression." In Kielholz, *Masked Depression*, 177–83.

Wallez, P. "Limitation de la sismothérapie dans les états mélancoliques
mineurs." Medical diss., Paris, 1947–48.

Wauters, A. "Les troubles de l'humeur: implications de la sérotonine,
applications thérapeutiques." In *Entretiens de Bichat Psychiatrie*, 82–4.
Paris: Expansion scientifique française, 1983.

Wessley, S. "Le syndrome de fatigue chronique." *L'Encéphale* 20, no. 3,
special issue, "Syndrome de fatigue, neurasthénie, psychasthénie,
thymasthénie, dysthymies" (1994): 581–95.

Whybrow, Peter C. *A Mood Apart: Depression, Mania, and Other Afflictions of the Self.* New York: Basic Books, 1997.

Widlöcher, Daniel. "L'échelle de ralentissement dépressif: fondements théoriques et premiers résultats." *Psychologie médicale* 13B (1981): 53–60.

– "Fatigue et dépression." *L'Encéphale* 7, no. 4 (1981): 347–51.

– "L'hystérie dépossédée." *Nouvelle revue de psychanalyse* 17 (1978): 73–88.

– Introduction to *La Revue du praticien* 35, no. 27 (May 11, 1985): 1613–4.

– *Les Logiques de la dépression.* Paris: Fayard, 1983.

– *Les Nouvelles Cartes de la psychanalyse.* Paris: Odile Jacob, 1996.

– "Le psychanalyste devant les problèmes de classification." *Confrontations psychiatriques* 24 (1984): 141–56.

– ed. *Traité de psychopathologie.* Paris: PUF, 1994.

Widlöcher, Daniel and F. Binoux. "La clinique de la dépression." *La Revue du praticien* 28, no. 39 (1978): 2953–60.

Widlöcher, Daniel and L. Colonna. "L'Évaluation quantitative du ralentissement psychomoteur dans les états dépressifs," *Psychologie médicale* 12, no. 13 (1980): 2725–9.

Widlöcher, Daniel and J. Delcros. "De la psychologie du deuil à la biochimie de la dépression." *La Revue du praticien* 28, no. 39 (1978): 2963–72.

Wilde, M.I., and R. Whittington. "Paroxetine: A Pharmacoeconomic Evaluation of Use in Depression." *Pharmacoeconomics* 8, no. 1 (1995): 62–81.

Wilson, M. "DSM-III and the Transformations of American Psychiatry." *American Journal of Psychiatry* 150, no. 3 (1993): 399–410.

Wittgenstein, Ludwig. *Culture and Value.* Edited by G.H. Von Wright, with Heikki Nyman. Translated by Peter Winch. Oxford, UK: Basil Blackwell, 1980.

– *Philosophical Investigations: The German Text with a Revised English Translation.* Translated by G.E.M. Anscombe. Malden, MA: Blackwell Publishing, 2003.

World Health Organization. *The ICD-10 classification of mental and behavioural disorders: clinical descriptions and diagnostic guidelines.* 10th ed. Geneva: World Health Organization, 1992.

Wurtzel, Elizabeth. *Prozac Nation: Young and Depressed in America.* New York: Riverhead Books, 1995. Original Edition, Boston: Houghton Mifflin 1994.

Wyvekins, Anne. "Délinquance des mineurs: justice de proximité et justice tutélaire." *Esprit* March-April 1998, 158–73.

Young, Allan. *The Harmony of Illusions: Inventing Post-Traumatic Stress Disorder.* Princeton: Princeton University Press, 1995.

Zarifian, Édouard. Les jardiniers de la folie. Paris: Odile Jacob, 1988.

– "Médicaments anxiolytiques et inhibition," *L'Encéphale* 4, no. 5, suppl. (1978): 547–51.

– *Le Prix du bien-être: psychotropes et société.* Paris: Odile Jacob, 1996.

Zarifian, Édouard and Henri Lôo. *Les Antidépresseurs.* Paris: Laboratoires Roché, 1982

Zeldin, Theodore. *Intellect, Taste and Anxiety.* Volume 2 of *A History of French Passions,* 1844–1945. Oxford: Oxford University Press, 1993.

Zimmerman, F. "The Love-Lorn Consumptive: South Asian Ethnography and the Psychosomatic Paradigm," *Curare* 7 (1991): 185–95.

Zinberg, Norman. *Drug, Set and Setting.* Cambridge: Harvard University Press, 1984.

Zirkle, C.-L. "To tranquilizers and antidepressant: From antimalarial and antihistamines." In *How Modern Medicines are Discovered,* edited by F.H. Clarke, 55–78. Mt Kisco, NY: Futura Publishing Company, 1973.

Index